NEUROLOGICAL EXAMINATION IN CLINICAL PRACTICE

Neurological Examination in Clinical Practice

EDWIN R. BICKERSTAFF
MD (Birmingham), FRCP (London)
Honorary Consulting Neurologist to the Midland Centre for Neurosurgery and Neurology;
Formerly
Honorary Consultant Associate in Neurology to the Birmingham Teaching Hospitals;
Formerly
Senior Clinical Lecturer and Tutor in Neurology, University of Birmingham

JOHN A. SPILLANE
MD (London), MRCP (UK)
Consultant Neurologist to the Midland Centre for Neurosurgery and Neurology;
Honorary Senior Clinical Lecturer in Neurology, University of Birmingham

FIFTH EDITION

BLACKWELL SCIENTIFIC PUBLICATIONS
OXFORD LONDON EDINBURGH
BOSTON MELBOURNE

Editorial offices:
Osney Mead, Oxford OX2 0EL
(*Orders*: Tel. 0865-240201)
8 John Street, London WC1N 2ES
23 Ainslie Place, Edinburgh EH3 6AJ
3 Cambridge Center, Suite 208
Cambridge, Massachusetts 02142, USA
107 Barry Street, Carlton
Victoria 3053, Australia

First published 1963
Second edition 1968
Third edition 1973
Reprinted 1974, 1976
Fourth edition 1980
Fifth edition 1989

Japanese edition 1966
Portuguese edition 1975
Italian edition 1977

Typeset in Times by
Enset (Photosetting),
Midsomer Norton, Bath, Avon
Printed and bound in Great Britain
at The University Press, Cambridge

DISTRIBUTORS
USA
Year Book Medical Publishers
200 North LaSalle Street
Chicago, Illinois 60601
(*Orders*: Tel. 312-726-9733)

Canada
The C.V. Mosby Company
5240 Finch Avenue East
Scarborough, Ontario
(*Orders*: Tel. 416-298-1588)

Australia
Blackwell Scientific Publications
(Australia) Pty Ltd
107 Barry Street
Carlton, Victoria 3053
(*Orders*: Tel. (03) 347-0300)

British Library
Cataloguing in Publication Data

Bickerstaff, Edwin R. (Edwin Robert)
Neurological examination in clinical practice.—5th ed.
1. Man. Nervous system. Diagnosis
I. Title II. Spillane, John A.
(John Alban)
616.8′0475

ISBN 0-632-02397-X

Contents

Part VIII · Conclusion

Part IX · Appendices

Preface to Fifth Edition

In the ten years since the last complete revision of this book the actual techniques of neurological examination have not fundamentally altered, but the interpretation of the findings and the relative importance of certain physical signs have altered as methods of investigation, and their clarity in demonstrating pathology, have improved by what can only be called leaps and bounds. Indeed were this a book on the further investigation of neurological disorders it could do with a new edition every year, especially as regards neuroradiology. To those who work in highly specialised neurological and neurosurgical units some paragraphs may appear superfluous. However as one frequently acts as reviewer of new neurological textbooks, one cannot help being impressed by the apparent assumption by the authors that, world-wide, there is easy access to the most modern sophisticated methods of neurological investigation. This is simply just not true, and as many of our less fortunate nations have done me the honour of using this book, it is the intention still to describe and discuss the older inferences to be drawn from physical signs, and the older styles of investigation, indicating when and where modern thought and method will take over when available.

Even in this day and age the vast majority of patients with neurological disease or suspected neurological disease are not seen initially at a special centre or by a neurologist or neurosurgeon. It is therefore upon the non-neurologist that the responsibility of deciding if a patient requires the help of such specialities falls, and it is both for him and for the young neurologist in training that this book is mainly intended and will we hope continue to be of value.

When one has repeatedly revised and re-written a book over more than a quarter of a century one realises one is getting a bit long in the tooth, and new blood needs to be infused into its veins. Accordingly I am delighted to welcome to co-authorship of this edition John Spillane, my friend and colleague, already well-known for the excellent *Atlas of Clinical Neurology* written jointly with his father, and who has helped with the revision of the whole book, and completely re-written the chapters on speech disorders, the unconscious patient, the autonomic nervous system, and neurophysiological investigations. We decided between us that the chapter on the examination of small children no longer carried the authority that the speciality of paediatric neurology has brought to this field, and it has been omitted. A new chapter aims to make readers think critically about the whole subject of modern methods of investigation, and we would like to show that despite the enormous rate of advance of technology the clinician need not fear that he has been totally left behind.

We wish to express our thanks to Professor Ian Macdonald of the Institute of Neurology for allowing us to use an excellent NMR scan of multiple sclerosis and we are particularly grateful to the Oxford University Press, publishers of *The Atlas of Clinical Neurology* (first edition by J. D. Spillane 1968, second edition 1975, and third edition by J. D. and J. A. Spillane 1982) for permission to reproduce a number of their illustrations to replace the similar pictures in previous editions of this book which were beginning to look rather tired. This applies to Figs 10(a) and (b), 22(c) and (d), and Figs 24–42, 44–49, and 51–64. Per Saugman, Chairman of Blackwell Scientific Publications, and his co-director John Robson, have guided this book and its first author through all its editions, and have continued their invaluable help and advice, and we wish to thank also Karen McNaught for the sub-editing of the new manuscript, and Caroline Sheard and Sara Bickerstaff for their help and hard work in preparation of the index.

Computers may be fed with information and come up with diagnostic answers, but a computer is only as good as the information that is fed into it. This information is what an experienced physician considers significant, which may not be what the relatively uninformed patient thinks must be important. The personal contact between physician and patient with all its infinite variety of approach, of personality, of articulateness and of sympathy, empathy, or apathy on both sides, must surely be the saving grace of medicine in this technological era, and from now on, for all time.

Cornwall and
Birmingham, 1988

EDWIN R. BICKERSTAFF
JOHN A. SPILLANE

Preface to First Edition

Those of us who teach neurology to postgraduates soon find that most students have a general idea of the different parts of the neurological examination, but are uncertain of the best methods of carrying out the various tests, of the purpose that lies behind them, of the true meaning of abnormal findings, and of how to overcome technical difficulties and to avoid arriving at false conclusions. This book is intended to present in some detail those methods which have stood the tests of time, and to select from the newer methods those which are rapidly proving their value. It is not in any sense a textbook of neurology, nor one of neurological diagnosis. I think, however, that the reader who follows the instructions will become sufficiently conversant with examination technique to be able to approach a neurological case with that confidence which is so often lacking.

References have been omitted from the text to make for greater ease in reading, but a selected list of papers, reviews and monographs is given at the end of many of the chapters. These are recommended for further reading, and will be a source of a more detailed bibliography. I have personally drawn widely on the publications of those pioneers who have so greatly increased the accuracy of neurological diagnosis in recent years, and in particular I have abstracted the Medical Research Council publications on peripheral nerve injuries, and the unique work of André-Thomas and his colleagues on the examination of the new-born child. With the invaluable help of Dr Philip Moxon, an extensive section has been devoted to the wise use of the all-important neuroradiological services. I have had the help of several clinical photographers in obtaining the illustrations, but in this respect I must particularly thank Mr Gordon Gasser, FIMLT, Chief Technician in our own laboratory. Messrs Charles C. Thomas have kindly allowed the charts of sensory dermatomes to be reproduced from *Pain* by Wolff and Wolf, and Mr Per Saugman and Mr J. L. Robson of Blackwell Scientific Publications have been of the greatest help to me throughout.

This publication gives the opportunity of acknowledging gratefully the debt I owe to my former chief, Professor Philip Cloake, and to my senior neurosurgical colleague, Mr Jack Small, the two men who have most influenced my career, and to Drs Macdonald Critchley, Denny Brown and Raymond Adams, in whose wards and laboratories I spent so many happy and fruitful months.

Finally, the exacting task of typing and re-typing the various versions of the manuscript has fallen entirely on the shoulders of my wife, Claire, whose criticisms have often been potent, and always pertinent, and to whom I affectionately dedicate this book.

Birmingham, March 1962 EDWIN R. BICKERSTAFF

Part I
The Introductory Stages

Chapter 1
Approaching a Neurological Problem

Solving a neurological problem can be the most fascinating exercise in medical detection and logical deduction in the whole clinical field, yet there can be few branches of medicine, excluding, perhaps, dermatology, in which practitioners from other disciplines feel more un-informed, ill-trained, and even impotent. In order to overcome this one has to develop an organised line of thought in approaching each problem, so that the pieces of what, after all, is a diagnostic jig-saw can be specifically looked for, and, if found, fitted together to form a recognisable portrait of a disease. Those who feel they are doomed to fail diagnostically display a method of approach that soon rubs off on the patient, who loses confidence, and later may repeat a phrase so often heard in neurological consultations—'the other doctors didn't seem to know where to begin'.

Each case poses and demands an answer to four vital questions:

(*a*) Is there a lesion of the nervous system present? This is determined by analysis of the history and physical examination.

(*b*) Where does this lesion lie in the nervous system? Is it possible to locate it at one site, or must multiple sites be involved? This can only be worked out by relating the symptoms and signs to a basic knowledge of neuroanatomy—but there is no need to be scared by this—only rarely does this have to be very detailed.

(*c*) What pathological conditions are known to be capable of causing lesions at this site (or sites)?

(*d*) In this particular individual, first from careful analysis of the history and examination, and later by intelligent use of the ancillary services, which of these suspected conditions is most likely to be present?

Each step taken in the study of the case, from the first interview onwards, should aim at answering each of these questions in turn. Each examination or investigation should have behind it the planned purpose of including, or excluding, one specific member of the 'short-list' of suspected conditions. It is always the failure to have such an organised plan of approach that makes neurological problems so artificially difficult. Routine steps must, of course, be followed, but blind routine and blunderbuss investigations, 'just so as not to miss anything', show that such a plan has not existed. The more experienced one becomes, the more one recognises 'patterns' of disease, and it may appear to the juniors that diagnoses are often arrived at by inspired guess-work in which many corners have been cut. In fact it is that the experienced clinician moves that much more quickly over these basic questions while they still remain the foundation of his decision. Diagnosis purely by comparison with previous cases is reserved for the man who is very experienced, remembers his cases truly accurately, and follows them carefully and critically, and he is a rarity. The beginner will come nearer to diagnostic accuracy by logically reasoning out each step along the lines suggested.

There is however another psychological barrier to be overcome. The view is still widely held that the exact solution of a neurological problem doesn't matter all that much, as it will be of academic interest only, there being no useful treatment. Nowadays this is just arrant nonsense. It may be true that we know of no treatment for motor neurone disease; that we cannot cure the hereditary ataxias; and that we have not yet found a reliable method of preventing relapses in multiple sclerosis, but, contrary to many people's belief, these occupy a relatively small part of the neurologist's time. Think for a moment of the transformation in the last 40 years in the treatment of epilepsy, of meningitis, of neurosyphilis and of deficiency neuropathies; of the influence of ACTH and steroids in hypersensitivity states, and in the acute episodes of demyelinative disease; of the continuing progress in the drug therapy of certain facets of the migraine complex, of Parkinsonism, and of trigeminal neuralgia; of the enormous advances of neurosurgery in the great problems of intracranial haemorrhage, extrapyramidal disease, some types of epilepsy, and all forms of benign cerebral and spinal compression. This list includes only a few examples of the way in which neurological practice offers possibilities for therapy which compare very favourably with all other branches of medicine. Complete eradication of the pathological process may rarely be achieved, but this unhappily also applies in medicine as a whole. If, however, an exact diagnosis is not reached, it is important that this be admitted, and that the patient does not become firmly labelled with one of the differential possibilities (such as, for instance, multiple sclerosis), for this may result in any and every future neurological event being accepted as 'just another symptom of his old trouble' when in fact these are new developments giving the essential clue to the diagnosis of a much more remediable condition.

Finally remember that the solution of a neurological problem takes time. It cannot be rushed, and the examiner must never allow his approach to be influenced by exhortations from optimistic colleagues to 'just glance at this case while passing', or to 'just run over the nervous system, it won't take you five minutes'. It will. It always does, and so it should.

Chapter 2
Equipment

The instruments required for bedside neurological examination are relatively simple and, with one exception, inexpensive. There are, however, a few points of guidance which may help those planning their equipment.

The ophthalmoscope
A simple instrument is quite adequate provided it gives a steady, even, white disc of bright light shining in the plane of the examiner's visual axis when properly and comfortably held. Leak-proof batteries last longer and protect the casing. One may improvise many things for neurological examination, but nothing will replace a good ophthalmoscope.

The torch
Pocket-size torches giving a fine bright beam are better than the diffuse light of the larger variety.

The percussion hammer
The handle should be long and flexible, the ring of thick resilient rubber, without a heavy centre.

The pins
Sharp mapping pins with white heads are also useful for testing visual fields.

The two-point discriminator
Dealers may call this an aesthesiometer. Its points must be blunt, and besides its primary purpose it can be used for testing ocular movement and the superficial reflexes, while the prong can be inserted under a plaster case to test the plantar reflex—a not uncommon problem to be faced.

The stethoscope
Its end should be adapted to fit closely to the skull or orbit in order to hear intracranial bruits.

The examination couch
This should be warm and securely covered so that the patient is comfortable and not afraid of slipping, for this maintains muscular tension. Its headpiece

should be adjustable and its height such that one can reach easily over an obese patient's stomach and yet not have to kneel to examine his legs. It should not stand opposite bright light and it should be possible to reach both sides easily.

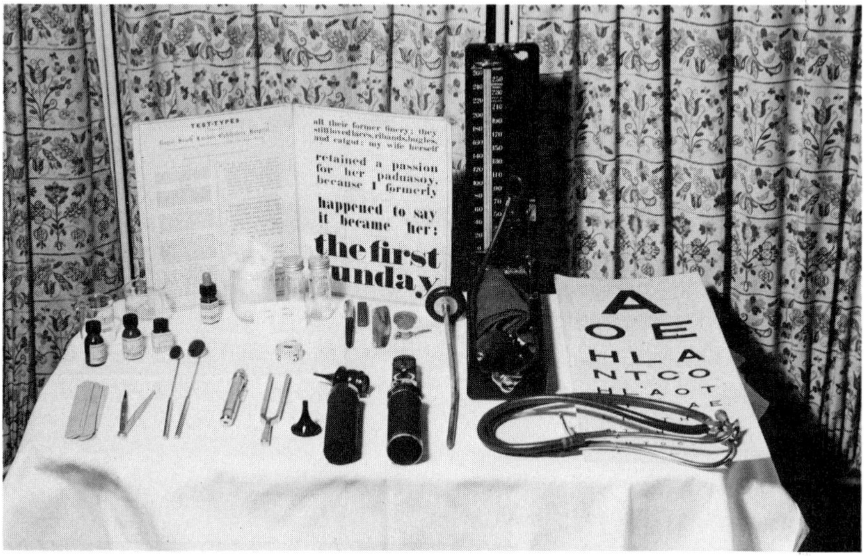

Fig. 1. Instruments required for neurological examination at the bedside.

The patient

Above all, one needs the patient preferably completely undressed or at the most wearing only short underpants. 'Shirt sleeves and socks' conceal diagnostic physical signs. Long pants in the elderly and modern trousers in the young should be removed, for if rolled above the knees they are efficient only as a tourniquet. Brassières and corsets may conceal a carcinoma of the breast, or a distended bladder or uterus, and these may have important bearing on diagnosis. (Yes—corsets *are* still worn.)

Chapter 3
The History

If a neurologist were in a group of people, stranded on a desert island, and if he were to be bereft of sight, arms and legs, but was still able to speak and hear, he would be able to take a history; and an accurate and detailed history is the supremely important part of the investigation of a neurological problem. By the time the history is complete, the physician should be three-quarters of the way towards the diagnosis, and, if he is not, then there is something wrong with the way in which it has been taken.

Experience of consultations has shown that this is almost invariably the weakest part in the presentation of a clinical problem. The modes of onset and progression of symptoms are ill-defined, the terms used are vague and woolly, and items of unhelpful information often predominate instead of the vital facts. The art of taking a good neurological history lies in paying particular attention to certain important points.

The age of the patient

Surprisingly enough, this is often omitted from verbal case reports, but it influences the management of the problem more than almost any other single factor. There is generally a fairly high degree of correlation between age and the most probable diagnosis. For example, at the age of 20, a very rapidly developing brain stem lesion is most likely to be due to demyelinative disease, whereas in the 60s it is probably due to basilar artery deficiency. A cerebellar tumour below the age of 12 is probably a medulloblastoma; in the late teens or early twenties, often an astrocytoma or ependymoma; between 35 and 50, usually a haemangioblastoma, while later on a metastasis becomes likely. Record the year of birth in the case notes, for records have a habit of perpetuating the age at which the patient first attended.

Clarifying the symptoms

It must be made absolutely clear what a patient means by his description of his symptoms. By all means put it down in his own words first, but do not be content with that. The term 'giddiness' may mean, to some, rotational vertigo; to others a sense of instability, ataxia of gait, disturbance of vision, loss of contact with surroundings, nausea, or the term may be used as a socially acceptable description of a full-scale epileptic convulsion. 'Black-outs' may mean loss of consciousness, loss of vision, loss of memory, or just loss of confidence. By explaining to the patient the great importance of the doctor knowing as well as he does what he means by the terms he uses, and if necessary giving illustrations of the way in which different people mean different things, these points can be clarified by careful insistence.

Having reached this stage, the patient must then be forced to be precise about the nature, position and duration of his symptoms. Do not be satisfied with generalisations and vague gestures. A note such as 'the patient complains of continuous pain in the right side of the face' is of very little practical value. 'Continuous' may mean truly continuous or frequently repeated. A pain in the right side of the face lasting continuously all day is not trigeminal neuralgia, but attacks of pain, each lasting a few seconds, but repeated every few minutes throughout the day, may very well be, yet it is likely that either will be described as 'continuous'. The patient should clarify the word 'pain'. Many use this word as the easiest in their vocabulary to describe some quite different sensation, such as tingling or even numbness. The character of the pain is important, whether it is aching, shooting, burning, searing, etc., and the patient should be asked to give an honest assessment of its severity. Adjectives such as 'agonising' slip off the tongue too easily.

Finally, and still taking the same example, the patient must be made to indicate with his forefinger the exact part of the face affected. Often by this method he may clearly trace out a sensory dermatome or the distribution of a peripheral nerve.

The mode of onset and progression of the symptoms

Most patients, if made to realise how important it is, will be able to say whether a symptom developed abruptly or gradually. As vascular accidents form so large a part of neurological work, this distinction is vital. It is still amazing how many patients with subarachnoid haemorrhages are admitted to fever hospitals with a diagnosis of 'meningitis' because the dramatic onset of the headache and neck stiffness is not appreciated. If the patient is persistently vague in this respect, he should be asked to compare the onset with either a clap of the hands or a gradually rising movement of the hand. In the same way, the progression must be clarified, whether it has been steadily worsening, worsening in a series of steps, or relapsing and remitting. Here again illustration by hand movement helps the inarticulate or the vague. Examiners must, however, constantly check themselves from putting words into their patient's mouth, for this is so easy a thing to do.

The chronological sequence of events

Sooner or later someone else is going to read the notes; someone, perhaps, who will have to rely on them entirely to formulate his opinion. They should, therefore, be easily intelligible, and the order of events in time be clearly documented, keeping the main complaints together and not interposing disorders in other systems unless of obvious relevance. It should be possible from rapidly glancing at a history for a newcomer to build up a clear mental picture of the development of the disease without having to go over each point again with the patient.

The value of negative information

From the symptoms the examiner will have formed a good idea of the general group of disorders into which the patient's case falls. Direct enquiry as to the absence of certain symptoms is often as helpful in differentiation as positive information.

Excluding irrelevancies

Every physician likes to form his own opinion; every patient likes to relate the opinions given to him by others. Patients delight in describing in detail the hospitals they have been to (with dates, usually accurate); the doctors they have seen (with names, usually inaccurate); the detailed conversations that they have had with them (with quotations, usually incredible); and the treatment ordered (with results, usually disastrous); together with a wealth of other information which contributes not one iota to the value of the history. These recitals must be checked and irrelevancies rigorously excluded, though an appendix giving previous hospital admissions may sometimes be of value if one wishes to obtain the results of previous investigations.

Drugs

Direct questions should be asked concerning medication, whether taken regularly, or at whim, and regarding exposure to habit-forming drugs, by mouth, by injection, or by inhalation. Many physicians, including neurologists, shy away from this question, and so, on occasions, may miss a vital cause of symptoms. Questions regarding prescribed medication apply particularly to anti-Parkinsonian remedies, to anticonvulsants, and to psychotropic drugs, taken singly or in combination, their type and their dosage. Special enquiry should be made as to the use of oral contraceptives, tactfully, but nevertheless at any age after puberty, and without regard to marital status, or religion.

Interviewing the relatives

While always wise to get an external observer's view of the story, in certain circumstances it is absolutely obligatory. These circumstances are:

(*a*) Where the patient is a child.
(*b*) Where he suffers from episodes of impairment of consciousness.
(*c*) Where there is obvious memory defect or mental change.

(*d*) When details concerning other members of the family need to be checked.

No case record should ever start with the words 'history unobtainable', even if the only history is what the policeman bringing in the patient can give.

In determining whether a patient is having epileptic attacks, and if so, whether these are focal or generalised, the need to interview a relative or witness would seem to be obvious. Yet at every clinic one sees a patient sent up entirely by himself, suffering from attacks of loss of consciousness of which he himself knows nothing until he comes round, with a request for a decision as to whether or not he has epilepsy, presumably in the pious, but misguided, belief that an EEG will answer the question.

Interviewing relatives will often give valuable insight into personal relationships in the family or household which the patient himself may be too embarrassed or too loyal to mention, but which may influence diagnosis and ultimate disposal.

Finally, the relatives may be able to give full details of birth, infancy and education; they may describe a voluntary or enforced change of handedness; and they may open up a whole new aspect to the case by confiding that one or other, or both, is or are not the true parents at all, so that a negative family history may be pure assumption.

Some extra details

Hospital residents should remember that the general practitioner is often able to clarify points confused by patients or relatives. A telephone call in time may save the patient numerous unrewarding investigations and the nation considerable expenditure. This applies particularly where the question of compensation following an injury may arise. 'I had never had any trouble with my back before' may turn out to be the understatement of the year.

In children, details of performance at school obtained from the school authorities will often show a recent deterioration not realised or not admitted by the parents, but having direct bearing on the clinical problem.

When the record of the history is completed it should be critically studied. If an intelligent layman, reading it for the first time, would end with a clear picture of the development of the case, then that history will probably be a good one. Remember, however, that it must also be an accurate one, and beware of the fallacy that the neat typing of notes, so perfected in some departments, guarantees their accuracy, as well as their legibility. It does not!

Chapter 4
First Impressions

To the experienced physician first impressions are invaluable, but if they are allowed to develop into spot diagnosis this will sooner or later lead to disaster. The purpose of this chapter is to emphasise that intelligent analysis of clinical observations made from the moment of first contact with the patient can give a wealth of information which may not be obtainable later under the somewhat artificial conditions of formal examination.

The circumstances differ when the patient enters the physician's room, and when the physician enters the patient's room, and they are dealt with separately.

PATIENT TO PHYSICIAN

Before the patient enters

Listen first to the patient's approach. Loud conversation outside the room usually indicates a patient well accustomed to attending doctors, one who is highly nervous and trying to prove to himself and others that he is not, one who has inco-ordination of the muscles of articulation such as in multiple sclerosis or one who has *recently* become deaf.

From the sounds made while walking towards the door, it should be possible to distinguish unilateral dragging of the foot in hemiplegia, bilateral dragging in spastic paraplegia, the double 'ker-lump' sound of the dropped foot, and the shorter, irregular, unsteady double sound of severe postural deficit, as in carcinomatous sensory neuropathy or in tabes. The Parkinsonian shuffle is a short, variable, accelerating sound and differs from the constant, short, even shuffle of the cerebral arteriosclerotic (marche aux petits pas).

Psychoneurotic patients, especially those with medico-legal problems, frequently arrive three-quarters of an hour or more before they are due to be seen but those coming for the umpteenth medico-legal report often arrive late, 'having had difficulty in finding the address'.

Coming through the door

The stooping, flexed, rigid attitude of Parkinsonism gives the impression that such patients are trying to come through the exact centre of a very narrow space (Fig. 2). Though they may smile, the facial immobility and absence of blinking often results in an appearance rather of startled surprise. They may appear to stick in the doorway, or come through the last few feet in a little run. Each turn is made by the body as a whole.

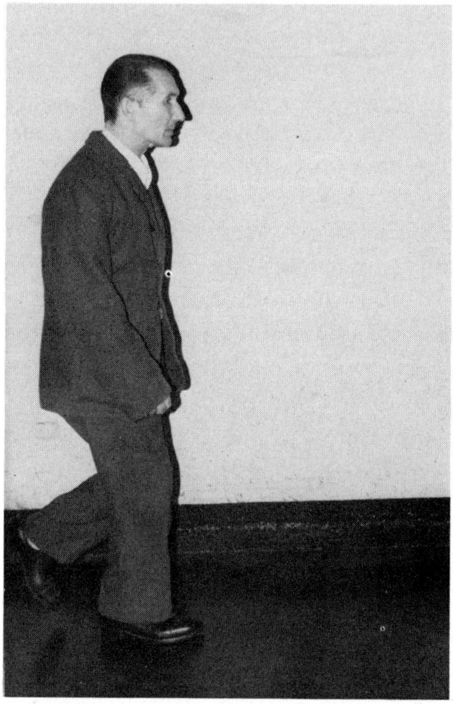

Fig. 2. A Parkinsonian patient enters the room. Note the stoop, the fixed expression, the flexed position of hands, arms and trunk.

Patients with cerebellar ataxia may reel into the door frame, but usually successfully fend themselves off. Those who hit it before they realise it, and then turn their heads apparently unnecessarily far round to see what they have hit, probably have a hemianopia. Those who reel only when they are within sight may be doing it especially for the examiner's benefit, but they nearly always forget on the way out.

The patient who reels explosively in on a broad base, stick thrust out forwards and sideways, an exaggerated, rather fatuous smile on his face, looking in the examiner's direction, but not exactly at him, and who begins talking equally explosively from the doorway, has almost always fairly advanced multiple sclerosis.

If the patient is both ataxic and has his head turned, as if deaf, towards the side of an obvious facial paralysis, it is probable that this is due to a cerebello-pontine angle tumour.

Moving from door to chair

The patient's chair should not be too near the entrance. In the few movements needed for him to reach it a great deal can be learnt.

THE SIZE AND SHAPE OF THE PATIENT

Note dwarfism, excessive height, obesity, wasting and obvious skeletal deformities. Look for an abnormal size of head such as in hydrocephalus, acromegaly, achondroplasia and Paget's disease. Mild degrees of acromegaly are not uncommon in the general population.

THE MODE OF DRESS

Note whether the dress is unkempt, as in the depressed and mentally deteriorated; over-cared for; too casual, often indicating an habitual patient, or merely a modern youth; or too voluminous (a warning to reorganise the next half-hour's work, for the patient is going to occupy the examination room for a very long time).

THE HAIR

The bedraggled hair style of the depressed female is very striking. This is also seen in women showing premature baldness associated with organic disease and is very obvious in dystrophia myotonica. A very sharp demarcation line between hair and scalp may suggest a wig, and suggest a history of alopecia with all its causative or attendant psychological stresses, or a previous cranial operation.

GAIT AND POSTURE

This is an ideal time to observe the gait. At the end of the examination it will be necessary to re-assess this when the patient is undressed, but now he is moving without realising that special observations are being made, and unnatural postures are less frequently adopted. The types of gait are dealt with in Chap. 18.

Look for the presence of kyphosis, scoliosis, torticollis, the short retracted neck of basilar invagination and the forward drooping neck of profound muscular weakness, such as in progressive muscular atrophy, myasthenia gravis, or carcinomatous neuropathy.

Shake hands with the patient, and compare the grip with the muscular development of the patient. A hand like a wet fish is common in psychoneurosis and those with an 'inadequate' personality. In those with non-organic states the grip is often strong under the automatic stimulus of a handshake, but during formal examination for strength may be almost non-existent.

On sitting down

Patients who ask to remain standing, or who collapse into a chair puffing, blowing and fanning themselves, do not very often have organic disease. Similarly those who sit on one buttock only should be viewed with caution.

Involuntary movements, tics, and habit spasms are now at their most obvious (see Chap. 19). A sudden distortion of one side of the face, to which the patient clasps his hand, probably holding a handkerchief, is almost pathognomonic of trigeminal neuralgia. The tremor of extrapyramidal disease appears as soon as the patient is settled, by which time, through force of habit, he may have attempted to conceal the affected limb.

Some Parkinsonian patients, unable to get comfortable, constantly change their position; others, due to intense akinesia, remain totally immobile and may be unable to rise when asked to do so. It is important for therapeutic reasons to recognise this akinesia.

Hearing aids indicate *bilateral* marked deafness and therefore make it very unlikely that the deafness is due to a cerebello-pontine angle tumour, which is a common query in the request for a neurological opinion.

In children and adolescents, a sudden pause, a stare into space, a flicker of the lids, a few mumbled words, and a little shake of the upper limbs, followed by an embarrassed smile, may illustrate a petit-mal attack before a word of history has been given. Other children will not sit down but continuously rush around the room, examining everything but concentrating on nothing. This *hyper*kinesia is often associated with epilepsy.

As the hands become visible, excessively long finger nails, particularly if painted unusual colours, often share with bizarre spectacle frames a method of drawing attention to an individual who might otherwise escape notice. Multiple burns suggest syringomyelia, but may be occupational. Note the presence of rheumatoid arthritis often associated with wasting of the small muscles.

THE FACE

Be on the alert to identify the plethoric, fat, hairy face of Cushing's syndrome; the round, smooth, hairless face with the yellowish pallor of hypopituitarism; or the sunken, wasted face with the brownish-yellow pallor of malignant cachexia. Note any scars. Exophthalmos and lid retraction occur in hyperthyroidism; gross exophthalmos with chemosis and ocular paresis in exophthalmic ophthalmoplegia. Watch the eyelids carefully for the drooping which varies from moment to moment in myasthenia gravis, or for the fixed bilateral droop with wrinkled forehead in ocular myopathy, or the fixed, unilateral droop of a IIIrd nerve palsy. A unilateral fixed ptosis may be part of a Horner's syndrome, when there will be enophthalmos and a small pupil. The combination of baldness, ptosis, downward drawn face and scraggy neck are typical of dystrophia myotonica (Fig. 3). Watch the patient's blinking. Absence of blinking is common in Parkinsonism. When there is a lower motor neurone facial paralysis the eyes turn up without the lids closing. Note any tremor of facial muscles, clonic spasm of orbicularis oculis and oris, and the flickering around the eyes of myokimia—which may also be seen in other parts of the facial musculature.

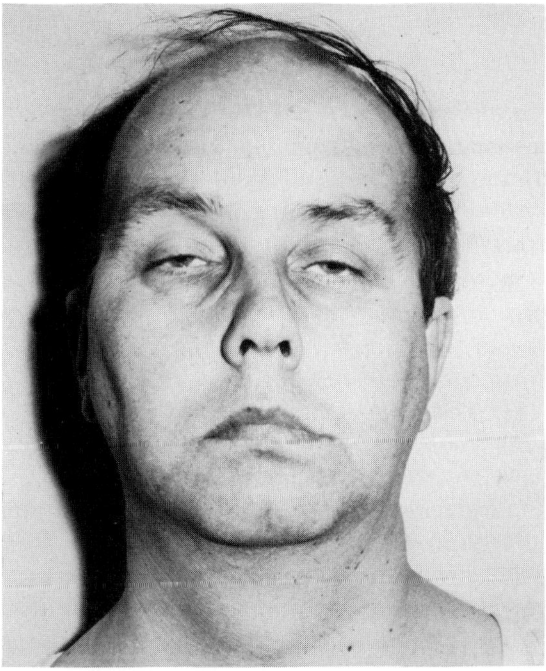

Fig. 3. Dystrophia myotonica. Baldness, ptosis, myopathic facies and absence of sternomastoids. See also Figs 19c and 20d.

THE VOICE

Listen to the volume of sound, the clarity of the words and the content of the speech. Disturbances of speech are dealt with in Chap. 28.

Patients with pseudobulbar palsy and occasionally with primary brain stem lesions often show 'incontinence' of emotion, laughing or crying involuntarily and irrelevantly.

Correlating the symptoms with the patient's condition

During the course of taking the history, the examiner must always ask himself 'Would this patient look or behave in this manner if he had the symptoms of which he complains?' Failure of correlation does not, of course, necessarily mean that the patient's condition is hysterical. It may be merely an indication that the exact nature of the patient's complaint must be clarified. A patient who says he has no use in the right leg and yet has just walked in, probably means that he has a disturbance of sensation in the leg. On the other hand, a patient who complains of unremitting and intolerable pain in the face, driving him to the point of suicide, and *present at that moment*, but who appears to be in no discomfort of any sort, is unlikely to be describing an organic condition. These are only two examples of comparisons too numerous to mention.

PHYSICIAN TO PATIENT

This is a rather different situation and arises when the physician approaches a bed in the ward, or enters the patient's room in his home. It is in the latter instance that clinical acumen is given its stiffest test, for before the physician leaves that room he will be expected to have formulated a complete analysis of the case.

The patient seated in a chair

Does the patient rise on one's entry? If not, note first the posture. It is easy to recognise the forward stooped immobility of the Parkinsonian; the lateral slump of the hemiplegic; the poorly focused, grimacing welcoming of the patient with multiple sclerosis; the grossly swollen legs that usually mean that the patient has been confined to that chair for many months.

Glance around at the rest of the room. Innumerable bottles and pillboxes suggest a demanding patient and probably a hypochondriacal one, and the stick close at hand for thumping the floor demonstrates the command that the patient has over his family. An empty room suggests a recent illness.

The patient in bed

In the home the state of the bedroom will show whether the patient is well accustomed to being there, or is an unwilling invalid. In hospital the environment of the ward is too standardised, and, apart from family photographs, one may obtain few clues from it.

Note the condition of bedclothes and nightclothes for evidence of cleanliness, vomiting or incontinence.

Next assess the patient's conscious level, using the methods dealt with in Chap. 27. If the patient is alert it can be seen by his drawn expression if he is in pain, or by his perfectly normal appearance that he evidently is not however much he may complain. Intense photophobia occurs in meningeal irritation, and migraine. However, do not confuse eye closure and turning of the head away from the light with blepharospasm, where the lids are forcibly, if tremulously, closed, this closure becoming tighter as one attempts to open them. The patient with vertigo lies still, not daring to turn. Patients with thyrotoxicosis usually sit upright and forwards, doing nothing; those with respiratory distress lean across a bedtable; those surrounded by writing materials are obviously not very ill.

The approach generally should be no different from that in the outpatient department. Accuracy of history is just as vital and in the home one usually has the unique opportunity of talking privately and unobtrusively to the relatives, and full advantage of this must be taken. There is, however, that subtle difference produced by the fact that it is the physician who is the visitor. In modern life, a doctor's visit is too common an event necessarily to make a deep impression, and to restore for him the position of control he must show confidence and precision both in history taking and in examination. This is not difficult if he knows the facts and features he must elicit and it is especially important for the young physician who may be visiting patients of an age and social position considerably more impressive than his own.

It is one of the saddest aspects of modern medical practice that consultants now visit patients at their homes in the absence of the patient's own doctor, whose knowledge of the background, hobbies, achievements, disappointments, may add so much to the clarification of puzzling symptoms, the need for which may not have been forseen in the preliminary conversation over the telephone.

Chapter 5
The General Physical and Mental Examination

So many neurological disorders form a part of general systemic disease that complete physical examination is absolutely obligatory in each case. To this must be added an assessment of the mental state. This need not be very elaborate, and indeed full mental examination is beyond the scope of this book. The paragraphs that follow are no more than very brief notes which help during routine examinations to detect organic mental disturbance. A suggested scheme for assessment of higher cerebral function is to be found in Appendix C p. 348. The remainder of this chapter lists relationships between general systemic diseases and nervous disease which may easily be forgotten.

THE MENTAL STATE

Co-operation

Unco-operativeness may be due to disturbance of conscious level, to confusion, suspicion, delusion, hallucination, aggressiveness or violence. It must be realised, however, that an apparent lack of co-operation may be due to dysphasia (See Chap. 28) and many unfortunate patients have found themselves admitted to mental hospitals for what is a wholly organic disturbance of speech.

Orientation

Determine whether the patient knows his name, age, address; the number and names of his children; the date, month and year; where he is, and who the doctors and nurses are. Disorientation may occur in time, place and person in organic dementias.

Memory

Test his ability to remember events of that day, the previous week, months and earlier years. Ask what actions he has recently carried out, how he came to the present building, where this building is and where he is going after he leaves. Find out if he has read the newspapers or watched television, and ask what have been the main news stories of recent days. If interested in sport see if he can recall items of topical sporting news.

Read out to him clearly and slowly a series of numbers for him to repeat. Start with three, and increase by one each time until he makes consistent errors. It is wise to have written out the groups of numbers beforehand. Avoid consecutive numbers; avoid emphasising any one number. Then carry out the test with different numbers asking him to repeat them in reverse order. Many people can repeat seven or eight forwards and four or five backwards correctly.

Many patients may fail these tests due simply to poor powers of concentration, but loss of recent memory and ability to retain and recall are common in all organic dementias, distant memory often being preserved.

In Korsakov's psychosis, recent memory and orientation in time and place are so disturbed that the patient makes up stories, often interesting ones, to fill in the gaps. This is termed *confabulation*, and may be so detailed as to convince an unwary examiner. Though classically associated with alcoholism, anterior hypothalamic lesions due perhaps to anterior communicating aneurysms or their surgical treatment can temporarily produce an identical picture.

Emotional state

Note if the patient is anxious, excited, depressed, frightened, apathetic or euphoric. Euphoria is apparently common in patients with multiple sclerosis, but often only when visiting the doctor. Some patients with frontal lobe disease repeatedly make fatuous remarks and treat all parts of the examination as something of a joke, a condition termed 'witzelsucht'. A somewhat aggressive euphoria commonly follows severe head injuries.

Incontinence of emotion, laughing or crying suddenly and often inappropriately, occurs in pseudobulbar palsy, usually due to bilateral cerebro-vascular disease.

Delusions and hallucinations

Listen to the flow of speech; is there evidence of delusions, and, if so, are they systematised or grandiose; does he appear to have auditory, visual or olfactory hallucinations, and can he describe them? Temporal lobe lesions produce well-organised hallucinations, sometimes terrifying; occipital lobe visual hallucinations are ill-formed. Patients with non-dominant hemisphere lesions are usually able to describe hallucinations more clearly and in greater detail.

Great assistance can be given by a qualified psychologist in psychometric examination, in assessing intelligence, educational state and capacity, and finding evidence of recent deterioration in organic cerebral disease. In children it may be difficult clinically to distinguish between mental deterioration and a pre-existing mental defect which has merely become more obvious as they grow older. Here serial recordings are important.

Tests for organic dementia are more than of academic interest these days for in the so-called low-pressure hydrocephalus beneficial therapy may be available for the appropriate few.

Tests for apraxia, agnosia and disorders of body scheme are dealt with in the appropriate sections (Chaps 29 and 30).

THE HEAD AND NECK

Note the size, shape, and position of the head; palpate, percuss and auscultate the surface.

Inspection

Gross degrees of *hydrocephalus* are obvious. To detect lesser degrees note that the hydrocephalic head and face resemble an inverted triangle, the forehead being large, bossed and bulging forwards over the orbits, the eyes being displaced slightly forwards and downwards.

In *microcephaly*, the head appears as a triangle the right way up, the forehead sloping backwards, the occiput forwards and the cranium coming to a rounded point.

In *craniosynostosis* the head is deformed in a manner which varies according to which sutures are prematurely fused. The fused sutures may be felt as hard ridges. The fontanelles are closed, the orbits are flattened and the eyes protrude, sometimes to an extreme degree. In these children there is often associated finger webbing, and also bronchiectasis.

In *acromegaly*, the size of the head is increased by elongation, with enlargement of the jaw, and of the ears and nose, while the teeth are separated, the skin coarsened and excessively folded around the eyes, and, of course, the hands and feet are also enlarged, the digits blunt-ended and spade-like.

The head in advanced *Paget's disease* is enlarged and appears unnaturally rounded, the scalp being red, warm and covered with dilated vessels.

In *basilar invagination*, the head appears to lie in extension on a shortened neck, the hair-line is low and movement is limited. It gives the appearance of being thrust downwards and backwards upon the cervical spine (Fig. 4).

Palpation

Feel the surface of the skull for bony irregularities or deficiencies. The latter are sometimes congenital, sometimes traumatic, often post-operative but may represent erosive lesions such as eosinophilic granulomata or xanthomata. Skull defects, like fontanelles, are normally concave and pulsating, but become convex and tense in raised intracranial pressure in very young children.

Localised bony lumps may lie over an exostosing meningioma, may be evidence of a sarcoma, or may be developmental abnormalities of no significance.

In infants the anterior fontanelle must be felt and measured. It is usually closed by 18 months, but this varies greatly. It is enlarged in hydrocephalus from any cause, but is tense and bulging in states of continued high intracranial pressure. It is prematurely closed in craniosynostosis.

Percussion

In children with hydrocephalus and separation of the sutures, tapping the skull with the finger tip produces a tympanitic, impure, and rather high-pitched note, the so-called 'cracked-pot' sound.

Auscultation

This is of utmost importance in all age groups. The stethoscope is placed on both frontal bones, on the lateral occipital regions and then on each closed eyelid in turn. In the last case, if the other eye is opened the noise due to eyelid flicker is reduced. Listen for a systolic bruit, which when present is

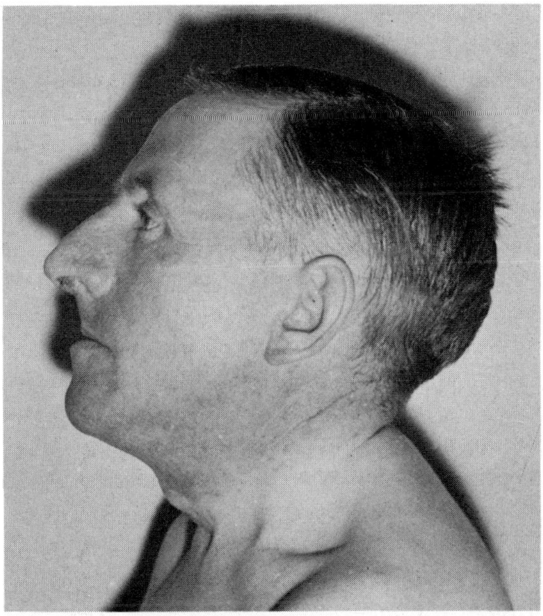

Fig. 4. Basilar impression. Note the short, retracted neck and low hair-line.

usually faint and distant, and may be heard only if the patient holds his breath. Bruits are heard:

(*a*) *In young children*, too frequently to be of value in diagnosis.

(*b*) *In arterio-venous communications*. This includes angiomata and carotico-cavernous fistulae, tumours of the glomus jugulare (best heard over the mastoid and jugular vein), and in advanced Paget's disease. It cannot be too strongly emphasised that intracranial bruits are very uncommon in berry aneurysms.

(*c*) *Over enlarged external vessels* supplying a vascular meningioma.

(*d*) *When conducted upwards from the neck*, such as in carotid stenosis or aortic stenosis.

(*e*) Sometimes for no very clear reason at all, investigation revealing no abnormality. This may be due to partial compression of a superficial vessel by the end of the stethoscope, so avoid areas where these are known to be present. They may occasionally occur with avascular intracranial neoplasms, possibly due to distortion of normal vessels.

Transillumination

In small hydrocephalic infants, transillumination of the skull in total darkness can give quite a good assessment of the size of the ventricles and the amount of residual brain tissue. Computerised scanning is useful, if available, because it will of course give much greater detail.

Neck movement and meningeal irritation

Place both hands under the occipital region and by flexing the wrists, gently raise the head forwards until the chin rests on the chest.

Neck ridigity occurs in meningeal irritation of any cause; in inflammatory and destructive disease of the cervical spine, and in cervical fusion; to some degree in cervical spondylosis and in Parkinsonism; and in high intracranial pressure it is a danger sign of tonsillar herniation. Extreme tenderness at the side of the neck over the course of the jugular vein is seen after extension of a lateral sinus thrombosis. Tenderness of scalp muscles is extremely rare in organic disease, but common in psychoneurosis, tension headache, and simulated head pains. In the same way persistent tenderness in neck muscles rarely has organic significance, yet is complained of for years after a potentially compensatable neck injury.

Now flex each hip in turn and then try to extend the knee. This is greatly limited in meningeal irritation (*Kernig's sign*), and not affected in the other conditions mentioned above.

Straight-leg raising

In suspected lumbar disc prolapse, the ability to raise the extended leg is limited on the side of the lesion (*Lasègue's sign*), and raising the normal leg may produce root pain on the affected side. In the rare high lumbar disc lesions, root pain may be reproduced by hyperextending the hip. Though similar to Kernig's sign, there is, of course, no neck rigidity. If the knee has been painlessly fully flexed, and then the hip flexed, and root pain is still claimed to be produced, one should be wary of the organic nature of the case.

THE SPINE

Spinal examination, normally carried out late in the examination, is described together with tests of stance and gait in Chap. 18.

THE PERIPHERAL NERVES

Palpate the ulnar nerve at the elbow, and the lateral popliteal nerve below the knee as it courses round the head of the fibula. Note if they are very superficial, for they are then prone to trauma, the ulnar nerve particularly if there is also cubitus valgus. Sometimes, especially after old injury, the ulnar nerve may be shrouded in thickened tissues at, or just below, the elbow. Thickening of nerves occurs in the hypertrophic forms of hereditary polyneuropathy (and differentiates this from similar physical signs caused by peroneal muscular atrophy)—and in leprosy. In the latter, the greater auricular nerve is almost always involved and patches of sensory loss and trophic changes are evident. Neurofibromata may be palpable along the course of a nerve. Following nerve injury, and during regeneration, tapping the point to which the nerve has regrown may produce paræsthesiæ in its distribution (*Tinel's sign*). Pressure at the wrist over the ulnar (and sometimes the median) nerve, may reproduce the patient's symptoms, especially if the nerve is compressed by a deep ganglion at this site.

GENERAL EXAMINATION

The ears

Auroscopy should be as much of the routine examination as examination of the heart and lungs. Most deafness is not due to VIIIth nerve disease. *Otitis media* must be most carefully looked for in any case of meningitis, meningism, facial paralysis, or if there are any other features suggestive of intracranial infection, such as rapidly spreading local fits, or a pleocytosis in the cerebro-spinal fluid.

In cases of unilateral lower cranial nerve palsies, a *polyp* in the middle ear seen behind the drum or extending into the external meatus may be the vital clue to the presence of a tumour of the glomus jugulare. Do not under any circumstances interfere with such a polyp; torrential haemorrhage may result.

The skin

Watch the skin carefully throughout the examination, for many features vary from moment to moment. Look in particular for:

(*a*) *Signs of vasomotor instability and peripheral vascular deficiency*, often associated with migraine, syncope and psychoneurosis.

(*b*) *Allergic lesions* and *dermatographia.*

(*c*) *Scleroderma.* Systemic sclerosis may present as muscle weakness and wasting, dysphargia and dysarthia, and resemble motor neurone disease.

(*d*) *Cutaneous von Recklinghausen's phenomena.* These include café-au-lait patches, mollusca fibrosa, subcutaneous and plexiform neurofibromata. These may be associated with spinal and intracranial neurofibromata and meningiomata, and may be familial.

(*e*) *Adenoma sebaceum.* In the early stages this consists of pink, globular, discrete spots on the cheeks, nose and chin, at first fading on pressure, but later darkening to deep red and coalescing. The spots almost spare the forehead and upper lip (Fig. 5b). This is associated with tuberous sclerosis.

(*f*) *Cutaneous angiomata.* Consider if they are distributed over a segmental

(a)

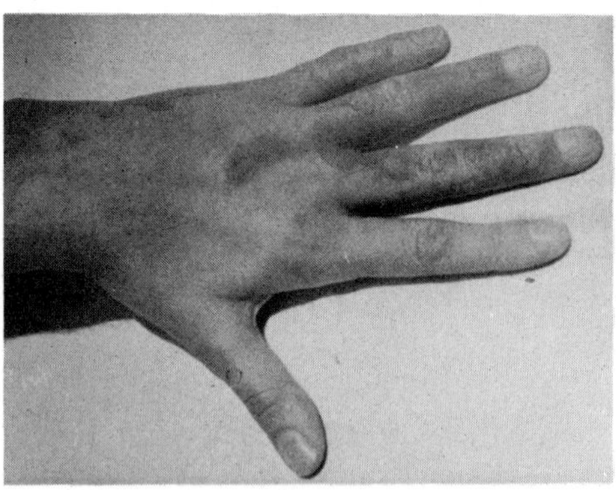

(b)

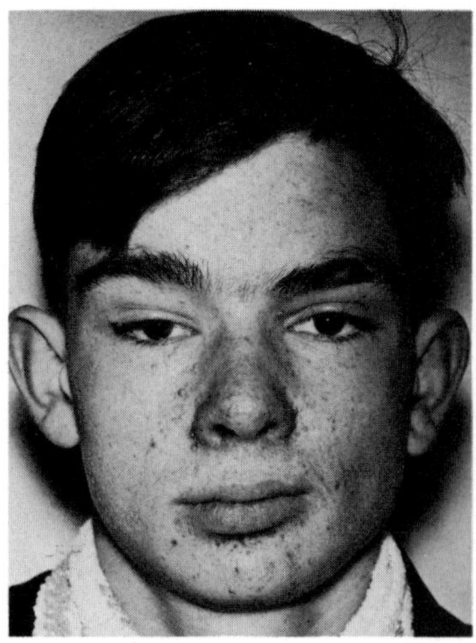

Fig. 5. (a) Segmental skin naevus. Naevus over C7, 8 dermatomes in a case of cervical syringomyelia. (b) Adenoma sebaceum. An early case of tuberous sclerosis with mental deficiency and retinal phakomata. The spots are still discrete and almost limited to the cheeks, nose and chin.

dermatome. Facial naevi occur in Sturge–Weber disease, and spinal segmental naevi with disorders of the neural crest, syringomyelia and spinal astrocytomata (Fig. 5a). Midline pink naevi centrally placed high in the neck are not uncommon in normal individuals, but may be very prominent in congenital spinal or cranio-spinal abnormalities. Spider naevi occur with hepatic cirrhosis and pregnancy, and in some normal people. In familial haemorrhagic telangiectasia, telangiectases may occur on the spinal arachnoid as well as on the skin.

(*g*) *Herpes zoster*. Apart from the disease itself, this type of eruption may occur at the segmental level of spinal lesions due to secondary deposits, multiple sclerosis and even trauma.

(*h*) *Herpes simplex*. Note this carefully, especially in children, for herpes encephalitis is now recognisable and treatable. Vesicles around the lips are common following surgical treatment of trigeminal neuralgia.

(*i*) *The common exanthemata* may be complicated by an encephalitis.

(*j*) A variety of *rashes* occur in the collagen diseases, in glandular fever and in drug toxicity.

(*k*) *Angular cheilitis* and *pellagra-like skin disorders* may be associated with deficiency neuropathies, and Hartnup disease (q.v.).

(*l*) *Skin malignancy*, in particular *melanomata*, may have multiple metastases in the nervous system and the primary may have been removed some years before.

(*m*) *Light-sensitive eruptions* occur in porphyria (polyneuropathy and mental changes with colicky abdominal pain).

(*n*) *Erythema ab igne* is common in the lonely and depressed.

(*o*) *Bed sores* are particularly prone to develop in anaesthetic areas.

(*p*) *Septic skin areas* often precede epidural spinal abscess formation.

(*q*) *Scars, burns, destruction of terminal phalanges* and all degrees of peripheral mutilation can occur in syringomyelia, leprosy, and hereditary sensory neuropathy.

(*r*) *Ulcers on the external genitalia, in the mouth*, and *eyes*, occurs in Behçet's syndrome, which may be accompanied by diffuse cerebral and spinal cord disease not unlike multiple sclerosis.

(*s*) *Tufts of hair* often overlie developmental spinal abnormalities, particularly a 'split cord'.

The heart

There are several ways in which cardiac abnormalities can be correlated with disease of the nervous system.

PULSE RATE AND REGULARITY

(*a*) A *very slow rate* occurs in increased intracranial pressure, in vasovagal seizures, and in complete heart block with Stokes–Adams attacks.

(*b*) A *very fast rate* is found in nervousness, systemic infections, thyrotoxicosis, paroxysmal tachycardia and severe haemorrhage.
(*c*) A *fibrillating heart* may produce cerebral emboli.
(*d*) *Changes in heart rate or rhythm*, including runs of *extra-systoles* (so often considered unimportant) may cause attacks of faintness or vertigo particularly if atheroma of the carotid, vertebral, or subclavian arteries is present.
(*e*) *Cerebral emboli* may follow any form of open heart surgery.

HEART SOUNDS
(*a*) *Cardiac murmurs* may be significant in patients with chorea.
(*b*) *Mitral and aortic disease* may be associated with cerebral emboli, especially if there is any suggestion of bacterial endocarditis.
(*c*) *Aortic stenosis* causes episodes of fainting.
(*d*) *Aortic regurgitation* may be associated with neurosyphilis.
(*e*) *Congenital cardiac lesions* predispose to cerebral abscess formation.
(*f*) *Subclavian stenosis* may result in a steal of blood from the vertebro-basilar system, especially on exercise. A subclavian bruit may be accompanied by a delayed radial pulse and a lower blood pressure in the affected arm.

The blood pressure

This must be taken in every case, both lying and standing, if the patient is fit enough to do so, and in both arms. *Hypertension* may be of the benign type in so far as it is not producing renal damage or retinal disease, but in the presence of a sudden loss of function of some part of the body, it may very well be of great significance. Transient postural hypotension is probably the commonest overall cause of attacks of loss of consciousness. The blood pressure is always an important feature in assessing both the wisdom of investigative procedures, such as arteriography and pneumoencephalography, and the future management of the case. Though difficult, the blood pressure can be measured in the legs, and coarctation of the aorta may be associated with cerebrovascular accidents in the young.

The lungs

Attention during examination should be paid particularly to any suggestion of:
(*a*) *Bronchial carcinoma*, for in the male this is the commonest primary site for intracranial or multiple neurological metastases.
(*a*) *Bronchiectasis*, a common origin for metastatic abscesses.
(*c*) *Tuberculosis*, when there are signs of meningitis.
(*d*) *Severe bronchitis and emphysema*, which can cause headaches, papilloedema, fluctuating consciousness, and involuntary movements ('asterixis').

(*e*) *A Pancoast tumour*. This usually presents as inexorable pain and marked sensory impairment in the distribution of the lowest cord of the brachial plexus.
(*f*) *Small oat-cell carcinomata* (and mesotheliomata) may be associated with inappropriate antidiuretic hormone secretion by the pituitary.

The abdomen
Carcinoma of the stomach, colon and *hypernephromata* may first declare themselves as metastases in the nervous system. Metastases from these tumours may manifest themselves years after removal of the primary growth. One of the senior author's cases developed signs from an intracranial metastasis 17 years after removal of a hypernephroma. Neuroblastoma in children may give rise to deposits in the orbit and frontal bones (Hutchinson's syndrome).

Hepato-splenomegaly is associated with cerebral disease in the lipoidoses of children, in sarcoidosis, reticulosis and leukaemia in adults, and in the older age groups may be further evidence of metastatic malignancies, or may accompany the neurological features of chronic alcoholism, such as polyneuropathy, Wernicke's encephalopathy and Korsakov's psychosis.

The pelvis
Malignancy of pelvic organs may cause lesions in the nervous system, most frequently by metastasis to the spine (e.g. in prostatic carcinoma) or by direct invasion of peripheral nerves (e.g. in carcinoma of the cervix). *Pregnancy* may be associated with psychological disorders, with chorea, with vascular accidents, and with enlargement of pre-existing unsuspected cerebral tumours. As induced abortion is now commonplace, and not necessarily always carried out by the most expert hands it must not be forgotten that fits, hemipareses, and coma, may follow, due to *air emboli*, or even *amniotic emboli*, usually in unskilled hands. A pituitary tumour can cause *amenorrhoea* and it is unwise to diagnose primary amenorrhoea or a very early menopause without X-raying the sella turcica.

The breasts
The *breast* is the second most common site of the primary tumour in cerebral or spinal metastases. Careful examination is essential in all cases of spinal or cerebral disease both in men and women. Evidence of *previous mastectomy*, even if very radical and with no signs of local recurrence, may be highly significant. Galactorrhoea is a symptom of prolactinoma. Premature breast development can occur in hypothalamic lesions.

The thyroid
Pay special attention to the thyroid, noting its size and consistency, the pres-

ence of any signs of *thyrotoxicosis*, or the presence of a recent *thyroidectomy scar*. These may be significant in the presence of:
(*a*) Exophthalmos with ophthalmoplegia.
(*b*) Muscle wasting and weakness; thyrotoxic myopathy is a rare possibility. A periodic paralysis can accompany thyrotoxicosis.
(*c*) Multiple lesions in the nervous system; the thyroid is a site of primary tumours.
(*d*) Tendon reflexes which are prolonged and relax slowly. These are a feature of myxoedema (see page 187).
(*e*) Thyroid enlargement, or a past thyroidectomy, may have caused recurrent laryngeal nerve paralysis.

The glands

Glandular enlargement, accompanying disease of the nervous system, directs attention particularly to the following possibilities:
(*a*) Metastatic carcinoma or possible Hodgkin's disease.
(*b*) Granulomata such as sarcoid, which may cause cerebral deposits and polyneuropathy.
(*c*) Lymphatic leukaemia or reticulosis, in which, terminally, there may be severe cerebral demyelination, or an encephalitis due to invasion by torula, or other organisms, especially if immunosuppressive therapy has been given.
(*d*) Glandular fever. A Guillain-Barré syndrome is a rare complication, encephalitis may occur and local pressure palsies are not unknown.

The teeth

Unsuspected *dental abscesses* are a possible source of cerebral abscesses especially if there is congenital heart disease.

Defective teeth, defective closure and *temporo-mandibular joint disease* can all cause facial neuralgic pain.

Gum hypertrophy indicates heavy epanutin dosage.

The tongue

For convenience abnormalities are classified together in Chap. 12.

The nails

Nail-biting commonly indicates tension and anxiety. Koilonychia should make one suspect severe anaemia. Clubbing may accompany congenital heart disease, chronic chest disease, bronchial malignancy and chronic hepatic disease.

Part II
The Cranial Nerves

Chapter 6
The First Cranial Nerve: The Olfactory Nerve

It is unfortunate that this is the first nerve, for tests of its function form one of the least satisfactory parts of the whole examination. At times, however, anosmia may give the vital clue to localisation of an intracranial lesion. Some may consider it too much devotion to routine to start the neurological examination here, but it is so easy to forget it when concentrating on other areas.

Function

To carry sensations of smell from the nasal mucosa to the olfactory bulb. The stimuli then pass through the olfactory tract and roots, especially the lateral root, running to the peri-amygdaloid and pre-piriform areas of the cortex, and probably not the hippocampus as usually thought.

Purpose of the test

To determine whether any impairment of the sense of smell is unilateral or bilateral, and whether it is due to local nasal disease, or to a neural lesion.

Method of testing

Small bottles are required containing essences of very familiar odours. These must indeed be familiar. Asafaetida and even musk are sometimes advised, but are useless. Coffee, almonds, chocolate, oil of lemon and peppermint are amongst the many that are suitable.

The cork, or a piece of wool held in tweezers, is moistened with the fluid. The patient must then compress each nostril in turn and, by sniffing through the other, show that the airway is clear. The test odour is then placed under one nostril while the other is compressed, and the patient told to take two good, but not over-exuberant, sniffs. He is then asked (*a*) if he can smell anything and (*b*) if he can identify the odour. The test is then repeated using the other nostril and he is asked (*c*) if the odour is the same in each nostril. After an interval to allow that odour to disperse, the test is then repeated with two further odours and, in addition to the above, he is asked (*d*) if he can distinguish the different odours.

Interpretation of results

Patients will fall into several categories:

(*a*) Those who recognise and name the odours quickly (usually women).

(*b*) Those who recognise, but cannot name them (usually men).
(*c*) Those who can detect a smell, and easily distinguish differences, but can neither recognise, nor name them.

(*a*), (*b*) and (*c*) should be accepted as normal.

(*d*) Those for whom each odour smells the same but is distorted and unpleasant—parosmia.
(*e*) Those who can smell nothing in one or both nostrils, or whose sense is much reduced on one side compared with the other. This represents true anosmia, but careful examination of the nasal passages is necessary to distinguish neural from local disease.
(*f*) Those whose responses are very vague and variable. This is probably going to be a long and tiring neurological examination, and to avoid impatience at this early stage it is wise to return to the problem later.

Commonest causes of anosmia

(*a*) Local acute or chronic inflammatory nasal disease; heavy smoking.
(*b*) Head injury—usually thought due to tearing of olfactory filaments. The trauma may be surprisingly slight and often occipital.

These are by far the most common causes, all others being relatively infrequent.

(*c*) Intracranial tumours, malignant or benign, compressing the olfactory bulb or tract.
(*d*) Atrophy of the olfactory bulbs.
(*e*) Chronic meningeal inflammation (e.g. syphilis) or infiltration (e.g. sarcoidosis).
(*f*) Hysteria.

Causes (*b*) and (*d*) may be accompanied by CSF rhinorrhoea.

Parosmia is not uncommon in incomplete olfactory recovery following head injuries. It also may occur in depressive states.

Difficulties and fallacies

This is a purely subjective test. The examiner has to take the patient at his word and unfortunately anosmia as a potential sequel to head injury is now a well-known symptom—well-known to litigants as well as to doctors. If an attempt is made to produce objective results by using substances such as ammonia or ether something other than the olfactory nerve is being stimulated as well. It is widely believed that an olfactory groove meningioma is a common cause of anosmia. It is certainly an important cause, but it is also a rare tumour, and if a tumour is present, an inferior frontal glioma is in practice more likely.

Chapter 7
The Second Cranial Nerve: The Optic Nerve

Though the optic nerve is the most important cranial nerve, it is not a peripheral nerve in the true sense of the word, but a forward extension of a part of the brain. As it can reflect conditions existing inside the cranial cavity, no amount of trouble is too great to ensure satisfactory examination. It is customary at this stage to include tests designed to detect lesions throughout the whole extent of the visual pathways.

Functions

To carry visual impulses from the retina to the optic chiasma and on in the optic tract to the lateral geniculate body; to act as the afferent pathway for the pupillary light reflex by means of fibres travelling to the superior colliculus of the mid-brain.

Purpose of the tests

(*a*) To measure the acuity of vision and to determine if any defect is due to local ocular disease.
(*b*) To chart the visual fields.
(*c*) To take the unique opportunity of inspecting directly a part of the nerve itself.

VISUAL ACUITY

Methods of testing

The standard Snellen's Type charts are used for testing distant vision and the Jaegar Type cards for near vision (see Fig. 1).

The Snellen's Type chart is placed, evenly illuminated, 6 metres (20 feet) from the patient, who covers one eye and is asked to read the smallest line he can see accurately. He should not close an eye, as this may make him partially close the other and give misleading results, especially in myopia.

Acuity is recorded as a fraction (e.g. 6/24 or 20/80). The numerator indicates the distance at which the patient has to be from the chart in order to read the same type that the normal person could read at a distance indicated by the denominator. 6/5–6/6 are within the average normal range.

The Jaegar Type card must be held one foot from the patient's eye and a similar test is then carried out. The different types are labelled as, for instance, J.4, according to their size. Average acuity lies between J.1 and J.4.

There are of course a number of other test types, but the general principles remain the same.

If visual acuity is severely depressed, hold up varying numbers of fingers to be counted with each eye. If unable to do this, see if hand movements can be detected.

Always equate the degree of visual deficit *claimed* with what you observe the patient to be able to do.

Loss of visual acuity

The commonest causes of visual failure lie in lesions of the eye itself. These are too numerous to list, but include all refractive errors, cataracts, vitreous opacities, etc. In all cases, and especially if routine inspection of the eye reveals no such lesion, the next stages are the examination of the visual fields and of the optic nerve head and the retina.

THE VISUAL FIELDS

Charting the visual fields is the most important method of locating a lesion in the visual pathways or of interpreting certain fundus appearances, yet in clinical notes it is often regrettably difficult to find evidence that any attempt has been made to examine them at all.

Purposes of the tests

To chart the periphery of the visual fields; to detect the position, size and shape of the blind spot and any abnormal scotomata; to compare any defects shown with those abnormalities known to be reproduced by lesions at specific points in the visual pathways.

Methods of testing

Do not underestimate the value of testing by confrontation. A surprising degree of accuracy is possible with a co-operative patient.

Confrontation

The patient and examiner face each other. The examiner covers (say) the right eye and the patient covers the left, either with a shield or with his fingers, taking care to avoid obscuring the nasal field of the other eye. He must fix carefully on the examiner's pupil while the examiner moves test objects of varying size (the whole hand, a moving finger, a white disc), inwards in each of the four quadrants from just outside the limits of his own field. The patient must say the moment he sees the object and whether it is of equal clarity in each quadrant, for 'greying' of vision often precedes a measurable defect. The central area of vision can be tested in order to map out the blind spot and any scotomata by using a disc of white paper about 5 mm in diameter attached to a rod or long pin.

Remember to move from blind areas to areas of vision, for it is easier to detect appearance than disappearance of objects.

When this is completed, both eyes are uncovered, the examiner holds both hands in the outer part of the fields, and, moving one or other hand, or both together, asks the patient to point to the hand moved. This will detect the phenomenon of visual inattention common in parietal disorders when though the fields tested in each eye separately are normal, only one object is appreciated when both are moved simultaneously (see Chap. 30). If a homonymous hemianopia is present this can also very quickly be picked up by this method.

PERIMETRY

In all cases of unexplained visual failure, suspected intracranial tumour, demyelinative disease, or if there have been any doubts on confrontation, the fields should be charted on a good perimeter and on the Bjerrum screen. The latter enlarges the central area (out to 30°), and so makes it easier to detect scotomata and to measure the blind spot.

Quantitative perimetry is essential. At least three objects of different size must be used. It is often possible to pick out an early defect with a 2 mm object which is missed with a 10 mm object (Fig. 6b), and, perhaps even more important, an apparently constricted field shown by a small object will almost always be explained when successively larger objects are used and diagnostic field defects may be demonstrated (Fig. 6a).

The *isoptres* are labelled according to the size of the object and the distance of the patient's eye from the fixation point, usually 330 mm for the perimeter and 2000 mm for the Bjerrum screen. Thus, a line marked 10/2000 indicates the points at which the 10 mm object is first seen using the Bjerrum screen. The visual angle can be worked out from the formula:

$$\frac{\text{Object}}{\text{Distance}} \times \frac{180}{\pi} \text{ (or 57.3).}$$

The colour fields. The field for red is smaller than that for white because the illumination of the red object is less. In this way, early defects may sometimes be detected, but in general greater value comes from the conscientious use of quantitative perimetry.

VISUAL EVOKED RESPONSES

See Chap. 39.

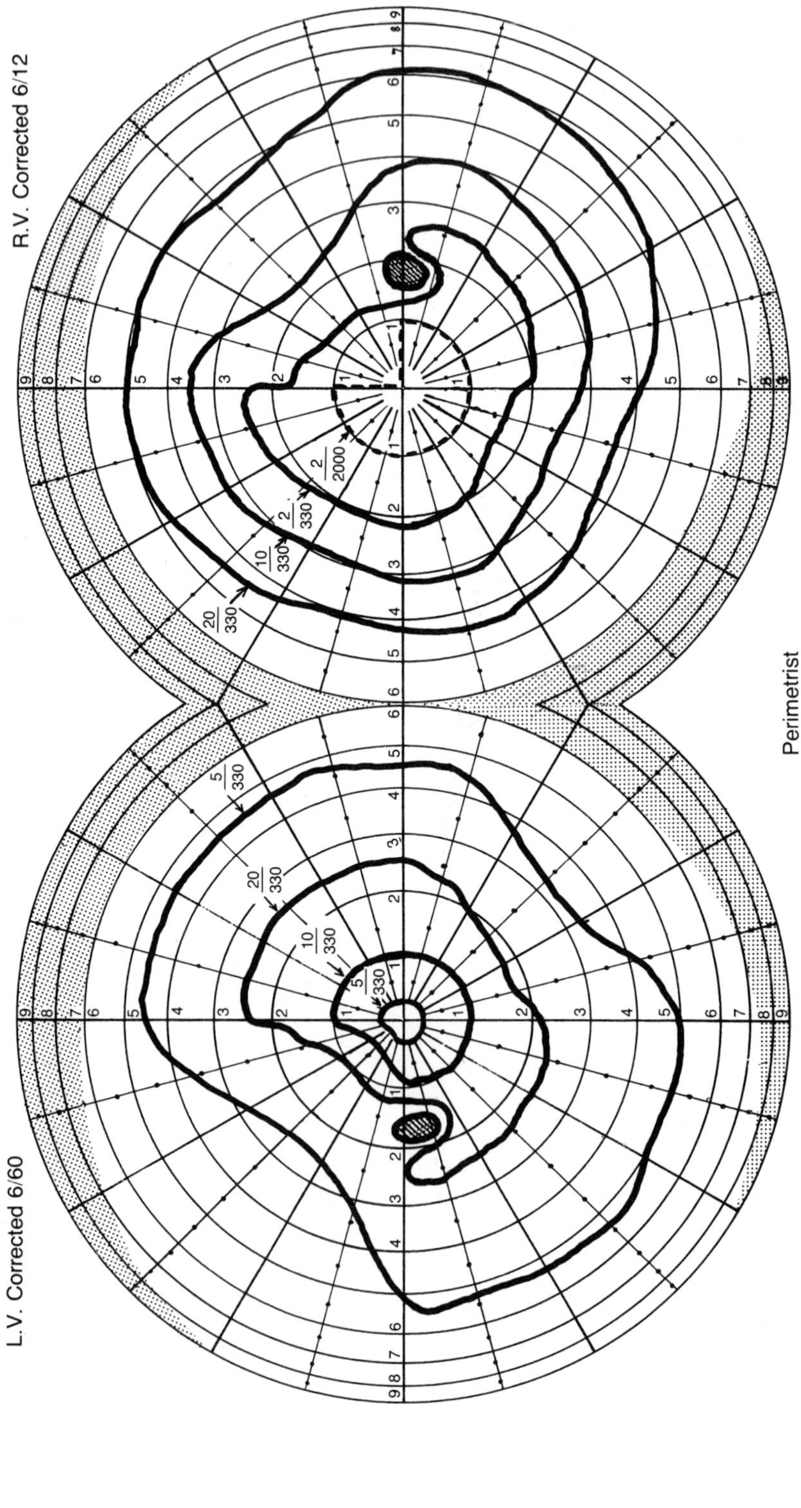

Fig. 6. Quantitative perimetery showing upper temporal quadrantic defects. In (a),

Visual field defects and their significance

So many and varied are the possible defects that one cannot describe them all, but the principles by which lesions are located are best illustrated by comparing a diagram of the visual pathways (Fig. 7) with the principal field defects (Fig. 8a–n).

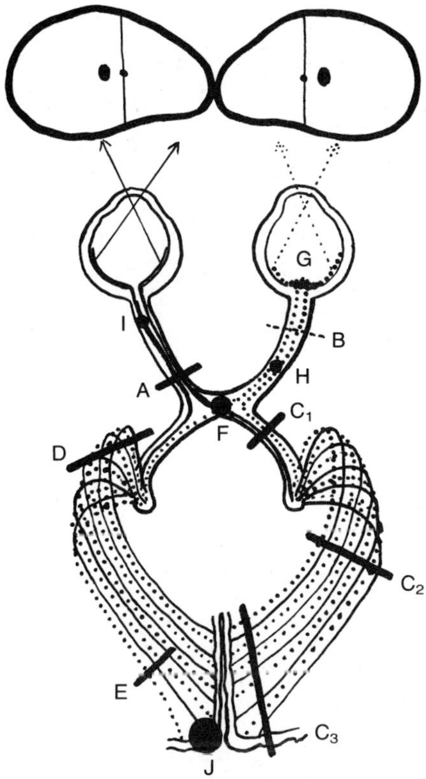

Fig. 7. Diagrammatic representation of the visual pathways. The common sites of lesions are lettered and the characteristic field defects so caused are illustrated in Fig. 8.

DIFFICULTIES AND FALLACIES

Curious bilateral defects of the upper fields or nasal fields can be produced by Mephistophelian eyebrows, or an over-generous nose. These can be avoided simply by tilting or turning the patient's head appropriately.

A patient with a central scotoma cannot fix on a central object. Two objects, placed just at the edge of the scotoma on the screen, can be held in their relative positions by a co-operative patient.

Always be suspicious of the accuracy of the small, concentrically constricted field *if visual acuity is adequate*. The real shape of the fields will be

Fig. 8. (a) to (n). Diagrammatic representation of common field defects to be studied in conjunction with Fig. 7.

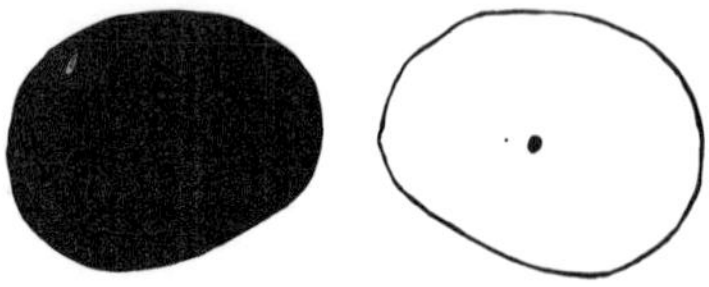
(a)

(a) **Total unilateral loss of vision.** A lesion of the optic nerve (Fig. 7 A).

Common causes: Injuries, retrobulbar neuritis, optic nerve compression.

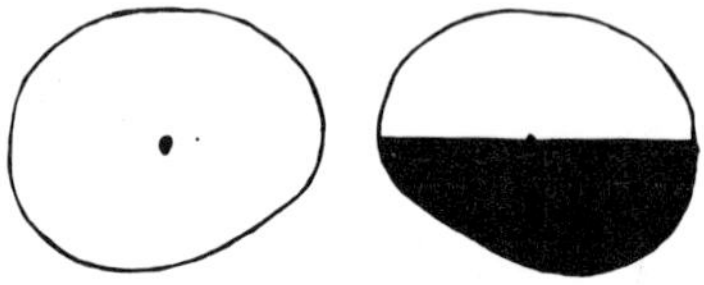
(b)

(b) **Altitudinous hemianopia.** A partial lesion of the blood supply to the optic nerve (Fig. 7 B).

Common causes: Trauma, vascular accidents.

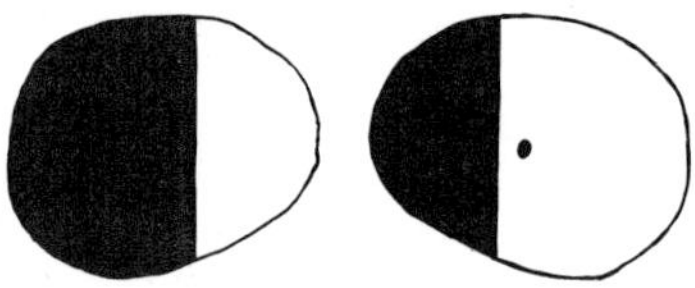
(c)

(c) **Homonymous hemianopia.** The commonest major defect; caused by a lesion anywhere from optic tract to occipital cortex. In the *tract* it is usually complete, incongruous, without macular sparing (Fig. 7 C1). In the *radiations* it is usually incomplete, congruous, with macular sparing (Fig. 7 C2). In the *calcarine cortex* it is usually complete, congruous and with macular sparing, but may show associated scotomata (Fig. 7 C3). Congruity and macular sparing are variable.

Common causes: Vascular accidents, cerebral tumours, vascular anomalies, injuries.

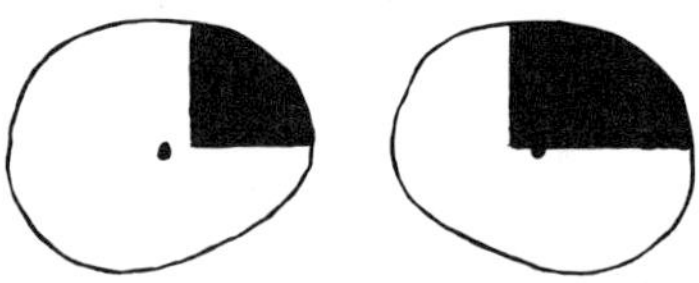
(d)

(d) **Upper quadrantic homonymous defect.** Temporal lobe lesions involving the optic radiations where they sweep round the temporal horn of the lateral ventricle (Fig. 7 D). Less commonly in lower calcarine lesions; occasionally in partial tract lesions.

Common causes: Cerebral tumours, vascular accidents, cerebral abscesses, injuries.

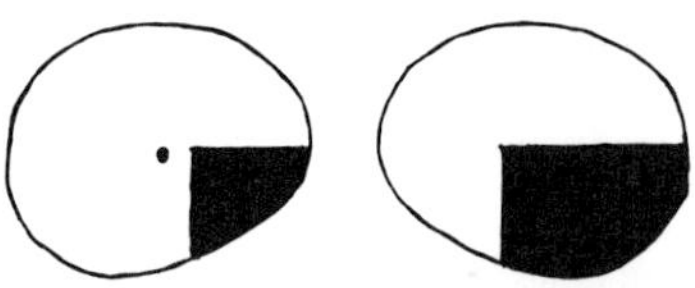
(e)

(e) **Lower quadrantic homonymous defect.** Lesions of the upper radiations or calcarine area (Fig. 7 E).

Common causes: Vascular accidents, injuries, tumours.

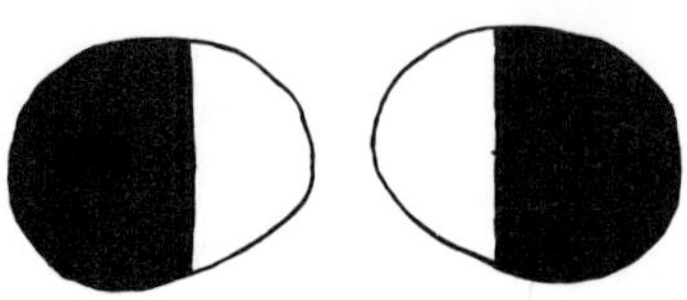
(f)

(f) **Bitemporal hemianopia.** Lesions at the optic chiasma (Fig. 7 F).

Common causes: Pituitary tumours, craniopharyngiomata, suprasellar meningiomata, midline aneurysms, hypothalamic neoplasms, gross IIIrd ventricular dilatation, optic chiasmal gliomata.

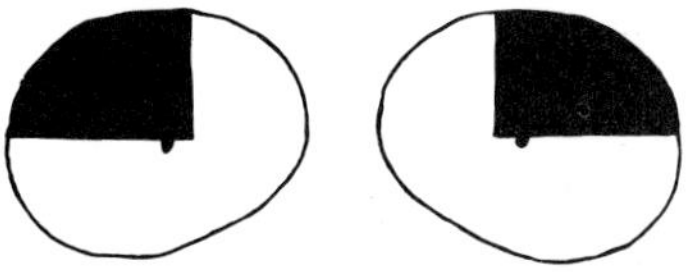

(g)

(g) **Bitemporal upper quadrantic defect.** The early stages of chiasmal compression from below (Fig. 7 F).

Common causes: Pituitary tumours.

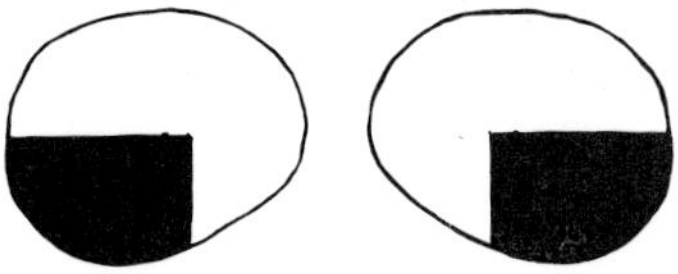

(h)

(h) **Bitemporal lower quadrantic defect.** The early stages of chiasmal compression from above (Fig. 7 F).

Common causes: Intrinsic tumours of the hypothalamus, suprasellar cysts or meningiomata. This is not a very common defect.

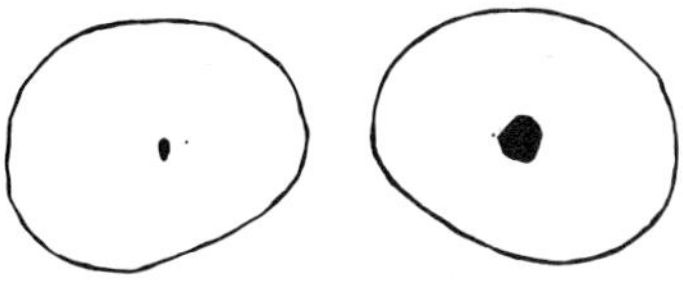

(i)

(i) **Enlarged blind spot.** Enlargement of the optic nerve head (Fig. 7 G).

Common causes: Papilloedema from increased intracranial pressure.

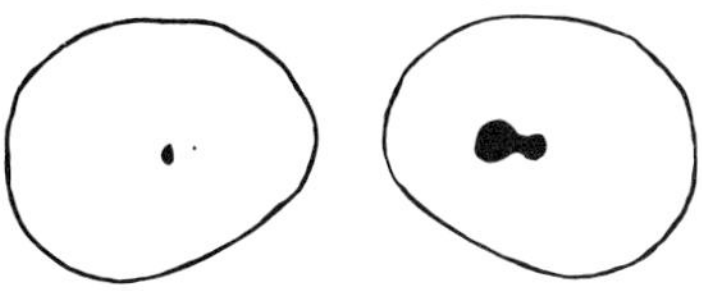

(j)

(j) **Central and centrocaecal scotomata.** Intrinsic lesions of the optic nerves between the chiasma and the nerve head (Fig. 7 H).

Common causes: Demyelinative lesions, optic nerve gliomata.

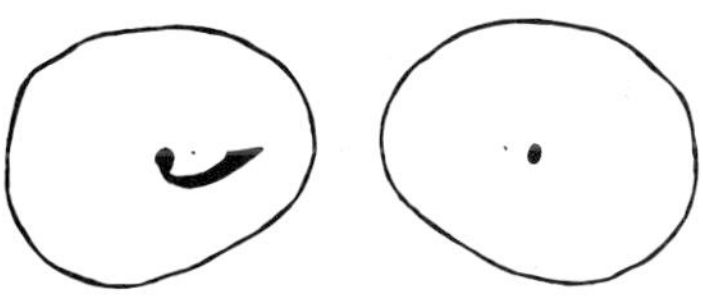

(k)

(k) **Fibre bundle defects.** Lesions of the optic nerve between the chiasma and the retina (Fig. 7 I).

Common causes: Vascular lesions, toxins, optic nerve gliomata, demyelinative lesions.

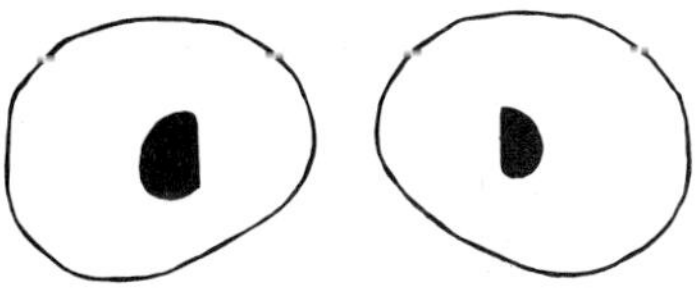

(l)

(l) **Bitemporal scotomata.** Chiasmal lesions. The peripheral field may be affected later (Fig. 7 F).

Common causes: The same as for bitemporal hemianopia, but with special reference to gliomata of the optic chiasma if in children.

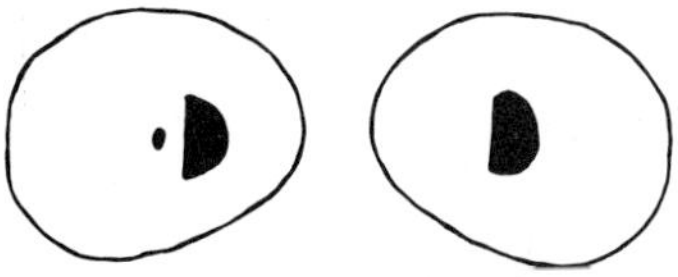

(m)

(m) **Homonymous scotomata.** Unilateral lesions of the tip of the calcarine cortex (Fig. 7 J).

Common causes: Injuries, tumours.

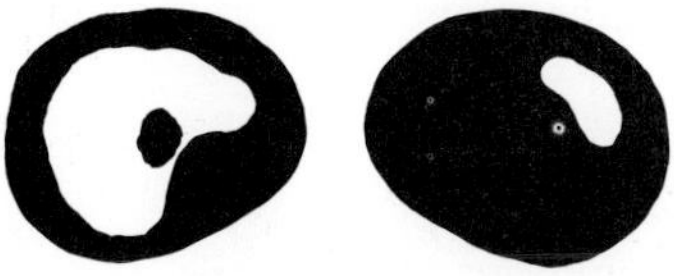

(n)

(n) **Purely nasal defects.** Though theoretically due to lateral chiasmal lesions, this is rarely the case.

Common causes: Glaucoma, and consecutive optic atrophy following papilloedema. In the latter the lower nasal field is first affected, then the upper nasal and lower temporal, so that finally only an island of vision is left in the upper temporal fields.

determined by using successively larger objects, unless the defect is of hysterical origin.

Poor co-operation in fixation can often be overcome simply by enlarging the object on which the patient is to fix. Modern perimeters however allow the perimetrists to view the patient's fixation directly while each point is tested, thus increasing accuracy, if not solving the problem.

Personal equations vary. Move the object slowly. It may take time for its appearance to register with the patient and for him to react.

EXAMINING THE FUNDUS

The fundus must always be carefully examined no matter what the patient's complaints may be. Only by inspecting the maximum possible number of fundi can that experience of the wide variation of normal be gained that makes it possible to detect early abnormalities, and quite unexpected abnormalities may be found which alter the whole aspect of the problem.

Methods of examination

To obtain a clear view of the fundus, there are certain requisites: (*a*) a good ophthalmoscope, (*b*) a large pupil, and (*c*) a still field.

In order to overcome the light reflex, diminish, if necessary, the illumination in the room; to overcome accommodation for near vision, instruct the patient to look at a *distant* point, which has been clearly defined for him, thus keeping the eye still. The temptation to look at the light of the ophthalmoscope is very great, and the patient must be warned not to do so.

Use the right eye to examine the right eye and then walk around the bed to examine the left eye with the left eye. Leaning over the patient is uncomfortable and prevents him from fixing on the distant object easily, while trying to use the wrong eye results in nasal collision.

If these measures fail, and especially when careful inspection of the periphery of the retina is important, it is perfectly justifiable to introduce a few drops of a quick-acting mydriatic. If homatropine is used it must be remembered that (*a*) the pupillary reflexes must be tested first, (*b*) it takes some time to achieve maximal dilation, and (*c*) it is followed by the use of eserine, otherwise the results of the examination will be unpopular, in the elderly dangerous, and in children the cause of a dilated, non-reacting pupil perhaps for several days. Quick-acting mydriatics are now readily available which avoid most of these problems.

Features to be examined

First find the optic disc. If the patient is carrying out instructions, this will immediately be seen; if not it will be the vessels first seen, and by following them to their point of convergence the disc will come into view. Note its colour, the clarity of its edges and the size of the depression in its centre, the optic cup. Next look at the vessels as they leave and enter the disc, the veins being the wider and darker; note the degree of curvature as they pass over the edge of the disc. See if the vessels are continuously visible or if they appear and disappear; if their curves are gradual or acute and tortuous. Now look at the points of crossing of the arteries and veins; note if one vessel appears to obliterate the other. Look next for haemorrhages, their size, shape and relationship to the vessels; and for exudates, their size, colour and texture. Finally inspect the retina itself, noting any deviations from the uniformity of colour. While doing this, ask the patient to look directly at the light, when the vessel-free macula area can be inspected. Mydriatics may be required for this.

The disc

PALLOR

Disc colour varies greatly, probably even in the same individual at different times, and only long experience makes it possible to assess minor degrees of pallor. There are three main varieties of marked pallor:

(*a*) The whole disc is quite white, standing out dramatically like a full moon against a dark red sky. This is the appearance often known as *primary optic atrophy*, usually due to local lesions of the optic nerve such as compression, injuries, toxins, the common demyelinative lesions, tabes dorsalis and certain familial disorders (e.g. Leber's disease). The same appearance sometimes can be seen a long time after severe papilloedema has settled down, and the word 'primary' is purely a visual description.

(*b*) The whole disc is pale, with a greenish tinge, but the edges blur off into the immediately surrounding retina. This is '*consecutive optic atrophy*' and follows previous severe swelling of the disc. It is, therefore, caused by any intracranial conditions capable of producing raised intracranial pressure.

(*c*) The disc is strikingly pale in a quadrantic or crescentic manner on the temporal half, the so-called *temporal pallor*, due to lesions principally of the papillomacular bundle. This is often seen in multiple sclerosis, but is neither constant in that disease, nor pathognomonic of it.

Difficulties and fallacies

The temporal side of the disc is usually paler than the nasal and in the absence of other signs, this alone should not be considered pathological. Optic atrophy is a description of what the examiner thinks he is seeing, and is not a diagnosis. One might just as well say a patient is suffering from an extensor plantar response. There is always an underlying cause for optic atrophy and failure to appreciate this has often led to patients being allowed to go blind from remediable optic nerve compression.

The myopic disc normally looks very pale, appears greatly enlarged and often has also a crescent of pallor immediately around it. Examine it through the patient's own spectacles to get the most accurate view.

The optic cup is sometimes so marked as to give an impression of optic atrophy. As this is especially the case in glaucomatous cupping, when seen the ocular tensions must be tested. Even here there is usually a rim of normal disc.

SWELLING

Normally the nasal edge of the disc is somewhat blurred. As swelling develops this blurring extends to the upper and lower margins first, the optic cup becomes less evident and the disc of more uniform colour with the rest of the retina. The temporal edges are the last to disappear. The area covered by the disc then enlarges, the margins cannot be defined and irregular radial streaks appear which give the disc an 'angry' appearance. The veins become swollen and engorged and the hump of the vessels entering and leaving the disc becomes very pronounced. The vessels appear and disappear as they course near the disc. Finally, small haemorrhages or large irregular ecchymoses appear usually near a vein. In addition, white streaks and patches of exudate appear near the disc margins and spread outwards towards the macula to produce the macular fan.

This is the appearance of papilloedema due to increased intracranial pressure from any cause. Despite the degree of swelling, vision may be well preserved, the visual fields showing only enlargement of the blind spot (Fig. 8i).

If the swelling is due to local lesions in the nerve (e.g. retrobulbar neuritis), there are important differences. The degree of swelling is usually slight and is usually unilateral, the veins are not engorged, the humping is only slight, the disc area is not greatly enlarged, and there are no exudates or haemorrhages. Despite this, however, vision is grossly disturbed due to large central or centro-caecal scotomata (Fig. 8j).

Note, however, that on rare occasions, especially in adolescence, very acute optic neuritis may give all the appearances of gross papilloedema and it is only the profound loss of vision at the onset which distinguishes it from papilloedema due to increased intracranial pressure.

THE FOSTER–KENNEDY SYNDROME

A tumour in the posterior inferior frontal region can cause optic atrophy on one side by compressing the optic nerve, and papilloedema on the other by obstructing venous return or causing raised intracranial pressure.

Difficulties and fallacies
The hypermetropic disc is pink and its edges appear blurred, but it is also a small disc and the vessels and fields are normal.

Swelling occurs not only in intracranial disease, but also in generalised vascular disease, severe emphysema, profound anaemia and in leukaemia. This emphasises the importance of the general physical examination.

Central venous obstruction causes an appearance similar to that of increased intracranial pressure, but it is usually unilateral, is even more dramatic and angry-looking, the onset is abrupt and the visual failure marked. Haemorrhages are larger and more extensive, they vary from day to day and may occur in the media.

Pseudopapilloedema is a disc appearance very similar to mild swelling, but without vessel engorgement, and symptomless throughout the patient's life. This term must not be confused with 'pseudo-tumour' now known as benign intracranial hypertension which is a syndrome where there is true papilloedema but not due to intracranial tumour.

Patients with a particularly fair skin and light (not necessarily blonde) hair may have disc appearances remarkably like mild papilloedema. The state of the veins and the optic cup must be carefully observed.

Obliquity of the optic nerves, Drusen bodies (small colloid bodies) near the nerve head, juxta-papillary choroiditis, and haziness of the vitreous may all give the appearance of disc swelling. Some of these can be distinguished by use of fluorescein (see p. 45).

The vessels
Arteries are lighter and narrower than veins and often have a central reflecting line, so that a 'silver wire' appearance can be quite normal. A very variable lumen, widening and narrowing throughout the course, is characteristic of arterial hypertension. The arteries are thin and scanty following consecutive optic atrophy, and very thin after ophthalmic artery thrombosis when there is corresponding retinal pallor. Minute emboli may be seen obstructing a retinal arteriole, while fragments of atheroma may be seen as refractile bodies blocking small vessels. These often indicate carotid artery disease.

If the arteries are thickened (arteriosclerosis) or under high pressure (hypertension), they compress the veins at points of crossing, obliterating them for a short distance, particularly on the side nearer the disc.

Veins become engorged in states of high intracranial pressure and in ophthalmic venous obstruction, such as in thrombosis of the central vein. Tortuosity accompanies severe engorgement and veins may appear and disappear rather like a sea-serpent.

N.B. It is important to correlate the degree of engorgement of the veins with the appearances of the disc—for a dubious papilloedema with quite normal veins, is probably either not papilloedema at all, or papilloedema that has subsided leaving blurred disc edges.

Both arteries and veins show gross tortuosity in angiomatosis of the optic nerve and retina producing bizarre appearances. An unusually tortuous artery should be traced to its periphery for it may lead to a retinal angioma, and retinal angiomata may be associated with cerebral angiomata, hamartomata, or cerebellar haemangioblastomata.

The retina

The number of possible abnormalities in the retina and choroid is so large that descriptions will best be sought in textbooks of ophthalmology. It is important to have a working knowledge of these appearances, for they may be the cause of visual failure or field defects thought to be of more central origin.

The important neurological features are described below.

HAEMORRHAGES

These occur as (*a*) small streaks, near the vessels, long and linear, or flame-shaped; (*b*) much larger ecchymoses capable of obscuring local vessels and retina. (*a*) and (*b*) occur in raised intracranial pressure and in venous engorgement of any cause; in hypertension, collagenoses and blood dyscrasias. In the latter they extend to the retinal periphery; (*c*) small rounded pin-head areas. These are now taken to be microaneurysms of the retinal vessels and occur in diabetes; (*d*) subhyaloid haemorrhages. Seen in subarachnoid haemorrhage, they appear as large effusions of blood related to and often below the disc, with crescentic inner and clear-cut outer borders extending forwards towards the lens.

EXUDATES

Fluffy, cotton-wool patches are seen in papilloedema, albuminuric retinitis and hypertension; hard crystalline streaks and dots in arteriosclerosis, chronic nephritis and the late stages of other exudative conditions. The appearances of exudates are not diagnostic and must be correlated with the appearance of the disc and vessels. Large exudative patches are seen in blood dyscrasias.

TUBERCLES

Choroidal tubercles appear, under ophthalmoscopic examination, much larger than tubercles as seen at post mortem. They are rounded, about half the size of the disc, yellowish at the centre, but with ill-defined pink edges, slightly raised and, if present for any length of time, surrounded by pigmentation.

PHAKOMATA

A phakoma is a collection of neuroglial cells appearing in the retina as a large white, or bluish-white, plaque with almost translucent edges, about one-half to two-thirds the size of the optic disc. Though on occasion seen in neurofibromatosis, they are most characteristically a feature of tuberous sclerosis.

PIGMENTARY ABNORMALITIES

Many choroido-retinal pigmentary lesions are not directly of neurological importance. Reduction of pigment in fair-haired people may allow choroidal vessels to be seen so clearly as to mimic an angiomatosis. Gross choroido-retinitis sometimes accompanies neurosyphilis.

In cerebro-macular degeneration there may be a cherry-red spot at the macula, surrounded by darker spots of pigment, sometimes a granular peppery appearance over a wide area, with retinal atrophy.

In toxoplasmosis large areas of pigmentary abnormality, irregularly oval in shape with clearly defined edges, are seen near the macula.

At the periphery the most important change is the spidery black 'bone corpuscles' pigmentation spreading towards the centre that is seen in retinitis pigmentosa, and to a lesser degree in several other heredo-familial disorders.

OPAQUE NERVE FIBRES

If myelinated nerve fibres persist in the retina a vivid white fan spreads from the disc, curving in the course of the nerve fibres. This is often mistaken for exudate, but the vivid whiteness and direction are quite different. The edges of such a patch are usually curvilinear and clear cut, while the peripheral edge gradually streaks off into the retina.

FLUORESCEIN AND FUNDUS PHOTOGRAPHY

Retinal photography has now become so advanced that it is almost standard procedure in many centres. The preliminary injection intravenously of a carefully sterilised solution of 10% fluorescein adds greatly to the interpretation of certain appearances. The dye does not escape from normal arterioles, but in hypertensive retinopathy areas of arteriolar necrosis are clearly seen; in retinal arterial occlusion the failure of filling is seen, and in central venous occlusion gross exudation will occur. This is also seen in true papilloedema, but is absent in pseudopapilloedema. In true optic atrophy, as opposed to doubtful disc pallor, the disc remains dark throughout serial photographs. The microaneurysms of diabetic retinopathy are seen earlier, and shown to be more extensive than ordinary ophthalmoscopy can detect.

There are problems yet to be overcome—e.g. Drusen bodies can cause confusion, and even the appearances of papilloedema can be mimicked by less serious conditions. To be of truly reliable value, the procedure needs to be carried out by someone doing it several times each week.

OPHTHALMODYNAMOMETRY

If digital pressure is exerted on the globe of the eye, by pressure on upper and lower lids near the inner canthus during the use of an ophthalmoscope, the retinal vessels can be seen first to pulsate, and then to empty. The veins obviously collapse first. When the intra-arterial pressure is high (hypertension), or the veins are engorged (increased intracranial pressure), greater than normal pressure is required. If ophthalmic artery pressure is low, as in internal carotid stenosis or thrombosis, only very slight pressure may be required to produce the same effect. This may be enough to cause transient impairment of vision if the ophthalmic artery supply is seriously embarrassed.

Digital pressure is, however, difficult to assess, and ophthalmologists use a dynamometer to exert graduated pressure. To get best results a mydriatic needs to be used. Differences in the two eyes can be accurately compared and unilateral low arterial pressure readings are of value in the diagnosis of carotid deficiency. In hypertensive retinopathy and encephalopathy the pressure may be raised out of proportion to the degree expected from the readings of systemic hypertension.

Chapter 8
The Third, Fourth and Sixth Cranial Nerves: The Oculomotor, Trochlear and Abducent Nerves

The actions of these nerves are so closely linked that they are considered together, and it is at this stage that abnormalities on inspection of the eyes are usually detected. Some of these relevant to neurological disease are mentioned in this section.

Functions
Control of all the external ocular muscles and the elevators of the lids. Autonomic fibres running in relation both to these nerves and the Vth nerve regulate pupillary muscles.

Purposes of the tests
(*a*) To inspect the pupils and determine if any abnormalities discovered are due to local disease, to a peripheral autonomic lesion, or to nuclear involvement in the brain stem.
(*b*) To examine eye movement and to determine if any defect is of local muscular origin, or due to lesions of the oculomotor nerves peripherally, their nuclei in the brain stem, or the pathways of supranuclear control.
(*c*) It is also convenient at this stage to detect and analyse nystagmus, though this is closely related to vestibular dysfunction.

Methods of examination

Preliminary inspection
While talking to the patient note the presence or absence of ptosis and squint, whether it is unilateral or bilateral, constant or variable. Compare the size of the palpebral fissures and note if the eyeballs are protruded (exophthalmos), or recessed (enophthalmos).

EXOPHTHALMOS
Assess protrusion by looking down on the eyes from above and behind the patient's head. Ocular prominence may be normal, but true exophthalmos, with lid retraction, occurs in thyrotoxicosis, and becomes severe, with injection and chemosis of the conjunctiva, oedema of the lids and oculomotor paralysis in endocrine exophthalmos (exophthalmic ophthalmoplegia).

Protrusion can become severe in craniosynostosis and may be associated with downward displacement of the globes in hydrocephalus.

Unilateral exophthalmos still most commonly dúe to thyroid dysfunction, may also be caused by orbital or retro-orbital neoplasms and granulomata, when the globe cannot be replaced by pressure, all eye movements may be limited, but the lid is normal. The exophthalmos, ptosis and oculomotor palsy becomes gross in tumours or thrombosis of the cavernous sinus, and if the globe pulsates and there is a bruit audible to patient and examiner, this is characteristic of a carotico-cavernous fistula.

Proptosis is a combination of ptosis and exophthalmos, both being capable of existence without the other.

ENOPHTHALMOS

Though most commonly part of a Horner's syndrome (q.v.) this may be due to a mal-developed eye. Do not be caught out by a well-fitting but recessed prosthesis, or by the true abnormality being prominence of eye or orbit on the other side.

HYPERTELORISM

Though not uncommon in normal individuals, this should make one alert to the possibility of intracranial congenital abnormalities.

Look next at the conjunctiva, cornea, and iris while the patient moves the eyeball in all directions. Note colours, pigmentary abnormalities, surgical or developmental defects.

THE CONJUNCTIVA

Subconjunctival haemorrhage is common following cranial trauma, and rare in spontaneous subarachnoid haemorrhage.

Telangiectases may be associated with skin telangiectases and cerebellar ataxia in the syndrome 'ataxia telangiectasia' (Louis–Bar syndrome).

Retro-orbital tumours may grow forwards as a red or grey felting visible on extreme deviation of the eyeball.

A *yellow tint* may be the only sign of liver disease and raise the possibility of metastatic or diffuse systemic disease.

An intense *inflammatory reaction* occurs in leptospira canicola infection, which also causes an acute meningitis, and during the migration of filaria (loa loa) which also may cause an encephalitis.

Conjunctival ulcers form part of the triad of Behçet's syndrome (q.v.).

THE CORNEA AND IRIS

Look particularly for different colouring of the two eyes; the pale atrophied iris of the tabetic; the arcus senilis; and the Kayser–Fleischer Ring.

ARCUS SENILIS

A pale bluish translucent ring overlying the iris, seen in the elderly and in those showing premature ageing, whose cerebral vessels may also be prematurely atheromatous.

THE KAYSER–FLEISCHER RING (Fig. 9)

This is a very characteristic golden-brown ring, lying just inside the limbus of the cornea, sometimes forming a complete circle, but at others merely a crescent at the upper and lower margins. It is seen most easily in light coloured eyes and is diagnostic of hepato-lenticular degeneration. If it is suspected its presence should be confirmed by slit-lamp examination. After treatment with penicillamine the vivid colour of the ring changes to a dull mottled brown.

(a) (b)

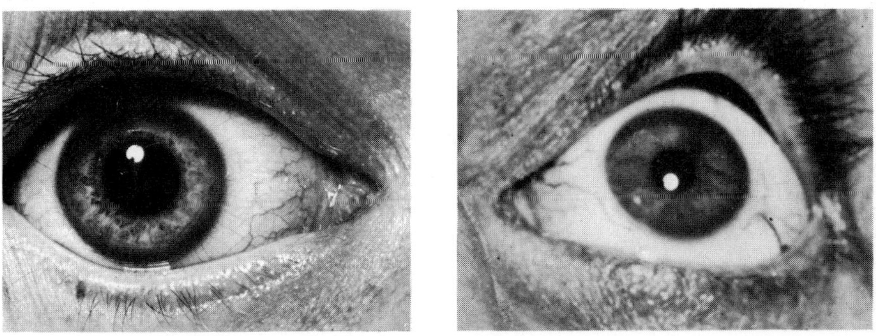

Fig. 9. Kayser–Fleischer rings, (a) as a complete circle, (b) as crescents most marked at the upper margin.

THE EYELIDS

Note the position of the lids in relation to the iris, and the width of the palpebral fissure. Then ask the patient to open the eyes widely and notice both the lid movement and the degree of movement of the frontalis muscle. Ask the patient to follow an object upwards and maintain forward gaze for at least 30–45 seconds without blinking.

PTOSIS

If the pupil is partly covered by the upper lid there is a slight degree of ptosis, which may be due to paralysis of the levator palpebrae superioris as a result of a IIIrd nerve lesion, or to weakness of the tarsal muscles due to a sympathetic lesion. In the latter, the lid can still be raised voluntarily, but in the former, the frontal muscles contract to overcome the drooping and there may be a permanent wrinkling of the forehead.

In myasthenia gravis, the degree of drooping of the lid varies from moment to moment, and may change sides. The lid will droop progressively on prolonged upward fixation, but a blink restores its position to normal.

In ocular myopathy the ptosis is fixed, the lids have a waxy appearance, and the head is often held extended in an attempt to see under the drooping lids.

LID RETRACTION

The lid is buried under the brow and the sclera is clearly visible above the iris in hyperthyroidism, after large doses of prostigmine, and in some normal patients.

THE PUPILS

Look at the size, shape, equality and regularity of the pupils. Correlate their size with the surrounding illumination, remembering that the pupil nearer a bright window is often smaller. It is normal for the pupils to be very small in early infancy, old age, during sleep and in bright light, and to be large in poor light, myopia and frightened children.

The reaction to light

It must be possible to see this reaction. If, therefore, the pupils are small, first darken the room, and give the patient the same instructions as for examining the fundi. A bright beam of light is then shone suddenly from slightly to one side of the eye (shining from directly in front may cause the patient to converge the eyes, when the pupils will contract anyway). The pupil should constrict briskly. Repeat the test for the other eye and compare the two reactions. Finally, shield one eye, shine the light in the other, and watch for the *consensual reaction* which is the constriction of the shielded pupil as well.

The reaction to convergence and accommodation for near vision
The patient should still be fixing on a distant object. Explain that he is about to be asked to look at a near object, and then place a pencil suddenly about nine inches in front of the *bridge* of the nose. This position prevents lowering of the lids which obscures the normal pupillary constriction, and the sudden movement emphasises it. Return the eyes then to the distant object, for the subsequent dilatation may be even easier to see.

Pupillary abnormalities

THE CONSTRICTED PUPIL (*Miosis*)
This indicates a lesion at some point in the very circuitous pathway taken by the sympathetic supply to the pupillary dilator muscle. Thus the lesion may be in the hypothalamus, brain stem, lateral aspect of the spinal cord as far down as the upper thoracic segments, the sympathetic chain, the cervical sympathetic ganglia, the peri-carotid plexus, or in the sympathetic fibres which run to the orbit by accompanying the ophthalmic division of the Vth cranial nerve. Pontine tumours or haemorrhages, primary or secondary tumours involving the cervical sympathetic chain, and vascular lesions of the carotid artery or its sheath, are the most common causes, but there are many others. Bilateral spontaneous sympathetic palsy almost invariably means an upper brain stem lesion. Remember, however, that a sleeping patient, even if his eyes are not closed, may have very small pupils which enlarge rapidly when roused.

Horner's syndrome
In its complete state this consists of miosis, ptosis, enophthalmos, and dryness and warmth of that half of the face (see Fig. 10c); cocaine will not dilate the pupil as it normally does, and adrenaline dilates it more than normally. This syndrome in its purest form is seen in lesions of the superior cervical ganglion in the neck, and of the fibres surrounding the carotid artery, but it can be seen in other lesions of the sympathetic supply, though usually with other physical signs to help localisation. It used to be common after carotid arteriography carried out by direct puncture. It may still occasionally be seen after carotid catheterisation. It occurs after many bouts of periodic migrainous neuralagia or cluster headache.

THE DILATED PUPIL (*Mydriasis*)
In practice this results from paralysis of the parasympathetic fibres, either at their origin from the pre-tectal nuclei and the Edinger-Westphal nucleus in the midbrain, during their course with the IIIrd nerve, or at the ciliary ganglion in the orbit. The possible sites of a lesion extend over a much

smaller distance than in the case of the sympathetic division. Most commonly such lesions are due to vascular accidents in the midbrain, tentorial herniation (due to cerebral space-occupying lesions), or aneurysms of the carotid artery. Never forget, however, that a very common cause of a dilated pupil is that someone has put in a mydriatic. When atropine was commonly used, one saw this in children for several days afterwards. Certain modern detergents may also produce pupillary dilatation; and it is seen sometimes after administration of mysoline. An eye that is *almost* completely blind may have a dilated pupil.

THE PUPIL THAT DOES NOT REACT TO LIGHT

This is due to a break in the pathways for the light reflex, and the lesion may lie in the afferent loop, i.e. the retina, optic nerve or chiasma; or in the efferent loop, i.e. the parasympathetic supply from the midbrain running with the IIIrd nerve. In the former, as no stimulus can be received there will also be no consensual reaction, but, if the lesion is unilateral (e.g. optic nerve injuries, retrobulbar neuritis) when the normal side is stimulated, *both* pupils will react. If the efferent loop is involved, however (e.g. causes as listed above), the affected pupil is unable to react no matter which side is stimulated. Bilateral failure to react, with intact vision, usually means a midbrain lesion. Bilateral blindness with non-reacting pupils must be due to a lesion between the retina and the first part of the optic tract, for after that the pupillo-constrictor fibres have left the visual fibres.

All these remarks assume that someone has not recently instilled a mydriatic to examine the fundi and omitted to record the fact.

THE PUPIL THAT FAILS TO ACCOMMODATE FOR NEAR VISION

This is most commonly due to a failure in the technique of the examination. If however, it is genuine, it usually results from failure to converge owing to upper brain stem lesions, such as tumours or encephalitis, or in Parkinsonism.

The Argyll Robertson pupil

Often incorrectly hyphenated, this name is given to a small irregular pupil, not reacting to light, reacting to accommodation, but responding poorly or not at all to atropine, physostigmine and methacholine. The pupil is, however, not always small and the two sides may differ. It usually is caused by syphilis, but may occasionally be seen in other midbrain lesions. The site of the lesion has never been fully determined. Some favour the tectum of the midbrain, others the ciliary ganglion, but bearing in mind the nature of neurosyphilitic lesions, multiple sites cannot be excluded.

THE MYOTONIC PUPIL (*Holmes–Adie syndrome*)
Correctly hyphenated, when this presents it is often in young women and is first seen as unilateral dilatation of one pupil with failure to react. However, if the patient is kept in a dark room for a quarter of an hour and the pupil then exposed to a diffuse light, a slight slow reaction may be seen. The most important feature, and one which is much less time-consuming to elicit, is the very slow constriction which occurs on maintaining convergence for 45 seconds or more. If the patient then looks at a distant object the dilatation of the myotonic pupil is similarly slow, so that there may be a stage at which the once larger pupil is now smaller than its fellow. As reaction to light is almost absent the myotonic response to convergence can often be better seen by illuminating the pupil at the same time with not too bright a torch. Minute doses of methacholine 2.5 per cent insufficient to affect a normal pupil, cause brisk contraction. Bilateral myotonic pupils may rarely occur. In the full syndrome the knee and ankle jerks are also absent and occasionally there is complete areflexia. The site of the lesion causing the pupillary abnormality is probably in the ciliary ganglion.

EXAMINING OCULAR MOVEMENT

The patient must look at a clear and definite point, such as the point of a pen or a fine point of light. The examiner then moves this point precisely and deliberately to right and left horizontally, upwards and downwards in the midline, and vertically when the eyes are deviated to one side. Do not attempt to make the eyes deviate beyond the point of comfort, and hold each deviation for at least 5 seconds. The aim is:

(*a*) To observe lagging of one or other eye.
(*b*) To analyse any diplopia the patient may describe (see below).
(*c*) To detect nystagmus.

The action of the ocular muscles
Complex though these are, one cannot understand the tests of ocular movement without learning a scheme of muscle action. This is a simplified form of considerable practical value.*

(A) *The External Rectus (VIth nerve)*. Moves the eye horizontally outwards.
(B) *The Internal Rectus (IIIrd nerve)*. Moves the eye horizontally inwards.

*Many earlier books give different actions for the superior and inferior recti, and for the obliques. This is due partly to the fact that no ocular muscle has an absolutely pure action, and also that some schemes are based on anatomical models rather than the actions *in vivo*.

(C) *The Superior Rectus (IIIrd nerve)*. Elevates the eye when it is turned outwards.

(D) *The Inferior Oblique (IIIrd nerve)*. Elevates the eye when it is turned inwards.

(E) *The Inferior Rectus (IIIrd nerve)*. Depresses the eye when it is turned outwards.

(F) *The Superior Oblique (IVth nerve)*. Depresses the eye when it is turned inwards.

The muscles paired together above act together. The vertical recti and obliques have other important actions, e.g. the vertical recti do, of course, turn the eye upwards or downwards, but it is only when the eye is in the positions mentioned that these muscles have the pure elevating or depressing action that is easiest to analyse.

If the action of one of the obliques is remembered, the others can easily be deduced.

OCULAR MUSCLE PARALYSIS

From this scheme the following general rules can be deduced.

(*a*) If an eye fails to move outwards, there is either a VIth nerve lesion, or a local lesion of the external rectus muscle (see A above).

(*b*) If the eye, when deviated inwards, will not then move downwards, there is either a IVth nerve lesion, or a local lesion of the superior oblique muscle (see F above).

(*c*) All other defects in movement are due to IIIrd nerve lesions, or a local lesion of the muscles.

In addition, however, when there is ocular muscle paralysis the unopposed pull of the normal antagonist will displace the eyeball. In *paralysis of the IIIrd nerve*, therefore, the eye is displaced outwards, and will not move inwards or vertically. There is accompanying ptosis and pupillary dilatation (Fig. 10a), though the latter may be absent if the lesion is recovering (Fig. 10b), or is incomplete.

In *VIth nerve paralysis* the eye is deviated inwards and will not move outwards beyond the midline, but will move vertically when deviated inwards (Fig. 10d).

Unfortunately, incomplete paralysis may show little visible abnormality and it is then that the diplopia produced must be investigated.

THE ANALYSIS OF DIPLOPIA

Diplopia can indicate ocular muscle weakness before it is evident to the examiner. The light rays fail to fall on exactly corresponding parts of the two

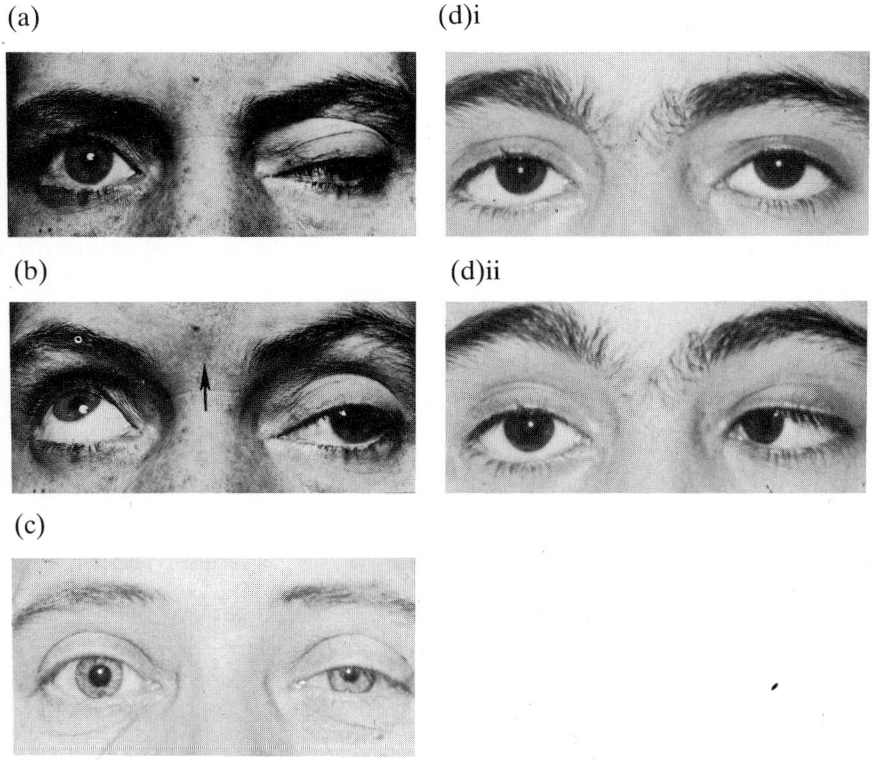

Fig. 10. Partial L. IIIrd nerve palsy; carcinoma of nasopharynx. (a) Ptosis and lateral deviation of left eye. (b) Upward gaze; slight elevation of L. lid reveals dilated pupil and paralysis of elevation of L. eyeball. (c) Horner's syndrome, ptosis, raising of lower lid, miosis, enophthalmos, but no overaction of frontalis. (di and ii) VIth nerve paralysis. The right eye is deviated inwards and will not move outwards across the midline.

retinae, and a false image is formed which is usually paler and less distinct. The rules governing the relationship of these two images are as follows:

Rule 1. Displacement of the false image may be horizontal, vertical or both.

Rule 2. Separation of the images is greatest in the direction in which the weak muscle has its purest action.

Rule 3. The false image is displaced furthest in the direction in which the weak muscle should move the eye.

Method of examination

Cover one of the patient's eyes with a transparent red shield and, using a point of light, move the object as above (p. 53). In each position ask the

patient:
(*a*) Whether he sees one object or two.
(*b*) If double, do the two images lie side by side, or one above the other.
(*c*) In which position are they furthest apart.
(*d*) Which is the red image.

Interpretation of results

If the images are exactly side by side, it will be only the external or internal recti that are involved. If they are one above the other, either of the obliques, or the superior and inferior recti, may be defective.

The muscle pair involved

It is the position in which there is maximum displacement which indicates which *pair* of muscles is involved (Rule 2 p. 55), e.g. if maximal displacement occurs when the eyes are deviated to the right and upwards, this is the movement carried out by the right superior rectus and the left inferior oblique (see C and D p. 54).

The individual muscle responsible

To determine which of the two muscles in each pair is at fault, the patient must say which of the two images is displaced furthest, the red or the white. Using the same example, if the red glass were over the right eye, and on looking to the right and upwards the red image is furthest displaced, then it must be the muscle moving the eye in that direction (see Rule 3 p. 55), namely the superior rectus, that is at fault. If it were the white image that was furthest displaced the fault would be with the left inferior oblique.

It is a good exercise to work out the situation in each direction for each possible muscle fault, and the more frequently this is done, the easier it becomes. In practice, of course, multiple faults occur, and, particularly when the IIIrd nerve is involved, it is at times easier to work out which muscles are acting normally.

Various charts exist for representing diplopia diagrammatically, of which the Hess chart and those used in orthoptic analysis are the most useful. They do not, however, offer better evidence than is afforded by carefully following the scheme of combination just described.

Common causes of oculomotor paralyses

The VIth nerve has such a long course that it can be involved in many conditions at or near the base of the skull. It can be paralysed in pontine lesions (often with a lower motor neurone VIIth nerve weakness if at the nucleus), neoplasms, vascular accidents, demyelinative lesions; in meningeal inflammation, acute or chronic; in tumours of the base of the skull; in posterior cerebral or superior cerebellar aneurysms; and very commonly as a false localising sign in generalised increase of intracranial pressure.

Isolated IVth nerve lesions are very rare, but may occur in lesions of the cerebral peduncles.

Isolated IIIrd nerve lesions occur in upper midbrain vascular accidents and demyelinative lesions, and peripherally due to compression by carotid and posterior communicating artery aneurysms, parasellar neoplasms, sphenoidal wing neoplasms, neoplasms of the base of the skull.

Total paralysis of all three nerves usually indicates a lesion in the cavernous sinus, most commonly a carotid aneurysm.

CONJUGATE OCULAR MOVEMENT

Normally, of course, the eyes do not move independently. For instance, each external rectus muscle contracts in conjunction with the opposite internal rectus, producing a movement so organised that the visual axes remain in the same relationship throughout and diplopia does not occur.

The centre for control of conjugate movement to, say, the right, is situated in the posterior part of the left frontal lobe and there is probably a further centre in the occipital region. The final common pathway for controlling this movement lies, however, in the brain stem and depends upon connections, running through the median longitudinal bundle, between the innervation of the left internal rectus and the right external rectus.

A lesion of the frontal lobe causes contralateral paralysis of conjugate gaze; a lesion of the brain stem causes ipsilateral paralysis of conjugate gaze.

Paralysis of the normal control of conjugate deviation to one side usually results in deviation of the eyes to the opposite side, which may be slight and transient, or marked and permanent.

Taking an example, it will be seen from these facts that deviation of the head and eyes *to the right* can result from several different types and positions of lesion.

(*a*) Destructive lesions (vascular or neoplastic), involving the supranuclear pathways between the *right* frontal lobes and the oculomotor nuclei, paralysing normal conjugate deviation to the left.

(*b*) Destructive lesions of the *left* side of the brain stem (vascular accidents or pontine neoplasms), also paralysing conjugate deviation to the left.

(*c*) Irritative lesions (focal fits), of the left frontal lobe, stimulating deviation to the right. Not theoretical—it occurs.

(*d*) Irritative lesions of the right side of the brain stem (encephalitis), also stimulating deviation to the right.

Failure of upward deviation follows an upper midbrain lesion due either to a vascular accident, compression by a tumour in the neighbourhood of the IIIrd ventricle, or tentorial herniation.

Fixed upward deviation is rare, but prolonged upward deviation occurs in the oculogyric spasms of post-encephalitic Parkinsonism, and following administration of the tranquilliser drugs, either in heavy dosage, or sometimes to a particularly sensitive individual.

As different sites of lesion can produce similar abnormalities of conjugate deviation, in order to distinguish them it is necessary to bring other neurological manifestations into the picture, and to test ocular movement on reflex fixation.

In the supranuclear destructive lesions the face and limbs are paralysed on the side opposite to the ocular deviation; in brain stem lesions, on the same side; but in the latter, if the face is paralysed it will be a lower motor neurone lesion on the side opposite to the hemiplegia. The situation is reversed for irritative lesions, but the deviation is spasmodic.

If the patient is able to co-operate and there is a failure of conjugate movement in any direction, he should be told to fix his eyes on a particular object while the examiner turns or flexes the patient's head passively according to the defect. If the defect is of supranuclear origin, the eyes will move throughout their full range on reflex fixation, even though voluntarily they cannot do so. If the lesion is at the level of the nucleus or peripheral to it, the eyes will still fail to move across the midline in the direction of the defect.

INTERNUCLEAR PARALYSIS

When there is a lesion of the brain stem involving the median longitudinal bundle (and so disrupting connections between one-third nerve nucleus and the opposite sixth nerve nucleus), there is disorganisation of the conjugate movement of the two eyes when looking laterally (Fig. 11). Internal deviation of the adducting eye is defective and 'out of step' with the external deviation of the other eye. A very marked nystagmus may develop (see 'ataxic nystagmus' p. 62).

DETECTING AND ANALYSING NYSTAGMUS

The balance of tone between opposing ocular muscles is influenced by impulses from the retina, the muscles themselves, the vestibular nuclei and their central and peripheral connections, and by proprioceptive impulses from neck muscles. It is normally so maintained that the eyes at rest remain in the midline. Any disturbance of this balance results in a drift of the eyes in one or other direction. If this drift is then corrected by a quick movement back to the original position, and this cycle is repeated frequently, nystagmus results.

It is intended here to describe nystagmus as it is actually seen by the examiner and to indicate the possible significance of the different varieties.

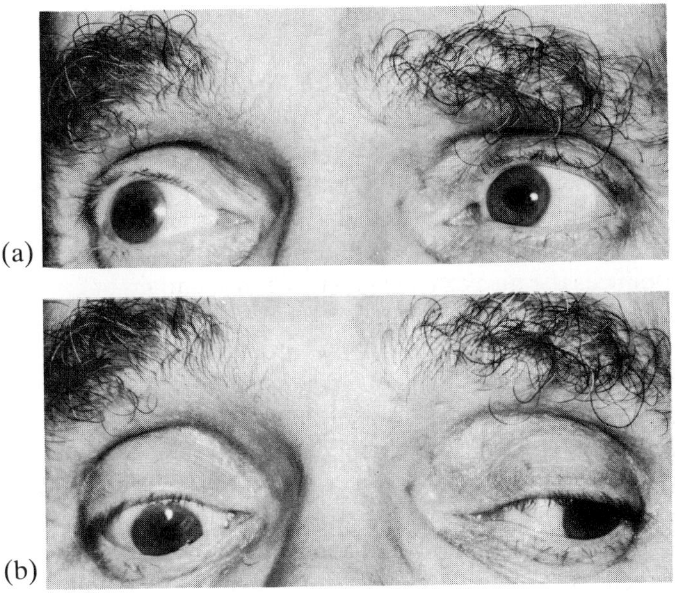

Fig. 11. Internuclear ophthalmoplegia. (a) Ocular deviation to the right is normal. (b) To the left, internal deviation of the right eye is defective and the eye turns downwards. External deviation of the left eye is dissociated, and accompanied by marked nystagmus.

Purpose of the tests

(*a*) To detect nystagmus.

(*b*) To determine its direction, rate and amplitude.

(*c*) To deduce from its character whether it is due to peripheral labyrinthine or central vestibular disease, to muscle weakness or to visual defects.

Methods of testing

Watch the patient's eyes while taking the history. Nystagmus on forward gaze can be noted at once. Note whether it is constant or occurring in bursts.

On direct examination, the patient must be told once again to look at a definite point, such as the tip of a pencil. Hold this object first in the midline, and then move it clearly and deliberately to left, to right, upwards and downwards. During this last movement, the eyelids should be held up by the other hand. Lateral deviation should be maintained for at least five seconds to give time for the nystagmus to occur and for it to be assessed. Note that the deviation should never be to the extreme of lateral movement. If the patient has to strain in order to see the object there is likely to be a spurious nystagmus in quite normal people.

Recording nystagmus

In describing nystagmus, the terms used must be quite clear. There is a great deal of confusion caused by different people meaning different things. The information required is:

(*a*) The position of the eyes when nystagmus occurs.

(*b*) The deviation which produces its greatest amplitude, usually to the side towards which the quick phase beats.

(*c*) The direction, in each oscillation, of the fast movement (not which deviation produces the quickest oscillation).

Custom decrees that the direction of nystagmus is described according to its fast movement (see caloric tests p. 81). To avoid confusion it is probably wise to be a little long-winded and describe what is seen, e.g. 'on deviation to the right, fine horizontal nystagmus, fast component to the right'.

Alternatively, especially useful in recording a changing clinical situation, the nystagmus can be described by 'degree'. Thus, when present only on deviation of the eyes, we speak of 'first degree' nystagmus; when also present looking straight forwards, 'second degree'; when visible even on gaze in the direction opposite to the fast beat, 'third degree'.

The presenting types of nystagmus

PENDULAR NYSTAGMUS

A rapid horizontal oscillation to either side of the mid-line, of equal amplitude, but variable speed, present and usually obvious on forward gaze, increased by fixation, but often losing its pendular character on lateral deviation. It is difficult to believe that any object is stationary to these patients.

Causes

Visual defects from earlier years including macular abnormalities, choroidoretinitis and albinism; high infantile myopia; opacities of the media. It may be seen in adults who have worked in poor illumination, e.g. the rare 'miner's nystagmus'. 'Congenital' nystagmus is also pendular, and horizontal, but becomes 'jerky' on lateral gaze, and remains horizontal on up gaze and down gaze. It is important to avoid unnecessary investigation in these patients.

'JERK NYSTAGMUS'

(*a*) *Horizontal nystagmus*

The rhythm of this common type of nystagmus is that of a slow drift in one direction and a fast correcting movement in the other. It may be present at rest, or only on ocular deviation; so coarse as almost to lose its characteristics, or so fine as to be visible only when using the ophthalmoscope. 'Jerk nystagmus' may also be vertical or rotary, the significance of which is described below, but note that 'horizontal' nystagmus is a *to-and-fro* movement in the horizontal plane, no matter in which direction the eyes may be deviated to demonstrate it.

Causes

Jerk nystagmus is produced by disturbances of the vestibular system. These may occur peripherally in the labyrinth, centrally at the nuclei, in the connections between these two (the vestibular nerve), or between the nuclei and the ocular muscles (the median longitudinal bundle); it is seen in lesions of the cerebellum (though probably because the type of lesion responsible usually involves the cerebello-vestibular connections) and in lesions of the uppermost cervical region.

In more peripheral lesions the quick phase is away from the lesion, and the amplitude is greater in the direction of the quick phase.

In cerebellar lesions, and disturbances of its brain stem connections, the quick phase and the greatest amplitude is towards the side of the lesion.

In cerebello-pontine angle lesions, there are both central and peripheral effects, but the amplitude is greater towards the side of the lesion.

Peripheral lesions usually have additional vertigo, tinnitus and deafness, such as in Ménière's disease, and acoustic neuromata, though the last produce central effects as well.

The more central lesions tend to be more chronic, may cause no tinnitus or deafness and vertigo is less constant. Examples include multiple sclerosis, vascular lesions, or tumours of the cerebellum, IVth ventricle and cerebello-pontine angles (when Vth and VIIth nerves may also be involved).

(*b*) *Vertical nystagmus*

This is *not* nystagmus on looking upwards, but nystagmus in which the oscillation is in an *up-and-down* direction, no matter what the position of the eye. It is never labyrinthine in origin, and the quick phase is most often upwards (upbeat nystagmus).

Causes. It is important to recognise this type of nystagmus because whereas horizontal nystagmus can arise from many sites in the vestibulo-ocular pathways, vertical nystagmus is essentially due to intrinsic disturbance of the brain-stem, such as in vascular accidents, encephalitis, multiple sclerosis, syringobulbia, and secondary to compression from cerebellar tumours, basilar invagination with tonsillar descent, and the Arnold-Chiari syndrome. However, drugs remain the commonest cause of vertical nystagmus which, when combined with a horizontal jerk variety, again always indicates a brain stem dysfunction. Benzodiazepines, barbiturates and phenytoin are often responsible.

(*c*) *Rotary nystagmus*
This type of nystagmus also has fast and slow components, but the oscillations are of rotary character.

Causes. It occurs both in labyrinthine and brain stem disease. In peripheral disorders it is usually at the acute stage, and is transient; if longstanding, it indicates disease of the vestibular nuclei, especially the inferior portion. Any of the disorders causing vertical nystagmus can be included here.

NYSTAGMUS OF DISSOCIATED RHYTHM IN THE TWO EYES
The so-called 'ataxic' nystagmus, in internuclear ophthalmoplegia. There is defective inward movement of the adducting eye with a fine nystagmus, accompanied by a coarse, irregular, rather dramatic nystagmus of the abducting eye, of dissociated rate and rhythm. 'Ataxic' nystagmus may be mimicked by asymmetrical muscle weakness in myasthenia gravis.

Causes
Lesions of the median longitudinal bundle. This most commonly, but by no means invariably, is caused by multiple sclerosis.

RARE FORMS OF NYSTAGMUS

SEE-SAW NYSTAGMUS
The name is self-explanatory. This is spontaneous nystagmus, one eye moving up while the other moves down, the movement being accompanied by a conjugate rotation. This rare phenomenon has most often been seen in lesions in the suprasellar region anterior to the third ventricle.

CONVERGENCE—RETRACTION NYSTAGMUS
Attempted upgaze, usually defective, provokes a jerk nystagmus with the fast phase inwards, in a convergent manner. Lesions of the upper midbrain near the pineal are responsible.

DOWNBEAT NYSTAGMUS
A vertical nystagmus, but here the fast phase is downwards and it is particularly provoked by lateral gaze. It is characteristic of lesions at the foramen magnum, commonly Chiari malformations and the accompanying symptom is oscillopsia, awareness of the apparent vertical movement of objects.

Difficulties and fallacies
(*a*) Misleading results come from failure to ensure that the patient understands what is required of him, from expecting the eyes to be able to deviate

as far as a chameleon's, and by not allowing the nystagmus time to appear.
(*b*) A patient with a hemianopia often has apparent difficulty in looking to that side. If told to look to the left, or towards the window, and to keep looking that way, an object on which he can fix can then be brought into his normal field and the results will be the same.
(*c*) Weakness of an ocular muscle, most often the external rectus, will give an impression of nystagmus, but is usually irregular, non-rhythmic and accompanied by diplopia. In myasthenia gravis, a very irregular nystagmus is often seen which will disappear on appropriate treatment.

Note that a patient either has nystagmus, or he does not. 'A few nystagmoid jerks' is a terminological escape-hatch for uncertain examiners.

Optokinetic nystagmus

Optic nystagmus is a normal phenomenon best observed when sitting opposite someone in a railway carriage. His eyes will follow a portion of passing scenery until they can follow no longer, when they will quickly move back to fix on a new object and follow that. The cycle is repeated regularly, so producing nystagmus and, as the quick phase is back towards the primary position, this is the reverse of all other forms.

The same effect can be obtained either by rotating in front of the patient's eyes a drum marked with alternate black and white stripes, or by passing before the eyes a tape marked with black and white squares, first in one direction, then in the other.

In deeply situated parietal lobe lesions the optokinetic response is absent or much reduced when the drum is rotated towards the side of the lesion.* The particular value of the test is that in patients with a homonymous hemianopia it is often difficult by other means to be certain whether the lesion lies in the optic tract or the temporal, parietal or occipital part of the radiations. Optokinetic nystagmus may, however, also be reduced in brain stem lesions, but there are usually signs of brain-stem disease, and no hemianopia.

The test can be employed on patients whose degree of co-operation is poor, or who are unable to understand commands, and being an involuntary movement depending on some degree of fixation, it is also of value in detecting the presence of vision in an infant thought to be blind, or in an adult thought to be *feigning* blindness. Its absence cannot of course be a proof of blindness.

---

*It is sometimes stated that optokinetic nystagmus is absent 'to the side opposite to the lesion'. This arises because nystagmus is described as being to the side of its fast component which is the side opposite the lesion. It is, however, easier to remember which way the drum is being rotated.

Chapter 9
The Fifth Cranial Nerve: The Trigeminal Nerve

The trigeminal nerve has a large sensory portion with extensive central and peripheral ramifications, and a small motor element which runs in close association with the mandibular division.

Functions

The important functions are:
(*a*) To carry all forms of sensation from the face, the anterior part of the scalp, the eye and the anterior two-thirds of the tongue.
(*b*) To give motor power to the muscles of mastication.

Purposes of the tests

(*a*) To determine which, if any, of the modalities of sensation are impaired.
(*b*) To decide from this whether the lesion lies in one of the peripheral branches, in the Gasserian ganglion or sensory root, or in the brain stem.
(*c*) To determine whether motor weakness is unilateral or bilateral, and of lower or upper motor neurone origin.

Methods of examination

SUPERFICIAL SKIN SENSATION

See Chaps 20 and 21 for general instructions regarding tests of sensation. Here, pain, temperature, and light touch are the main modalities examined. Six areas on each side are tested near, but not at, the midline: (*a*) the forehead and upper part of the side of the nose (ophthalmic division); (*b*) the malar region and upper lip (maxillary division); (*c*) the chin and anterior part of the tongue (mandibular division). The area and extent of any abnormality should be carefully charted and compared with the known distribution of the three divisions (Fig. 67). In addition, remember that:
(*a*) On the scalp, the areas supplied by the Vth nerve and the second cervical segment meet a little posterior to the vertex, but the exact point varies.
(*b*) The mandibular division supplies the anterior upper pinna.
(*c*) The skin over the angle of the jaws is supplied not by the Vth nerve, but by the upper cervical segments.
(*d*) All forms of sensation must pass to the Gasserian ganglion, sensory root and brain stem. Fibres serving touch enter the principal sensory nucleus in

the pons, cross and ascend to the thalamus. Pain and temperature fibres pass downwards to the second cervical segment, gradually entering the descending nucleus. Ophthalmic division fibres pass to the lowest level. From this nucleus all fibres cross the midline and ascend again in the quintothalamic tract.

Abnormalities of sensation

(*a*) *Total loss of sensation over the whole distribution of the nerve*. This indicates a lesion of the ganglion or sensory root, or an extensive lesion anterior to the ganglion, when the motor root is usually involved as well. Tumours eroding the base of the skull, large neurofibromata of the Vth and VIIIth nerves, epidermoids, chronic meningeal lesions such as sarcoid or syphilis, and basal injuries are the commonest causes. There is an 'idiopathic' form of trigeminal sensory neuropathy, with pathological changes rather like a lupus or granulomatous syndrome in the Gasserian ganglion found in a very few. If this sensory abnormality is merely part of a total loss down the whole of that side of the body, the lesion is in the neighbourhood of the opposite thalamus.

(*b*) *Total sensory loss over one or more of the main divisions*. This can also be found in partial lesions of the ganglion (e.g. herpes zoster), or of the root (acoustic neuroma). More peripherally, the ophthalmic division is involved in the cavernous sinus by carotid aneurysms, and in the orbital fissure by tumours. The maxillary division is rarely involved alone except as a result of local trauma, but it is also affected in the cavernous sinus, while basal tumours involve the mandibular division, usually affecting the motor root as well.

(*c*) *Touch only is lost*. This is a pontine lesion affecting the principle sensory nucleus, and is usually due to vascular disease, to pontine tumours, or to brain stem displacement by large tumours.

(*d*) *Pain and temperature are lost, but touch preserved*. Dissociated anaesthesia results from a lesion of the descending root and occurs in syringobulbia, foramen magnum tumours or anomalies, and bulbar vascular accidents. Traditionally a thrombosis of the posterior inferior cerebellar artery causes ipsilateral loss of pain and temperature sensation on the face and contralateral loss on the rest of the body. In practice, however, this syndrome is usually caused by a vertebral artery deficiency, particularly if there is anomalous development of the two posterior inferior cerebellar arteries in relation to each other. High cervical lesions can cause loss in the ophthalmic division but this is quite rare.

(*e*) *Hyperaesthesia over all or part of the distribution of the nerve*. Apart from indicating an irritative rather than a destructive lesion, it gives little localising value, but is most common in vascular lesions and herpes and least common in syringomyelia. This is rather different from the trigger zones of trigeminal neuralgia. Here a light touch on certain points—often the corner of the upper lip, the ala nasae, just in front of the jaw joint, or just below the lower lip—will produce an intense spasm of pain in the related division of the Vth nerve. In men these areas may be left unshaven.

The corneal reflex

This test must first be explained to the patient, who will otherwise undoubtedly flinch if some pointed object is suddenly thrust towards his eye. It must be the cornea, and not the lids, lashes or even the conjunctiva, that is stimulated. In order to widen the palpebral fissure as much as possible, the patient is told to look upwards as far as he can, and a piece of cotton wool teased to a point is touched just lateral to the pupil on either side. A little puff of breath on one cornea, while shielding the other, is a quick alternative method of value. Normally there is a *bilateral* blink whichever side is tested, the facial nerve forming the efferent loop of the reflex arc.

REDUCTION OF THE CORNEAL REFLEX

If there is no response on one side this may be due to a breach of the sensory or motor sides of the reflex arc, i.e. the ophthalmic division of the trigeminal nerve or the facial nerve.

In Vth nerve lesions there will be no response from *either* lid when the abnormal side is stimulated, and a normal response from *both* lids when the normal side is stimulated.

In VIIth nerve lesions there will be no response from the side of the facial paralysis no matter which side is stimulated, but, providing the Vth nerve is intact, there will be a blink on the normal side even when the abnormal side is touched and both eyeballs can be seen to turn upwards.

Loss of this reflex may be the first and only sign of a Vth nerve lesion and is of great value in early cerebello-pontine angle tumours, and in aneurysms and tumours in relation to the cavernous sinus and orbital fissure.

Difficulties and fallacies

All the difficulties which surround sensory testing are, of course, encountered here (Chap. 21). Some people have very insensitive corneae, especially if there is some degree of exophthalmos. If no response is obtained on either side, ask the patient if he can feel the touch and if it is equal on both sides.

The cervical segmental supply to the angle of the jaw is very variable and may sometimes extend quite far up on to the cheek. This emphasises the importance of testing near the midline.

In the presence of a simple facial paralysis the skin sometimes seems less sensitive and may give a false impression of a concomitant trigeminal lesion.

Sensory loss can be simulated, but the curious features of anatomical distribution are not reproduced. In particular, the area supplied by the cervical segments is too unexpected as, not unnaturally, to be included in an alleged Vth nerve loss.

Remember loss of facial sensation may be part of a total hemianaesthesia, which, if genuine, indicates a lesion high in the stem or in the region of the opposite thalamus.

The motor function of the Vth nerve

The temporal muscles, masseters and pterygoids are tested. Note the symmetry of the temporal fossae, and the angles of the jaw, and then palpate the muscles while the patient clenches his jaws. The muscles can be compared as they stand out as hard lumps. Next place the hand under the jaw and instruct the patient to open his mouth.

MOTOR ABNORMALITIES

Wasting of temporal muscles and masseters due to a lower motor neurone or local muscular lesion produces hollowing of the temple and flattening of the angle of the jaw. This may be caused by nuclear lesions as in motor neurone disease (bilateral), a peripheral nerve lesion, as in compression of the motor root (unilateral), or muscular dystrophy.

Pterygoid weakness causes the jaw to deviate towards the paralysed side on opening as a result of the action of the normal muscle.

If the jaw keeps falling open, but closes satisfactorily after rest, this indicates myasthenia, but not necessarily myasthenia gravis, for this symptom is common in the myasthenia associated with a carcinoma.

The jaw jerk

This is a very important reflex which sadly is often ignored. To obtain it the patient is told to let his jaw sag open slightly, but not to push it open and not to open it wide. The examiner then places the left forefinger below the lower lip and taps it in a downward direction with the percussion hammer (Fig. 12). There may be a slight palpable upward jerk immediately after the purely percussive effect is over, but in many normal people no response is obtained.

ABNORMALITIES

An absent jaw jerk is rarely helpful, but in lesions of the upper motor neurone above the level of the pons, great exaggeration, even amounting to jaw clonus, may be found. This is commonly the case in pseudobulbar palsy, motor neurone disease, and quite often in multiple sclerosis. When a patient has pathological exaggeration of all tendon reflexes in arms and legs, an exaggerated jaw jerk shows that the lesion must be higher than the cervical spine. Be on guard however, not to be misled by emotional hyper-reflexia,

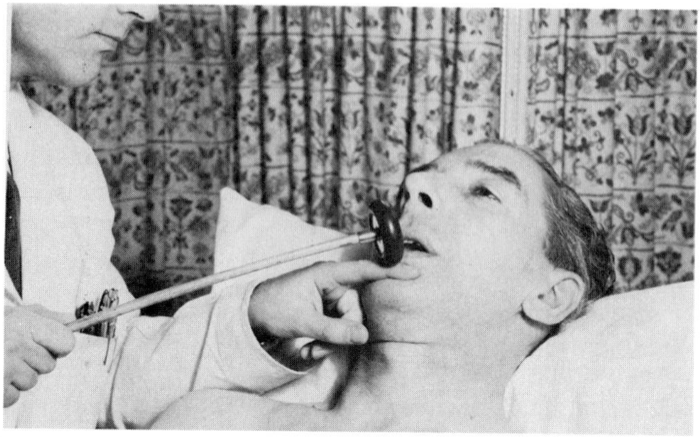

Fig. 12. The jaw jerk. A gentle tap is essential or the mechanical effect of the percussion will confuse the responses.

which will be generalised, and without any other signs of cortico-spinal tract abnormality.

Trophic changes

Erosion of the ala nasae and surrounding skin can follow severe sensory loss; this is occasionally seen after trigeminal ganglion injection for tic douloureux, and in the idiopathic trigeminal neuropathy.

Corneal ulceration, infection, and panophthalmitis may follow profound ophthalmic sensory loss but it would suggest the VIIth nerve was involved as well so that the cornea was inadequately protected.

Chapter 10
The Seventh Cranial Nerve: The Facial Nerve

Owing to the close anatomical relationship between the facial nerve and the nervus intermedius, they are considered together, though their functions differ greatly.

Functions

For the purpose of neurological examination the important functions are the motor innervation of the muscles of expression and facial movement, including platysma, and of the stapedius.

The intermediate nerve carries secretory fibres to the lachrymal glands through the greater superficial petrosal nerve and to the salivary glands through the chorda tympani, which also carries the sensation of taste from the anterior two-thirds of the tongue.

Purposes of the tests

To determine whether any weakness of the facial muscles detected is unilateral or bilateral, and whether of upper or lower motor neurone origin. If of peripheral origin, to determine by association with other abnormalities the site of the lesion along the course of the nerve. To detect impairment of taste.

Methods of examination

Inspection

Everything in this part of the examination is a matter of symmetry and asymmetry as seen while first talking to the patient. Observe:

(*a*) The face as a whole.

(*b*) The wrinkles of the forehead and the naso-labial folds.

(*c*) Blinking, and whether the eyeballs can be seen to turn up with each blink. (This of course happens normally, but is hidden by efficient closure of the lids.)

(*d*) Movements of the mouth while talking, smiling, etc. Note also the presence of twitching, tremors, or other involuntary movements in the facial muscles (see Chap. 19).

Motor functions

It is common practice to say to the patient 'show me your teeth'. This often results in a tedious explanation that they are false, or the more eager patients may actually take them out and show them. These undesirable experiences may be avoided if the examiner bares his teeth himself and asks the patient to copy him. This also helps edentulous patients to overcome a curious difficulty in making this particular movement. Note the symmetry of the movement and of the naso-labial folds. Next ask the patient to open his mouth and compare the naso-labial folds. Be on guard, however, for deviation of the *jaw* due to motor Vth nerve weakness.

The upper facial muscles are tested by telling the patient to close his eyes (noting whether he can do so), then to screw them up tightly and to resist attempts to open them. The orbicularis oculis is normally powerful enough to overcome this even in a puny child.

Ask the patient next to bare his teeth and open the mouth at the same time; this enables the platysma to stand out in the young and not too well covered.

Other movements such as whistling, blowing out the cheeks, etc., can be used as confirmation of strength or weakness, but do not usually give additional information.

Examination of taste

This shares with the tests of the sense of smell the most unsatisfactory part of the examination. There are four primary tastes only, sweet, salt, sour and bitter; all others are flavours, their appreciation depending upon an intact sense of smell. The tests are carried out with sugar, salt, vinegar and quinine in that order. The patient must protrude the tongue to one side, keep it out throughout the test and not talk. The four possible tastes are written on a card. The tip of the tongue is held gently with a piece of gauze and the side of the tongue is moistened about an inch from the tip with a little of the test substance. The patient should indicate the taste by pointing to the card. In between each test he must swill out his mouth with water.

If two flat leaves of copper and zinc are soldered at one end and the free ends touched by the examiner or the patient on the tongue, a small electric current, and a metallic taste, is produced. This is simple and avoids the need for elaborate apparatus.

Secretory functions

The flow of tears on the two sides can be compared by giving the patient ammonia to inhale.

The flow of saliva is compared by placing a highly spiced substance on the tongue and asking the patient to raise the tip.

These tests are not often required and the patient will usually be able to describe any defects spontaneously.

The types of facial weakness

These are dealt with in the order in which they are usually appreciated.

UNILATERAL FACIAL PARALYSIS

(*a*) A deviation of the mouth on smiling, which disappears on voluntary movement, constitutes the so-called *emotional facial weakness*. This occurs in deep-seated lesions of the opposite thalamus, or its connections with the frontal lobe.

(*b*) Deviation of the mouth and deepening of the naso-labial fold but with normal strength of the orbicularis occurs in an *upper motor neurone facial weakness* (Fig. 13). This is due to a lesion at some point between the opposite cortex and the facial nucleus in the pons. The upper facial muscles on each side are controlled by *both* cerebral cortices, so that if one supranuclear pathway is damaged the other is still capable of performing its function. An associated hemianopia will mean a hemisphere lesion; any hemiplegia will be on the *same* side.

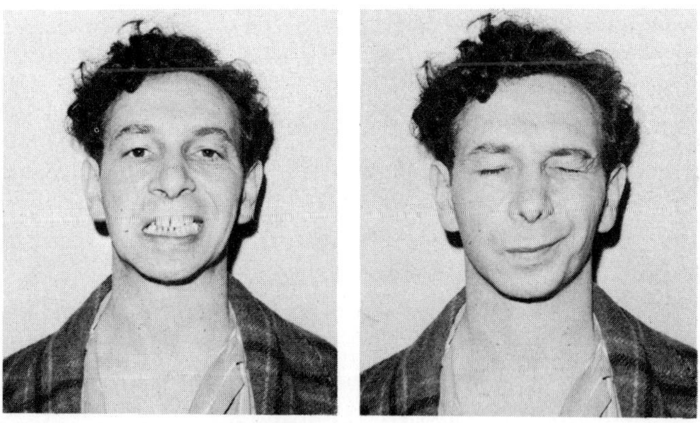

(a) (b)

Fig. 13. Upper motor neurone facial paresis. (a) The weakness of the lower part of the face is very much greater than the upper. (b) In this case associated movements of the right lower facial muscles were also affected.

(*c*) Both upper and lower parts of the face may be paralysed. The eye cannot be closed or can easily be opened by the examiner, the eyeball is seen to turn upwards on attempted closure, the patient does not blink on that side and the normal wrinkling on that side of the forehead is absent (Fig. 14). This is a *lower motor neurone weakness*, occurring when the final common pathway between the nucleus and the muscle is interrupted, cutting off all stimuli to both upper and lower facial muscles. The lesion may lie, *on the same side*, at any point along the course of the facial nerve, and it is necessary to consider associated abnormalities to decide on its exact site.

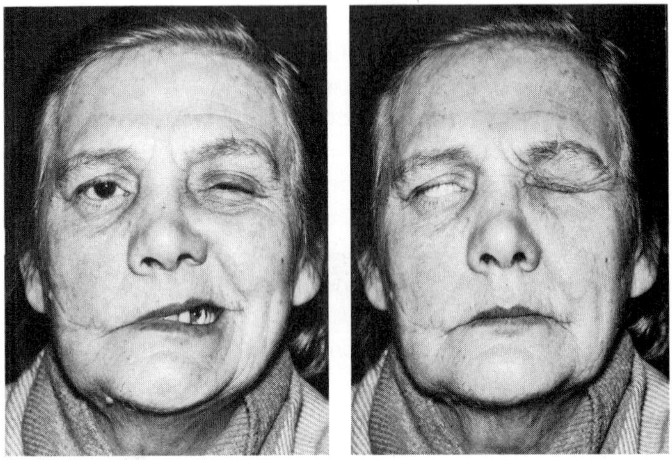

Fig. 14. Lower motor neurone facial paralysis. Both upper and lower parts of the face are equally involved. Note absence of wrinkling of R. forehead and visible sclera on screwing up eyes.

1 If the VIth nerve is also involved the lesion is in the pons. Any hemiplegia will be on the *opposite* side.
2 If the Vth and VIIIth nerves are also involved the lesion is in the cerebello-pontine angle.
3 If taste, salivation and tear production are affected the lesion lies between the brain stem and the departure of the chorda tympani in the middle ear. Distortion of sound due to stapedius palsy is also present.
4 If taste and salivation are involved, but the secretion of tears is normal, the lesion is in the middle ear after the departure of the superficial petrosal branch, but before the departure of the chorda tympani.
5 If nothing other than motor weakness is present the lesion may, in fact, be anywhere along the route of the nerve, but is usually either at the nucleus, or in the facial canal peripheral to the departure of the chorda tympani.
6 If only some of the facial muscles are paralysed and especially if only the upper part, the lesion is usually very peripheral and often in the parotid gland, or in the muscles themselves. Perineural spread of certain skin malignancies or infratemporal fossa tumours characteristically produce a gradually extending lower motor neurone type weakness.

BILATERAL FACIAL PARALYSIS

This often causes difficulty in detection, because symmetry may be maintained. In *bilateral emotional facial palsy* there is a mask-like face, complete lack of the normal play of expression, and diminished blinking, yet when it occurs it is normal, and there is transformation when the patient smiles. In *bilateral upper motor neurone palsy* the masking is not so marked, blinking is little affected, but the mouth cannot be moved on command, yet often appears to move quite well during ordinary conversation. In *bilateral lower motor neurone palsy* there is a flattening of all normal folds, the corners of the mouth sag, all attempts at voluntary movement fail, and the whites of the eyes are seen when the patient attempts to close them or to blink (Fig. 15). The patient talks as if he were protecting a very sore mouth.

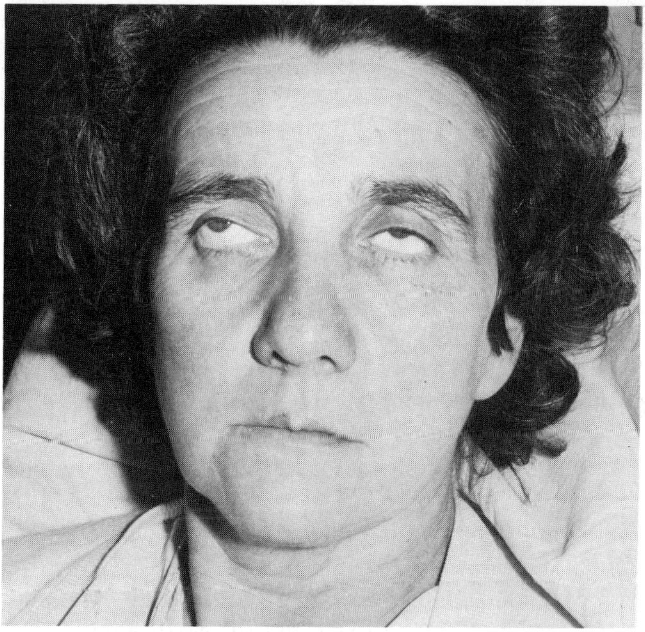

Fig. 15. Bilateral lower motor neurone facial paralysis. The patient is trying to close her eyes. The eyeballs move upwards, but are uncovered; the lower part of the face is flattened and expressionless.

Long after a facial palsy there may be aberrant re-innervation. If this is bilateral the whole face wrinkles when any expression is attempted, and the result may be quite inappropriate for the emotion being expressed and as unexpected to the onlooker as it is embarrassing to the patient (see Fig. 16). Spontaneous twitching is also common during re-innervation and often interpreted by the patient as a sign of potential recurrence.

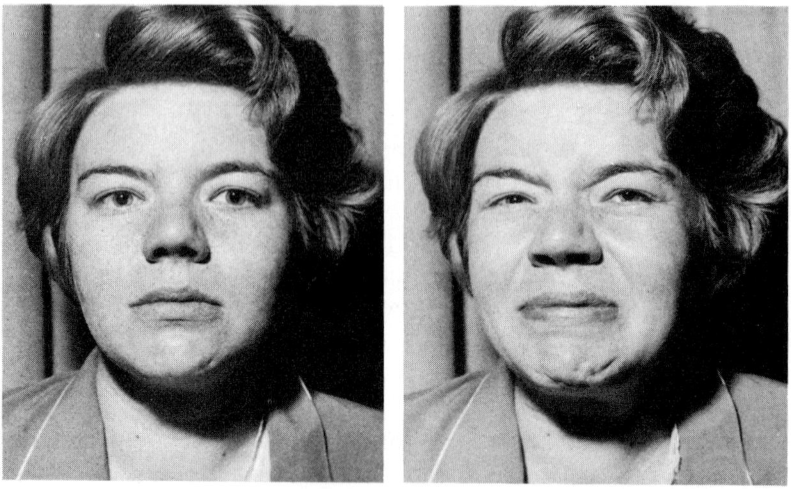

(a) (b)

Fig. 16. Old bilateral lower motor neurone facial paralysis with aberrant re-innervation. (a) at rest, (b) on smiling.

PRIMARY MUSCULAR DISORDERS

In myasthenic states facial expressions are markedly diminished, the muscles are weak, particularly in the upper part and there is usually associated ptosis and oculomotor paresis. These features are returned to normal by injection of neostigmine or edrophonium chloride (Tensilon)—see Figs 65 and 66.

Myopathies are characterised by a sagging of the whole facial musculature, downward drawn lines at the corners of the eyes and mouth, generalised weakness of the muscles, inability to raise the corners of the mouth in smiling. The whole face is given an abnormally long thin appearance (see Fig. 3).

In dystrophia myotonica (myotonic dystrophy) when the patient closes the eyes and is told to open them quickly, they remain closed for a measurable interval. Similarly, an expression such as a smile will persist after that emotion is, in fact, over. This is rare in myotonia congenita.

Loss of taste

Unilateral loss of taste, without VIIth or lingual nerve abnormality, is very rare, but could occur in middle ear lesions of the chorda tympani. More peripherally, lesions in the lingual nerve cause loss of common sensation over the anterior two-thirds of the tongue as well. Bilateral 'loss of taste' usually is a loss of flavours, due to anosmia, the primary tastes remaining intact when tested. Occasionally true bilateral loss occurs in demyelinative or vascular lesions of the brain stem involving the nucleus of the solitary tract but this is usually temporary.

Difficulties and fallacies

Natural facial asymmetry can usually be overcome if the problem is explained to the patient with the aid of a mirror.

If a patient does not smile, asking him to whistle will often result in a successful smile, if an unsuccessful whistle.

In long-standing lower motor neurone lesions contracture occurs and may suggest a contralateral palsy. This error is corrected when the patient makes a voluntary movement.

In very severe upper motor neurone lesions the upper part of the face may be so weak as to mimic a lower motor neurone lesion. Even here, however, there is a far greater paralysis of the lower facial muscles and almost invariably a hemiplegia on the *same* side whereas it would be on the opposite side if the paralysis were truly of lower motor neurone origin, for the neighbouring pyramidal fibres if involved would shortly be decussating in the medulla.

Common lesions of the facial nerve

Unilateral emotional paralysis

Neoplasms and vascular accidents affecting the thalamus and thalamofrontal connections.

Bilateral emotional paralysis

Parkinsonism, pseudobulbar palsy.

Bilateral upper motor neurone paralysis

Cerebrovascular accidents, early or late, neoplasms, demyelinative lesions.

Bilateral upper motor neurone paralysis

Diffuse cerebrovascular disease producing a pseudobulbar palsy. Motor neurone disease.

Unilateral lower motor neurone paralysis

Bell's palsy is by far the most common cause. Others include pontine neoplasms and vascular accidents; cerebello-pontine angle tumours; petrous epidermoids (gradual onset), tumours, infections and operations in the middle ear; fractures of the petrous bone; trauma to the jaw and parotid regions; parotid tumours or sarcoid.

Bilateral lower motor neurone paralysis

The Guillain–Barré syndrome; progressive muscular atrophy (exaggerated jaw jerk); brain stem encephalitis. Certain muscle disorders involve the facial muscles and mimic lower motor neurone paralysis.

Chapter 11
The Eighth Cranial Nerve: The Auditory Nerve

Synonyms: the acoustic nerve, the stato-acoustic nerve

Unilateral total loss of hearing may easily be overlooked, both by the patient, who is either not aware of it or has grown to accept it (always using the telephone on the other ear), and by the doctor who has not carried out any appropriate examination. Disturbances of the vestibular function are however so dramatic in their effects rarely to be ignored by either, though the bedside tests of cochlear function are much the simpler of the two.

Functions

(*a*) *The cochlear nerve*. This carries impulses of sound from the hair cells of the organ of Corti, through the spiral ganglion in the cochlea, to the cochlear nuclei in the pons. Most fibres cross, run in the lateral leminiscus to the medial geniculate body and are relayed to the superior temporal gyrus. But there is some uncrossed upwards transmission, so that deafness from a unilateral cerebral cortical lesion is virtually precluded.

(*b*) *The vestibular nerve*. Impulses arise in the labyrinth by displacement of endolymph affecting the hair cells in the ampullae of the semi-circular canals, and the otoliths in the saccule and utricle. Fibres run to the vestibular ganglia and on in the main trunk of the nerve to the vestibular nuclei in the medulla. These nuclei have connections with the cerebellum, the oculomotor nuclei, the nuclei of the upper cervical nerves, the spinal cord and the temporal lobes.

Purposes of the tests

To determine whether any deafness is bilateral or unilateral, and whether due to disease of the middle ear, or of the cochlear nerve.

To determine whether disturbance of vestibular function originates in the labyrinth, the vestibular nerve, or the brain stem.

EXAMINATION OF HEARING

A deaf patient turns his head to bring the unaffected side nearer. Hearing aids may be cunningly concealed, but if present, efficient or inefficient, silent or singing, they almost invariably mean marked bilateral deafness, which considerably reduces the chances of it being due to intracranial disease—reduces, but by no means excludes.

A simple bedside test of hearing is carried out as follows:

Place a finger in the patient's external meatus on one side and move it constantly in order to produce a masking noise. Position the head so that lip-reading is impossible, and ask the patient to repeat the words said to him. In order to produce a standard volume of sound, breathe out, and at the end of expiration whisper a few numbers, e.g. 26 or 68 to test high tones, and 42 or 100 to test low tones. If nothing is heard, the force of the whisper should be gradually increased and the two sides compared. Do not be surprised if the patient whispers back.

If deafness is present, the auroscope must be used to exclude the presence of wax and any disease of the middle ear and drum.

The type of deafness

Conduction of sound through the air to the drum and bony ossicles is the normal method of hearing and is about twice as efficient as conduction through bone.

Rinne's test

Strike a tuning fork gently, hold it near one external meatus, mask the other, and ask the patient if he can hear it. Place it then on the mastoid, ask if he can still hear it, and tell him to say 'now' the moment the sound ceases. When he does so at once place the blades of the fork near the meatus again. Normally, the note is still audible.

In middle ear deafness, this will not be so. In nerve deafness, both air and bone conduction are reduced, but air conduction remains the better, and the note will still be heard. Further information must now be obtained from Weber's test.

Weber's test

The fork is placed on the centre of the forehead. Ask the patient if he can hear the sound all over the head, or in both ears, or in one ear predominantly.

In nerve deafness, the sound appears to be heard in the normal ear, but in chronic middle ear disease, it is conducted to the abnormal ear.

NOTES ON TERMINOLOGY

'Conduction deafness' means middle ear deafness. 'Perception deafness' means nerve deafness.

'Rinne's positive' is the normal response, which occurs also with nerve deafness. 'Rinne's negative' indicates reduced air conduction and middle ear deafness.

CAUSES OF CONDUCTION DEAFNESS

This includes all diseases of the external meatus, middle ear, and Eustachian tubes, none of which come directly within the sphere of neurological disease. Detection of middle ear infection is of course of paramount importance in suspected intracranial infection, and certain middle ear tumours extend intracranially (e.g. tumours of the glomus jugulare).

COMMON CAUSES OF PERCEPTION DEAFNESS

(*a*) *At cochlear level*

Ménière's disease, advanced otosclerosis, deafness due to drugs, internal auditory artery occlusions, prolonged exposure to loud noise.

(*b*) *In the nerve trunk*

Old age, post-inflammatory lesions, toxic lesions, meningitis, cerebello-pontine angle tumours, trauma.

(*c*) *In the brain stem*

Severe pontine vascular lesions, severe demyelinative lesions, occasionally tumours.

Deciding the level of the lesion is by no means easy. If deafness occurs as a result of a brain stem lesion it is usually gross and profound neurological disability is present. If it is due to cerebello-pontine angle tumour, the Vth and VIIth nerves are also involved, but other lesions of the nerve trunk may be difficult to separate from cochlear lesions. Various additional tests of greater or less sophistication have been devised, none of which is specific, but a combination of which can help to distinguish between cochlear and neural deafness.

PURE TONE AUDIOMETRY

This is a quantitative measurement of hearing particularly important in detecting early nerve deafness. Musical notes of varying pitch are produced by an electric oscillator, and the intensity of the sound is increased until the patient can hear it and then decreased until the sound disappears. One ear is examined at a time while the other is masked. Naturally, if hearing is impaired, the intensity of a particular note will have to be increased more than is usual for it to be heard, and the degree of loss of hearing is plotted against the frequency of the note on special charts. High tone loss is characteristic of nerve deafness and low tone loss of middle ear deafness (Fig. 17).

Speech discrimination audiometry

Speech is employed, instead of pure tones, and discrimination of speech is

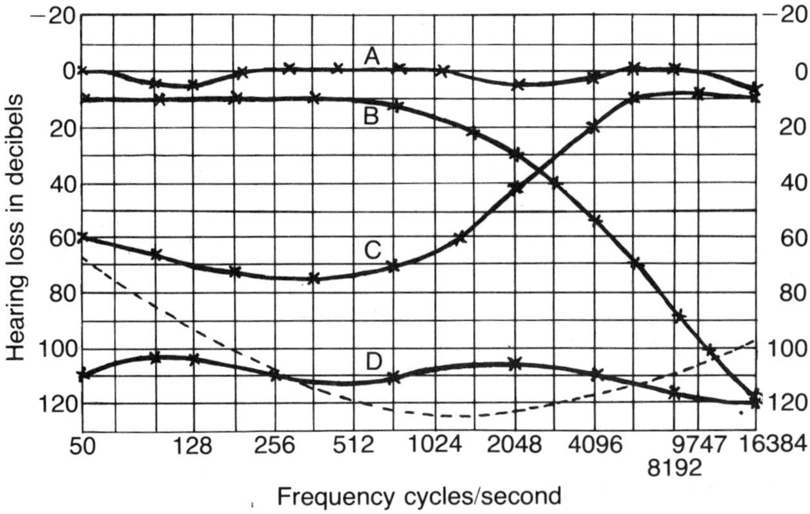

Fig. 17. Audiogram. (A) Normal curve. (B) Nerve deafness—loss of high tones. (C) Middle-ear deafness—loss of low tones. (D) Gross loss of hearing.

more affected in about 75 per cent of VIIIth nerve tumours.

Loudness recruitment

Normally, as the intensity of a sound of a fixed frequency is increased, it is heard equally well in either ear. Under certain conditions of unilateral deafness, appreciation of a sound of low intensity may be diminished in the affected ear, but when the same sound reaches a high intensity it may be heard equally in both ears. The deafness of the affected ear is reduced at higher intensities of the same frequency. This is termed 'loudness recruitment' and occurs when there is a lesion of the hair cells in the organ of Corti. As it is found in Ménière's disease and otosclerosis and not as a rule in acoustic neuromata or other lesions of the nerve trunk or its entry to the brain stem, it is a useful adjunct to the differentiation of causes of perceptive deafness.

Tone decay

With time the intensity of a pure tone signal has to be raised appreciably to remain audible to a patient with an VIIIth nerve tumour. Decay of some degree occurs in cochlea lesions but the need to raise the intensity by over 20 dB in less than 3 minutes suggests a nerve lesion.

Békésy Audiometry

This is a method of showing a mixture of hearing threshold, loudness recruitment and decay. Either interrupted or continuous tones of different frequency are automatically presented to the patient who controls their intensity to remain just audible, and the intensity is graphically recorded. A continuous tracing falling abruptly away from a pulsed tracing is highly suggestive of a nerve lesion.

Even more sensitive tests include measuring response of the stapedius muscle to sounds, both determining threshold response, and decay to long-continued stimulation (acoustic reflex measurements) and direct measurement of the electrical output of the cochlea (electrocochleography) but these tests require great experience both in performance and interpretation.

No one test gives a certain localisation, but taking the cochlear tests together with vestibular tests can offer a high degree of probability.

Auditory evoked responses

See Chap. 39.

TESTS OF VESTIBULAR FUNCTION

All vestibular tests make use of the fact that disturbances of the balance of vestibular function result in vertigo, nystagmus, past pointing and falling. The varieties of spontaneous nystagmus are discussed under the oculomotor nerves.

By stimulation of the vestibular system, usually the labyrinth, these features can normally be produced at will, and defects may be detected which are helpful in localising the lesion.

The rotational test

The patient is seated in a chair which can be rotated, with his head well supported and fixed in a head rest.

To test the horizontal canals, the head is flexed 30° so that the eye/external meatus plane is horizontal. To test the vertical canals, the head is flexed to 120°. The chair is then rotated ten times in 20 seconds. Normally, when rotation to (say) the right has stopped, the endolymph continues to flow in that direction. This results in nystagmus with its slow phase to the right, this always being in the direction of the current. There is also past-pointing and falling to the right, and vertigo with apparent movement of objects to the left. Unfortunately, this test stimulates the labyrinths on both sides and for neurological purposes the caloric tests are of greater value.

The caloric tests

Many people find difficulty in understanding these invaluable tests. If the patient lies supine with the head flexed 30°, the horizontal canals lie in the vertical plane, with the ampullae at the highest point. In this position, warming or cooling the endolymph will produce currents upwards or downwards respectively. This movement stimulates the ampullae of the canal, producing nystagmus. For example, if, with the head in this position, one runs warm water into the right external ear, a current flows upwards in the right horizontal canal toward the ampulla. The position of the head makes no difference, however, to the fact that this is really the horizontal canal, and if such displacement of endolymph took place when the canal was in its normal plane, the flow would be in an arc curving forwards towards the left. The nystagmus, therefore, has its slow phase towards the left, this phase always being in the direction of the flow. Tradition, however, makes it more complicated by decreeing that nystagmus is always named after its quick phase, which in this case is to the right. Therefore, irrigating the right ear with warm water produces nystagmus to the right; with cold water, to the left. Similarly, irrigating the left ear with warm water produces nystagmus to the left; with cold water to the right.

During the test about 250 ml water is irrigated through the external auditory meatus over a period of about 40 seconds, first using water at 30°C and later at 44°C. The patient fixes his eyes on a given point immediately above his head and, after ceasing the irrigation, the time in seconds is measured during which nystagmus on forward gaze persists. The test is repeated on the other ear and the results are charted as shown (Fig. 18). Normally all four durations are of approximately the same value.

If equivocal results are produced at 30°C a much lower temperature may be used. If the drum is perforated, air at a controlled temperature can be blown in, instead of water irrigation.

CALORIC ABNORMALITIES

If there is no response, or a much diminished response, to both warm and cold water on one side, this is termed canal paresis. It is caused by lesions of one labyrinth (Ménière's disease), or vestibular nerve (e.g. acoustic nerve tumour, or vestibular neuronitis, the former showing deafness, the latter no deafness), or lesions of the vestibular nuclei.

If the response is always reduced for irrigations producing nystagmus in the same direction (e.g. cold water in the right ear and warm water in the left), there is said to be *directional preponderance*, which in this case would be to the right. This is a sign of imbalance between the two sides of the vestibular system, normally held in a state of equilibrium. This balance can be disturbed by lesions of the peripheral or central vestibular apparatus or of the cerebellum and cortico-fugal fibres deep in the temporal lobe.

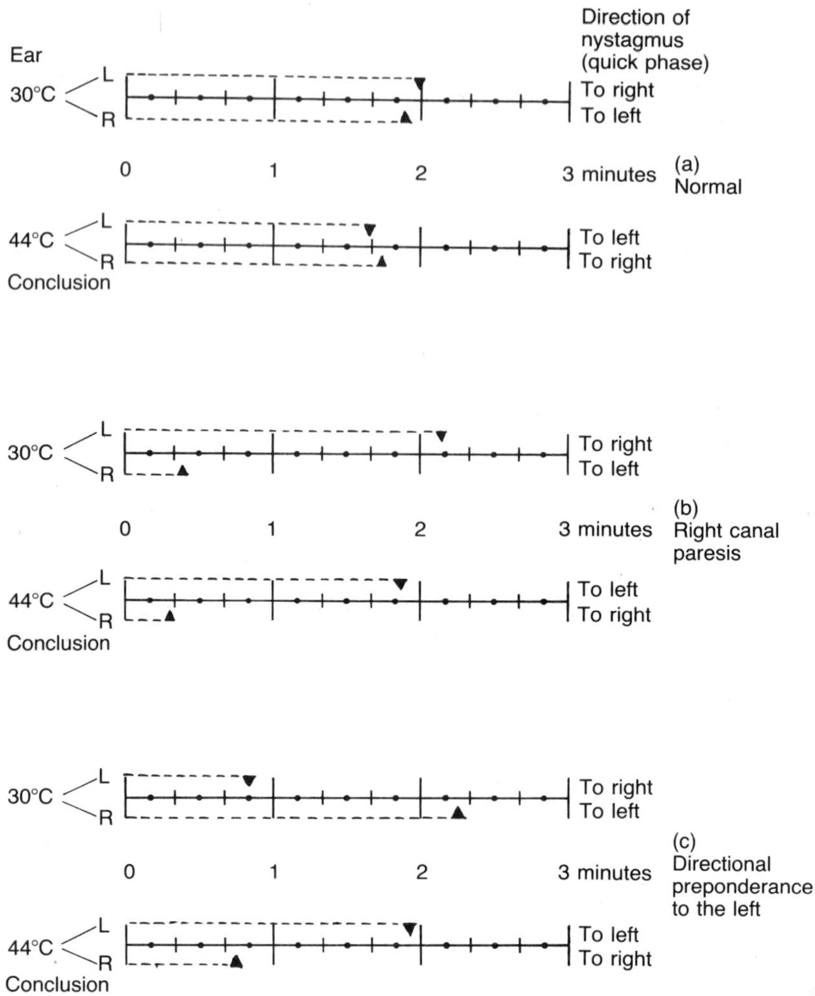

Fig. 18. Caloric responses. The broken line marks the time in minutes for which nystagmus on forward gaze persists after the end of irrigation. The temperature of the water is indicated on the left, the direction of the nystagmus on the right. (a) Normal response, (b) right canal paresis in a case of acoustic neuroma, (c) directional preponderance to left in a case of L. posterior temporal lobe tumour.

Combinations of these two types of abnormality may at times be seen in lesions of the vestibular nerve or labyrinth. This emphasises, therefore, that the caloric tests must be interpreted in conjunction with audiometry and, of course, the clinical picture.

ELECTRONYSTAGMOGRAPHY

As the eye is surrounded by an electric field, probably originating from the pigment epithelium of the retina, changes in potential difference produced by movement of the eyeball can be recorded graphically between skin electrodes on opposite sides of the eye. This enables the nystagmus to be measured at leisure, is not so dependent upon a subjective impression, and though neither simple nor without drawbacks, can be an adjunct to caloric testing. In addition, eye movement can be measured in darkness, with the eyes shut, without fixation, and this constitutes much of the importance of the examination for fixation diminishes spontaneous nystagmus of peripheral origin, but increases it when the lesion is supranuclear, so the method has localisation value. These differing effects of eye closure and darkness on spontaneous nystagmus allows recognition of characteristic patterns emerging from lesions peripheral to the vestibular nuclei, at nucleus level, or above.

POSITIONAL VERTIGO AND NYSTAGMUS

Seat the patient on a couch, grasp the head, turn it 30–40° to one side, and then lower the patient backwards until he is supine with the head over the end of the couch and 30° below the horizontal. A patient with positional vertigo will, after a short latent period, develop both nystagmus and vertigo, the fast phase of the eye movement being towards the lower ear. Adaptation rapidly occurs, and these features cannot usually be elicited again within 10–15 minutes. This is the benign paroxysmal type, thought to be due to a utricle lesion, and common after infective or vascular lesions, and following head injury. Such patients experience transient vertigo on movement of the head and neck.

If nystagmus appears at once, adaptation does not occur, nystagmus reappears immediately on reassuming the position, and its direction is altered by varying the head posture, then this is the central type and may indicate deeply situated posterior fossa lesions—though will not say what type. Such patients may also have vertigo on movement but it is likely to be more prolonged and prostrating. Unfortunately, in practice, this distinction between 'benign' and 'central' does not always hold true. The clinical and even electronystagmography findings may suggest a peripheral lesion, only for the CT scan to reveal a cerebellar infarct or tumour.

Common causes of spontaneous vestibular disturbances

At labyrinthine level. Ménière's disease, motion sickness, streptomycin toxicity.

In the vestibular nerve. As for perception deafness, but add also 'vestibular neuronitis'.

In the brain stem. Vascular deficiency, especially vertebro-basilar artery disease; cerebellar and IVth ventricular tumours, acute demyelinative disease, migraine.

In the temporal lobe. As an epileptic manifestation, especially in children, or as an ischaemic lesion in the elderly.

Chapter 12
The Ninth and Tenth Cranial Nerves: The Glossopharyngeal and Vagus Nerves

Clinically, and even anatomically, it is so difficult to separate the actions of these two nerves that it is customary to consider them together.

Functions

From the very widespread functions of the vagus and glossopharyngeal nerves the following are of most importance in neurological examination:
(*a*) To carry common sensation from the pharynx, tonsils, soft palate and posterior one-third of the tongue.
(*b*) To carry the sense of taste from the posterior one-third of the tongue (probably almost purely by the IXth nerve).
(*c*) To give motor supply to the palatal and pharyngeal muscles.
(*d*) To give motor supply to the vocal cords (purely the vagus).

Purposes of the tests

(*a*) To determine the integrity of the reflex arc for the gag reflex.
(*b*) If abnormal, to differentiate between a breach on the sensory side by testing sensation in the pharynx and palate, and on the motor side by testing elevation of the palate and contraction of the pharynx.
(*c*) To examine the movements of the vocal cords.

Methods of examination

Preliminary observations

Notice the pitch and quality of the patient's voice, and of his cough, and whether there is any difficulty in swallowing his saliva. Ask if there has been any nasal regurgitation of fluids.

A high-pitched, hoarse voice may mean vocal cord paralysis; a nasal tone which increases if the head is bent forwards means palatal paralysis when lying back, this can become almost normal. If the patient chokes over his saliva while talking, there may be both palatal and pharyngeal weakness, and if any of these features increase towards the end of each sentence, this may be due to myasthenia gravis.

Motor functions

Ask the patient to open his mouth wide. A few moments' wait, allowing the tongue to rest in the floor of the mouth, will usually make it possible to see the palate without the use of the unpopular tongue depressor. The patient is then asked to say 'Ah' while breathing out, followed by 'Ugh' while breathing in. In each case the palate should move symmetrically upwards and backwards, the uvula remaining in the midline, and the two sides of the pharynx should contract symmetrically. He should then be asked to phonate several times in succession and the palate is watched to see if any defect worsens with repeated use.

Sensory functions

Common sensation

It is normally only the sense of touch that is tested, relying on its ability to stimulate a reflex arc.

A throat swab, with the cotton wool safely attached, is passed to one side of the back of the throat, while the tongue is gently and slowly depressed. Touching any part of the palate, tonsil or the back of the tongue will normally result in contraction of the pharynx, elevation of the palate and retraction of the tongue. This is called the gag reflex, and varies in sensitivity from individual to individual.

Taste

Testing taste on the posterior part of the tongue is so difficult by normal means that it is hardly worth spending much time over it. Using a galvanic current of 2–4 mA, and touching the tongue in this area with the anode on either side, will produce a metallic taste which the patient should be able to detect if not define, and allows the two sides to be compared, but the simple device described on p. 70 can be more easily applied to this area than any of the conventional methods.

Abnormalities

On inspection

The uvula lies to one side of the midline due to:

(*a*) Simple asymmetry of the palate. In this case, movement on phonation is normal.

(*b*) Swelling in the tonsillar region. This will be visible. Take this opportunity to detect other naso-pharyngeal swellings, so easily overlooked, and yet so vital in cases of lower cranial nerve palsies.

(*c*) Unilateral muscle paralysis.

A constant rhythmic vertical oscillation of the palate, sometimes also involving the pharynx, is called *palatal nystagmus*, due to a lesion in the central tegmental tract. A more extensive form has been referred to as *palatopharyngolaryngooculodiaphragmatic myoclonus*, a name which if alphabetically uneconomical, is, at least, self explanatory. Palatal fasciculation can be seen in motor neurone disease.

On phonation

The palate moves up and over to one side when there is paralysis of the opposite side, owing to the pulling movement of the unopposed normal muscle. In pharyngeal paralysis, the muscles will also appear to move towards the normal side, so resembling a flat sheet being drawn across that it is called the 'curtain movement'. These features are caused by a lower motor neurone lesion of the vagus.

If there is no movement of the palate and pharynx there should also be dysphagia, nasal regurgitation and nasal speech, and this usually indicates either a bilateral medullary nuclear lesion, or a bilateral upper motor neurone lesion as seen in pseudobulbar palsy. These two groups of symptoms may be combined, however, in motor neurone disease.

Repeated phonation can demonstrate the fatiguability which occurs in myasthenia gravis.

This is a time to note the high arched palate of patients with Marfan's syndrome, which may be associated with intracranial vascular disorders and a cleft palate, which may be associated with other congenital malformations.

On testing sensation

Unilateral absence of the gag reflex may be due to loss of sensation, of motor power, or both. Phonation will have shown if one side is paralysed. If due to loss of sensation alone, stimulation of the normal side will produce a normal symmetrical reflex. This rare event would be due to a glossopharyngeal lesion.

If the defect, however, is due to combined motor and sensory paralysis, stimulation of the normal side will cause the palate to be pulled towards that side. This more common finding indicates a combined lesion of glossopharyngeal and vagus nerves.

No reaction on either side, but normal movement on phonation, is practically never due to organic disease, though theoretically it might possibly occur in syringomyelia or tabes dorsalis.

A combination of bilateral anaesthesia and bilateral motor paralysis indicates a severe medullary lesion and is usually associated with other lower cranial nerve palsies.

Difficulties and fallacies

Some people have intensely sensitive fauces and pharynx and are unable to tolerate any touch. Others appear to have complete insensitivity. In these watch spontaneous movements on phonation and inspiration, and ask them to attempt to swallow with the mouth open. A great deal of information can be obtained in this way without touching at all.

In children, these tests are best left to a late stage or one may never regain the 'rapport' required for the rest of the examination.

Hysterical insensitivity of the pharynx is not uncommon and may be associated with hysterical hoarseness, but movements on sudden respiratory intake are normal, even if phonation is not attempted.

If local anaesthetic has been used to enable good visualisation of the vocal cords, it is important to know when this was carried out. Patients vary greatly in the length of time that local anaesthesia lasts, and apparent sensory loss may be misleading.

EXAMINING THE VOCAL CORDS

This examination, while not carried out routinely, should be included in any case where hoarseness is present, or where it is suspected that there is a neurological lesion responsible for palato-pharyngeal abnormalities and further evidence is required in support.

The patient should sit upright, and open the mouth wide. A laryngeal mirror is passed rapidly through a flame to minimise misting, and is then carefully introduced into the back of the throat without touching the palate or pharynx. This requires a great deal of practice and it is best left, if possible, to an experienced examiner if the information required is of vital importance. If the patient gags, the instrument must be withdrawn at once. Any mirror which is easily detachable from its parent rod is not recommended for this examination.

If a good view is obtained, the movements of the cords are first watched during inspiration and expiration, and the patient is then asked to say a long 'Ah'. Normally the cords abduct during inspiration and come together during phonation.

Abnormalities of the vocal cords

As laryngoscopy may reveal a great deal more than vocal cord paralysis, full details should be obtained from a textbook of laryngology. In neurological disease the most common lesions are those producing *unilateral abductor paralysis* and *total unilateral paralysis*. In the former the affected cord remains in the midline at rest and on inspiration, but during phonation may move slightly towards the normal side. It is due to a lesion of the recurrent laryngeal nerve. In the latter, the cord lies in mid-abduction, but is pulled over to the normal side on phonation, and this is due to a severe lesion of the vagus. In both, phonation remains possible, though the sound may be hoarse.

In *bilateral total paralysis*, both cords are immobile in mid-abduction and no phonation is possible. This indicates a bilateral lesion of the vagus. In *bilateral abductor paralysis*, both cords lie together, are immobile on inspiration, with the result that respiratory obstruction is severe. This occurs in bilateral recurrent laryngeal nerve lesions or occasionally in nuclear lesions in the brain stem.

Common lesions of the glossopharyngeal and vagus nerves

Unilateral pure motor paralysis. Poliomyelitis; toxins, e.g. diphtheria, botulism.

Unilateral sensory loss. Very rare as an isolated finding.

Unilateral motor paralysis and sensory loss. Vascular accidents in the medulla; syringobulbia; posterior fossa tumours; vascular or bony anomalies; trauma, tumours or glandular enlargement at or below the jugular foramen.

Bilateral upper motor neurone paralysis. Bilateral cerebrovascular disease (pseudobulbar palsy); advanced Parkinsonism; amyotrophic lateral sclerosis.

Bilateral lower motor neurone paralysis. Poliomyelitis, toxins, progressive bulbar palsy.

Fatiguable motor paralysis. Myasthenia gravis.

Palatal nystagmus. A vascular lesion interrupting the central tegmental tract.

Common lesions of the recurrent laryngeal nerve

Unilateral. Mediastinal tumours, primary or secondary aortic aneurysms, enlarged cervical glands, malignant disease of the thyroid, trauma, including surgical operations on the neck.

Bilateral. Enlarged cervical glands, including the thyroid, trauma.

Chapter 13
The Eleventh Cranial Nerve: The Accessory Nerve

It is the spinal root of the XIth nerve that is examined here, the cranial root joining the vagus after leaving the brain stem and being considered part of that nerve.

Functions
To supply motor power to the upper part of the trapezii and to the sternomastoids, and so to influence the posture and movements of the head and shoulder girdles.

Purpose of the tests
To detect wasting and weakness, unilateral or bilateral, of these muscles; to decide if the lesion is nuclear, in the nerve trunk or its branches, or due to local muscular disease.

Methods of examination
When the patient is first seen severe trapezius weakness may be suspected if the head falls forwards, and sternomastoid weakness if it falls backwards.

Sternomastoids
Place one hand against the right side of the patient's face and ask him to turn (not bend) his head against it. The left sternomastoid will stand out clearly (Fig. 19a). Repeat this in the opposite direction and compare the two sides for bulk and strength. Then rest a hand on his forehead and ask him to bend his head forwards. Both sternomastoids will stand out together and are easily compared (Fig. 19b). Now ask the patient to sit up. Normally the head leaves the pillow first and the movement is easy.

Trapezius
Go behind the patient and compare the line and curve of the trapezii and the position of the scapulae, making certain that he is sitting symmetrically upright. Then ask him to raise his shoulders towards his ears. (Asking patients to 'shrug their shoulders' often produced a most unnatural convulsive movement.) Now try to depress the shoulders forcibly. Even the most feeble patient is normally able to resist the manœuvre.

Abnormalities

When the sternomastoids are wasted or absent the neck appears elongated, thin, scraggy and poultry-like, the thyroid cartilage and gland standing out abnormally.

In bilateral sternomastoid weakness, when the patient sits up, the head seems to be left behind on the pillow and then is raised with difficulty (Fig. 19c). The platysma may stand out even to the extent of drawing the mouth downwards, the resultant grimace making the whole movement look most unpleasant.

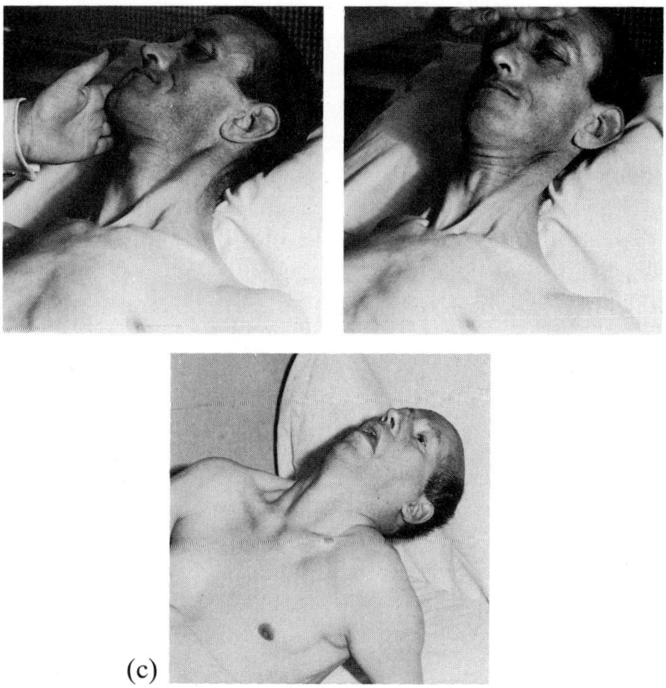
(a) (b) (c)

Fig. 19. The sternomastoids. (a) Turning the head against resistance brings the opposite sternomastoid into action. (b) Raising the head forwards against resistance brings both muscles into action. (c) Typical result of bilateral sternomastoid weakness. On sitting up the patient's head lags behind and overaction of platysma draws the mouth downwards.

In unilateral sternomastoid weakness the patient will fail to turn his head against resistance to the opposite side. The muscle will not stand out clearly either then or when the head is flexed forwards against resistance. Do not overdo this latter test, for it may put the anterior neck muscles into painful cramp.

Trapezius weakness results in the shoulder dropping on one side and the scapula being displaced downwards and laterally, giving a steeper gradient to the contour of the neck. Shrugging of that shoulder may be weaker, though not absent, for part of the trapezius is supplied by cervical nerves.

Fasciculation in these muscles means a nuclear lesion, as in motor neurone disease, but coarse twitching of the trapezius is seen in irritative and compressive lesions of the nerve trunk near its origin.

Upper motor neurone lesions of the accessory nerve rarely produce much demonstrable abnormality unless the paralysis is very profound, when the face and arm at least are likely to be grossly affected.

Difficulties and fallacies

These tests are very simple. The main problems arise from variations in muscular development. Muscles with very little bulk may, nevertheless, be very strong, and the symmetry of their size and their strength is of most importance.

Common lesions

Bilateral sternomastoid paralysis. Usually in muscular dystrophy, especially dystrophia myotonica; in nuclear lesions, such as motor neurone disease; poliomyelitis; or in polyneuritis.

Bilateral trapezius paralysis. Motor neurone disease; polyneuritis; poliomyelitis.

Unilateral lesions. Trauma in the neck or base of skull; virus diseases including poliomyelitis; tumours at jugular foramen level; bony anomalies at base of skull; syringomelia.

Chapter 14
The Twelfth Cranial Nerve: The Hypoglossal Nerve

The twelfth nerve contains only motor fibres and all tests applied to it are truly objective.

Functions
To control all movements of the tongue, and certain movements of the hyoid bone and larynx during and after deglutition.

Purposes of the tests
To inspect the surface of the tongue; to detect wasting, weakness and involuntary movement; to examine voluntary muscle control; to detect myotonia.

Method of examination

If the patient opens his mouth, the surface, size, shape and position of the tongue can be inspected before his attention is drawn to it. Then ask that it should be protruded in the midline. When the jovial comments which accompany this traditionally impolite gesture have been accepted with good humour and the movement achieved, repeat these observations and note any difficulty in performing the movement, any deviation from the midline and any involuntary movement.

If dystrophia myotonica is suspected tap the tongue sharply with a blunt point, such as the hooked end of a two-point discriminator.

Abnormalities

On inspection and protrusion
Many deviations from normal are irrelevant to neurological diagnosis. The tongue is enlarged in cretins and mongols. It will show corrosion after ingestion of caustic fluids. In vitamin deficiencies the papillae atrophy and the tongue appears shiny, smooth and translucent with shallow, irregular, reddened ulcers flanked by desquamating tissue. It looks small though there is no muscle loss. This is particularly important in pernicious anaemia, Vitamin B_{12} deficiency and multiple deficiencies of the B group of vitamins.

If there is unilateral muscle wasting, the longitudinal folds on that side

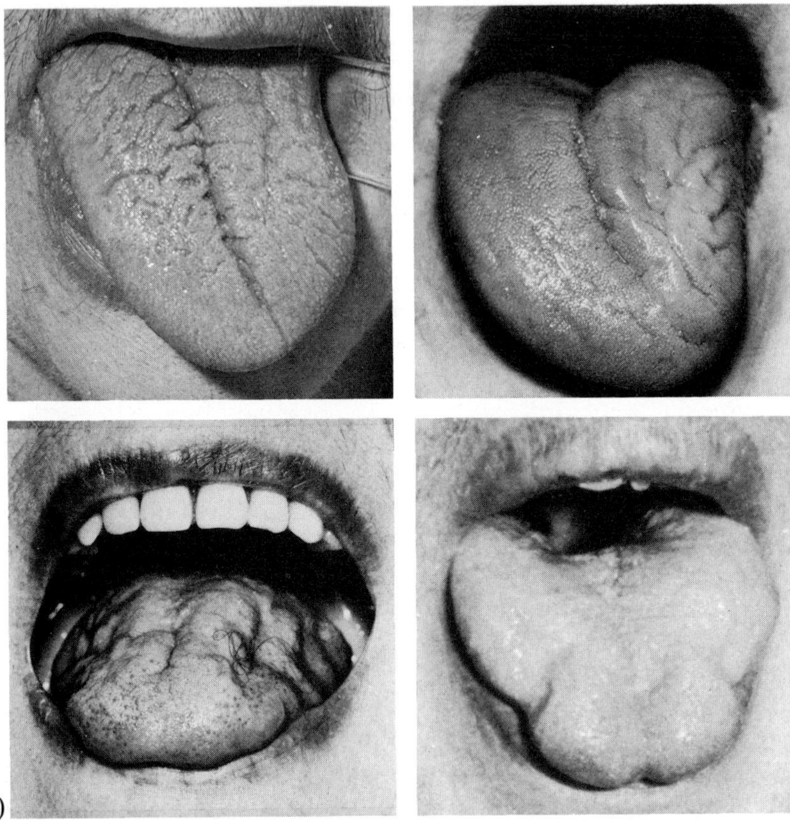

(a) (b) (c) (d)

Fig. 20. (a) Early, and (b) advanced, lower motor neurone paralysis of tongue. Note reduction in size of affected side, excessive ridging and wrinkling, and curve of tip and median raphé towards the side of the lesion. (c) Bilateral wasting and spasticity in motor neurone disease. Note restricted protrusion, surface indentations and reduction in size without deviation. (d) Myotonia. Note characteristic prolonged dimpling after percussion of tongue.

are greatly exaggerated and the tip and median raphé curve round towards the affected side on protrusion, owing to the unopposed pushing action of the normal genioglossus (Figs. 20a, 20b). There may be fasciculation, but speech is little affected. This is the result of an ipsilateral lower motor neurone lesion.

When such wasting is bilateral the tip and median raphé remain central, the tongue is greatly reduced in size, there may be difficulty in protrusion and speech is grossly disturbed. Fasciculation is marked if the lesion is nuclear (Fig. 20c) as in motor neurone disease.

If a normal-looking, symmetrical tongue moves constantly to one side, this can be due to a contralateral upper motor neurone lesion, but would then usually be part of a profound hemiplegia. As an isolated feature it is more commonly due to faulty performance of the test and can be corrected.

A small, tight, compact-looking tongue, lying in the floor of the mouth like a nut in an open shell, its surface little altered, but almost incapable of protrusion and with gross disturbance of speech, is the result of bilateral upper neurone lesions. The jaw jerk will be exaggerated.

The features of nuclear and upper motor neurone lesions co-exist in varying proportions in motor neurone disease. The tongue may become immobile.

A coarse, trombone-like tremor on protrusion may be seen in neurosyphilis and some cases of Parkinsonism. An up and down flapping movement with alternate protrusion and retraction is common in chorea. Dystonic movements of the tongue follow high and prolonged dosage of chlorpromazine derivatives. Other involuntary movements are described in Chap. 19.

On percussion

Normally the dent formed will disappear immediately. In myotonia it persists and may enlarge for a few seconds in a linear manner. Tapping the tongue on one side will produce a dent on both sides (see Fig. 20d).

Difficulties and fallacies

Apraxia of the tongue may prevent it from being protruded, but it will probably move normally during automatic speech, licking of lips, etc., and there is likely to be other evidence of apraxia. The patient may have failed to understand the directions due to receptive dysphasia. A very short frenulum holds back the tip, which curves downwards so that the centre of the tongue appears to be somersaulting forwards on protrusion.

If there is a facial paralysis the tongue may appear to deviate to one side owing to the asymmetry of the mouth. This is overcome by drawing back the corner of the mouth into its normal position and comparing the position of the median raphé with the central incisors.

Many tongues have corrugated edges and deep clefts. These are not necessarily significant. Little muscular movements frequently occur on the surface, which must not be confused with fasciculation, for they are inconstant and not associated with wasting. Most people, of both sexes, are unable to keep their tongues still for long, so that great care should be taken before deciding that involuntary movements are present.

Common lesions

Unilateral lower motor neurone lesions. Syringomelia, poliomyelitis, tumours at or near the jugular foramen, angiomas of the stem, trauma, tumours or glandular enlargement high in the neck, and early motor neurone disease. Possibly also long after unsuspected virus infections in infancy.

Bilateral lower motor neurone lesions. Progressive bulbar palsy, syringomyelia, occasionally foramen magnum anomalies.

Unilateral upper motor neurone lesions. Profound hemiplegia due to vascular accidents or deep-seated neoplasms.

Bilateral upper motor neurone lesions. Bilateral vascular accidents producing a pseudobulbar palsy, amyotrophic lateral sclerosis.

Part III
The Motor System

Chapter 15
Development and Wasting

Normal movement depends upon the correct functioning of normal muscles, their motor neurones and the bones and joints that they have to move, any of which may develop primary disease processes. To help in distinguishing the neurological lesions, careful preliminary inspection is essential.

Preliminary general inspection

The aim is to compare the size and shape of the limbs and to detect deformities.

Examine the patient lying, sitting and later standing, placing the limbs in symmetrical positions. Any apparent differences in size must be checked by careful measurement. If definite asymmetry is confirmed, try and decide if this is due to:

(*a*) *Congenital maldevelopment*. This will include absence of muscles or parts of a limb, webbing of fingers and toes, polydactyly, etc. The possibilities are too numerous to mention in detail.

(*b*) *Long-standing neurological lesions*. Lesions of the lower motor neurone in infancy, such as obstetric paralysis or poliomyelitis, cause marked retardation in limb growth with wasting and absence of reflexes. Following infantile cerebral lesions, such as birth trauma, acute infantile hemiplegias, and sometimes with vascular anomalies, there is again retardation in growth, but of lesser degree, with little wasting, a hemiplegic posture, and exaggerated reflexes. 'Old polio' used to be much too casually diagnosed in such patients.

(*c*) *Acquired lesions of local structures*. This includes deformities of bones, joints and muscles, surgical operations, wounds, osteoarthritis or rheumatoid arthritis and Dupuytren's contracture.

Examination of joint movement

Each joint should be put gently through its full range of movement. In *Charcot's joints*, once mainly seen in tabes dorsalis, but now more commonly in other forms of sensory neuropathy, especially syringomyelia, there is swelling, abnormal motility, often alarming crepitus, associated effusion, but usually practically no pain on movement. In the '*frozen shoulder*' the arm cannot be abducted or rotated, the joint is tender and all movement is very painful.

Local inspection of muscle

Next inspect the muscles of the shoulder girdles, upper arms, forearms, hands, hip girdles, thighs and calves, the aim being to detect wasting, hypertrophy and fasciculation.

Measure the circumference of the limbs at clearly stated places, e.g. 10 cm (4 inches) above or below the olecranon; 18 cm (7 inches) above the patella; 10 cm (4 inches) below the tibial tuberosity.

If wasting is observed, inspect the groups affected individually to decide which of the component muscles is involved. Compare the muscles with their fellows on the other side, with experience of the normal for that build of individual, and observe if related structures are uncovered, e.g. the prominence of the tibia when the anterior tibial muscle is wasted, or of the spine of the scapula with wasting of the supra- and infra-spinati. In the hands note if rheumatoid arthritis is obvious, for small muscle wasting is often associated.

Hypertrophy may be physiological, when the muscles are merely big and powerful, their texture being normal. In the pathological pseudohypertrophy of muscular dystrophy, which most frequently involves the calves, buttock and thighs and the shoulder girdles, the muscle is abnormally globular, has a tense rubbery feeling due to excessive deposition of fat, and is weaker rather than stronger than normal.

Dropping of the shoulders due to trapezius wasting may give a false impression of enlargement of the shoulder girdle muscles.

Look at the palms of the hands—Dupuytren's contracture is not too uncommon in prolonged anticonvulsant medication.

Fasciculation is discussed in Chap. 19.

TYPES OF MUSCLE WASTING

Generalised wasting

Though commonly the result of systemic diseases such as malignancy, or thyrotoxicosis, wasting is also seen in the very advanced stages of many crippling neurological diseases, but particularly myopathies and motor neurone disease. In the latter, fasciculation and exaggeration of reflexes may persist to a late stage, when both will disappear. By this time, however, the tongue will almost always be markedly affected and the jaw jerk exaggerated, features not seen in the myopathies. The slow progress of the myopathies allows deposition of fat, so that superficially the limbs may not appear wasted. Sometimes loss of subcutaneous tissue is mistaken for muscle wasting.

Proximal muscle wasting

Wasting diseases cannot be clearly divided into those affecting proximal and those affecting distal muscles, but *in the early stages* it is common to find one or other predominating in certain conditions.

MUSCULAR DYSTROPHIES

It must be realised that the end-stage of all muscular dystrophies can be similar. It is the early signs that differentiate the types and so are invaluable in prognosis.

(*a*) *Facio-scapulo-humeral dystrophy*. The face and shoulder girdle are involved, the lesions are asymmetrical, hypertrophy is rare and the remainder of the body is not involved until late. A scapulo-peroneal dystrophy occurs in which these muscles are affected almost in isolation in the early stages of the disease.

(*b*) *Proximal limb girdle dystrophy*. Both shoulder and hip girdles may be involved, there may be asymmetry, but the face is spared. Several different conditions can be grouped under this heading, including the relatively benign Kugelberg–Welander syndrome, late onset Werdnig–Hoffman disease, and a proximal myopathy that accompanies cryptogenic carcinoma especially when seen in men over the age of 50. Polymyositis and a number of metabolic myopathies also present in this way. The diagnosis was originally a very valuable differentiation from other myopathies. It is now seen to be a mixture of several disorders. Providing this is realised, and the term is used as a description of what one is seeing, rather than a diagnosis, then it is worth retaining.

(*c*) *Pseudo-hypertrophic muscular dystrophy* (*Duchenne*). The distribution is also patchy, affecting arms and legs and including the calves. Some muscles retain the rounded, rubbery hypertrophy to a late stage. Almost confined to boys, few living to full adult life. Its rare appearance in girls runs a somewhat longer course, and a similar but benign dystrophy in adults (the Becker variety) is now known to exist.

(*d*) *Dystrophia myotonica* (myotonic dystrophy). The face, sternomastoids and quadriceps femoris are the main proximal muscles involved. The myotonia is present mainly in the peripheral muscles and tongue.

(*e*) *Thyrotoxic myopathy*. The muscles show fasciculation, may be painful, reflexes may be brisk instead of absent and thyrotoxicosis is present.

MOTOR NEURONE DISEASE

Wasting and fasciculation may often be marked in the shoulder girdles when distal muscles appear normal. Never be content with examination of hands or forearms only. Tendon reflexes are usually, but not always, exaggerated.

SYRINGOMYELIA

Often starting in the shoulder girdles, there is dissociated sensory loss to pain and temperature with relative preservation of touch, affecting several spinal segments, and often including the occipital region. The reflexes in the upper limbs are absent.

INFLAMMATORY LESIONS

(*a*) *Neuralgic amyotrophy*. Usually, but not invariably, unilateral, this starts as a painful condition about 10 days after an illness, injury or inoculation, and is followed by marked wasting of the shoulder girdle muscles and impairment of sensation limited to the area supplied by the circumflex nerve (Fig. 21). Wasting may not appear for 2–3 weeks and may progress for months, but recovers over years. Wasting may extend beyond the shoulder girdle. Relapses are not uncommon.

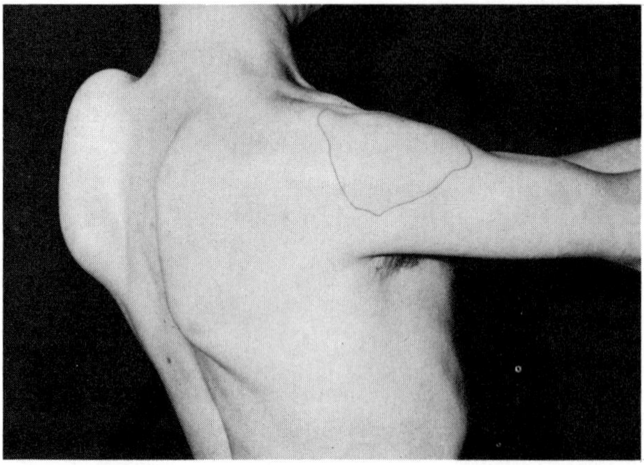

Fig. 21. Neuralgic amyotrophy. Note prominence of bony parts due to wasting of supraspinatus and deltoid, winging of scapula and area of sensory loss (rather higher than usual).

(*b*) *Old poliomyelitis*. Muscles having the same segmental supply are involved, there is no sensory loss, and the history of the onset is typical.

(*c*) *Myositis*. The muscles may be tender, correspond to no one segment or nerve distribution, there is no sensory loss. The skin over the muscles may appear bound to deeper tissues. The sedimentation rate may be high, and the serum muscle enzymes may be raised. The words 'may be' are repeated advisedly in this paragraph, because this is a very difficult diagnosis to make without muscle biopsy.

COMPRESSIVE LESIONS

Spondylotic or neoplastic compression of the lower cervical roots, usually the 5th or 6th, is accompanied by segmental pain and sensory impairment over the outer aspect of the arm.

Cauda equina lesions, due to neoplasms, massive disc prolapse, or arachnoiditis cause wasting of the buttocks, loss of sensation in the saddle area and loss of sphincter control. These signs may also be found in long-standing ankylosing spondylitis but there will be no signs myelographically of cauda equina compression.

Peripheral muscle wasting

Nearly all the conditions mentioned already, if severe enough, will affect the periphery of the limbs as well. In the early stages, however, certain diseases may be confined to the distal muscles. One must again stress the difference between diagnostic early features, and common end-results.

THE FOREARM AND SMALL MUSCLES OF THE HAND

Wasting results from a lower motor neurone lesion affecting principally the segmental distribution of C7–T1. This may occur at many levels, (*a*) the anterior horn cell (*poliomyelitis, motor neurone disease, syringomelia, cervical cord tumours*), (*b*) the anterior root (*cervical spondylosis, cervical tumours*), (*c*) the brachial plexus (*injuries, cervical ribs, cervical glandular enlargement, superior pulmonary sulcus tumour*), (*d*) traumatic lesions of the *radial, median* and *ulnar nerves*.

In addition the *median* nerve is often compressed in the carpal tunnel. This causes wasting of the thenar eminence and slight sensory loss. If the *ulnar nerve* is damaged at, or just below, the elbow, there is wasting of most of the small muscles except opponens pollicis and abductor pollicis brevis, and marked sensory change (Fig. 22). Injury at the wrist, or compression by a ganglion, may spare the hypothenar eminence and sensation, though pressure at the point of the lesion can produce paraesthesia over the ulnar distribution.

Muscular lesions include dystrophia myotonica, those due to advancing age, and rheumatoid arthritis. Very occasionally wasting occurs in contralateral parietal lobe lesions without necessarily marked paralysis.

THE LOWER LEG

Isolated peripheral wasting is much less common than in the arm. It occurs as part of an extensive cauda equina lesion, as part of a polyneuritis and in peroneal muscular atrophy. It will follow poliomyelitis and peripheral nerve trauma, especially to the exposed lateral popliteal nerve, e.g. by an inadequately padded plaster, or by skin traction techniques. The anterior muscles of the lower leg waste following the acute 'syndrome of the anterior tibial compartment' when usually after unaccustomed exercise, pain and swelling occur, causing muscle necrosis—the exact aetiology being uncertain.

(a) (b)

(c) (d)

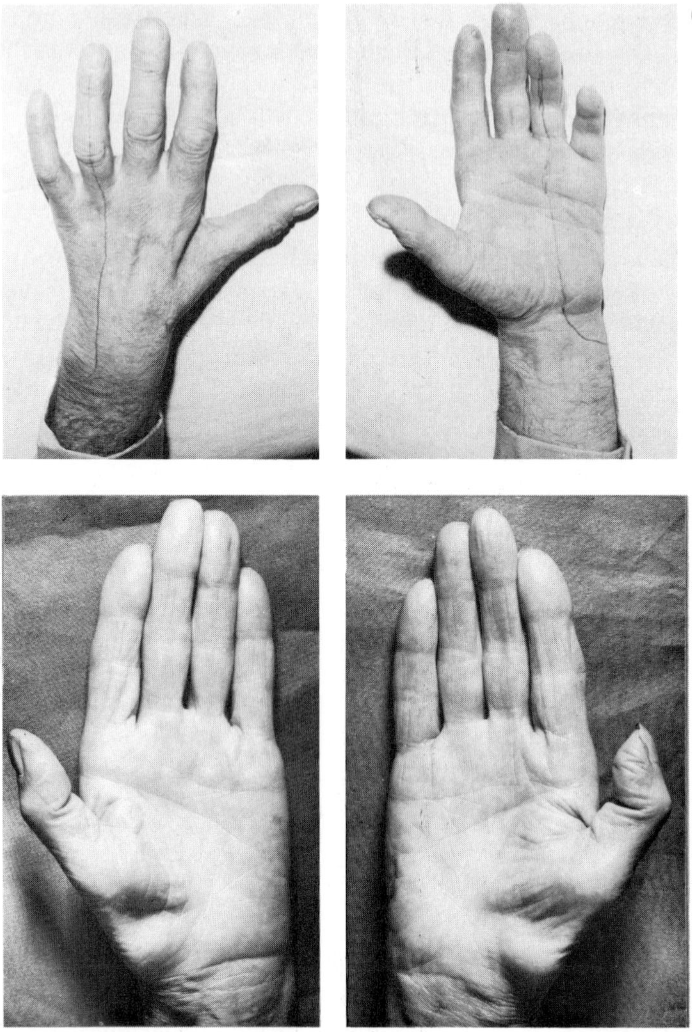

Fig. 22. Wasting of small muscles of hand and sensory loss due to ulnar nerve lesion at the elbow. Note (a) marked wasting of interossei, and (b) preservation of opponens pollicis (median nerve); (c) and (d) Bilateral carpal tunnel syndrome showing typical severe wasting of both thenar eminences.

Peripheral wasting in both upper and lower limbs

Peripheral wasting in all four extremities is rare except in two conditions:
(*a*) *Peroneal muscular atrophy. (Charcot–Marie–Tooth disease)*. Here there is a transverse demarcation between normal and wasted muscle, often at mid-thigh level, giving the limbs the characteristic inverted bottle appear-

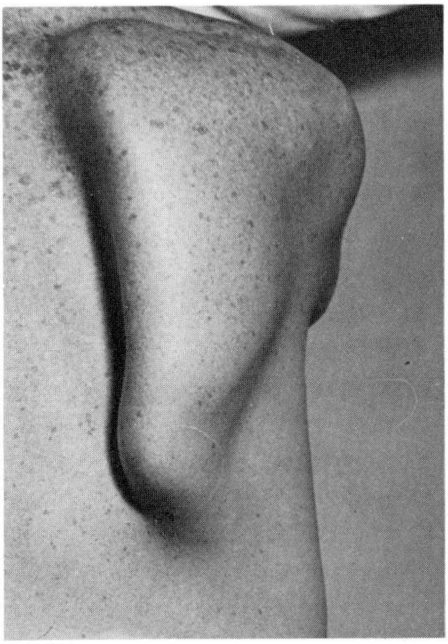

Fig. 23. Winging of the scapula due to isolated paralysis of right serratus magnus (compare with Fig. 28).

ance, with similar but less striking appearances in the upper limbs. In addition, there are pes cavus, absent reflexes, trophic and vasomotor changes, and often peripheral sensory disturbances such as impaired pain and vibration sense. Despite all these features, disability is remarkably slight.

(*b*) *Chronic polyneuritis*. This can be very similar in appearance, but the history is shorter; the transverse demarcation is not marked; pes cavus is absent; sensory loss is greater; there is no family history, and the degree of disability is usually considerably greater.

To these must be added Werdnig-Hoffman's disease in childhood, the later stages of the Kugelberg-Welander syndrome, and the rare distal myopathy of Gowers.

Individual muscle group and muscle wasting

(*a*) *A compressive or traumatic lesion of the nerve root.* Wasting is often slight, sensory changes are almost invariable, but correspond to a lesser area than the segmental supply of the root, due to overlap from neighbouring segments.

(*b*) *A traumatic or vascular lesion of the peripheral nerve*. Both wasting and sensory disturbances in the distribution of the nerve are marked, but overlap again occurs.

(*c*) *Peripheral nerve lesions in metabolic* (e.g. diabetic) or *toxic* (e.g. lead) neuropathy. As in (*b*).

(*d*) *Presumed infective lesions*. This is assumed to cause the isolated paralysis of the long thoracic nerve with wasting of the serratus magnus (Fig. 23).

(*e*) *The syndrome of the anterior tibial compartment* (see above).

(*f*) *Local trauma to muscle*.

Chapter 16
Muscle Tone

Tone, most simply defined as the degree of tension present in a muscle at rest, is not easy to assess because of the variations which take place from one examination to another. The patient must be warm, comfortable, and have confidence in the examiner, and this is where kindness and precision prove to be so important in producing relaxation. Using the local phrase for the relaxed state will be much more successful than peremptorily ordering the patient to 'relax' for this usually induces a state of boardlike rigidity.

Testing tone in the upper limb

First pick up the patient's hand and forearm as if to take the pulse, holding his fingers in the right hand. The fingers should now be submitted to an undulating flexion-extension movement passing proximally from the terminal phalanges to and including the wrist. Such movements can be carried out before the patient realises that it is not simply an examination of the pulse, a gesture so much to be expected that there is no danger of muscular tension. Similar movements are then applied to the proximal muscles. Finally, hold the patient's chest and shake his shoulders gently. All movements must be gentle. Vigorous and violent movements are quite useless.

Now raise each arm in turn and let it fall back on to the bed, comparing on the two sides the checking movement which usually breaks the fall. This is of value in stuporose and unco-operative patients as well.

Testing tone in the lower limbs

First gently roll the limbs with the palms of the hands on the shins. This not only gives one an initial assessment of tone in the hip girdle muscles, but in some curious way it also encourages relaxation, and the examination can then proceed to passive flexion and extension of the hip, knee and ankle.

Then flex the hip, raise the lower leg until it forms more than a right angle at the knee, and allow it to fall, noting once again normal checking movements.

Finally, with the flat of the fingers, flap the calf muscles on each side.

Loss of tone

The muscles are lax; they assume a pendulous shape when allowed to hang freely, offer diminished resistance to passive movement and so widen the range of movement at a joint; they have difficulty in maintaining the position of a limb, allow it to be displaced easily and do not check its sudden release. The tendon reflexes (q.v.) are decreased or absent.

In complete relaxation tone is at its minimum, a state attained so easily by children that their limbs often appear hypotonic. Muscles out of use for long periods also become atonic. In neurological lesions, however, hypotonicity is produced by (*a*) a breach in the reflex arc; (*b*) cerebellar disease; and (*c*) cerebral or spinal 'shock', i.e. very soon after a vascular accident or trauma.

Common causes of hypotonia

Lesions of the motor side of the reflex arc. Poliomyelitis, polyneuritis, peripheral nerve injuries.

Lesions of the sensory side of the reflex arc. Tabes dorsalis, carcinomatous neuropathies, herpes zoster.

Combined motor and sensory lesions. Syringomyelia, cord or root compression, gross cord destruction.

Lesions of the muscle itself. Myopathies, benign infantile hypotonia, myasthenia gravis. In pseudohypertrophic muscular dystrophy, though the limb is hypotonic, the muscles themselves have a rubbery texture. In periodic paralysis, during an attack, the muscles, though paralysed and areflexic, feel tense, swollen and entirely different from the flabby flaccid feeling in other hypotonic states.

States of neurological 'shock'. The earliest stages of a severe cord lesion, or a profound hemiplegia. This is temporary unless destruction is extreme.

Cerebellar lesions. Ipsilateral hypotonia is common, but rarely very marked, and the reflexes are prolonged and pendular rather than lost.

Chorea. In Sydenham's chorea, the involuntary movements are associated with marked hyperextensibility of the joints, especially the wrists and fingers, but reflexes are often retained.

Increase of tone

There are three main types of hypertonicity:

(*a*) Tone and resistance is greater in one group of muscles (e.g. the quadriceps) than in the antagonists (e.g. the hamstrings). The resistance is usually most noticeable when the movement is first made and then is suddenly overcome, producing the so-called '*clasp knife*' spasticity, most easily demonstrated at the elbow and knee. Affected muscles are compact at rest, feel firm, do not flap on palpation and tend to form contractures.

This is a sign of an upper motor neurone lesion and is usually more marked in the flexor muscles in the upper limb and the extensor muscles in the lower limb.

(*b*) In the second type, there is equal resistance in both agonists and antagonists at any point, with the result that the same degree of hypertonicity is felt throughout each movement—the so-called *plastic* or *'lead-pipe' rigidity*. When this becomes very marked a state of true rigidity is reached in which the muscles, though not greatly altered in appearance, hold the limb in complete immobility.

Though this may be seen in extreme spasticity from upper motor neurone lesions, it is a characteristic feature of a lesion of the extra-pyramidal system.

(*c*) In the third type, the agonists and antagonists contract alternately, rapidly, and regularly during the movement, producing the so-called *'cog-wheel' rigidity*. This may be present only during the first moments of testing, and perhaps only at the wrist, *so that the examiner must be on the alert for it from the very outset*. It is a valuable sign of extra-pyramidal disease, and may be felt in the absence of any visible tremor, though it is much increased when tremor is present.

Clonus

Sudden stretching of hypertonic muscles produces reflex contraction. If the stretch is maintained during the subsequent relaxation, further reflex contraction occurs and this may continue almost indefinitely, unless the stretch stimulus is released. It is most easily demonstrated by dorsiflexing the foot or by sharply moving the patella downwards, but it may be present at any joint. There is nothing diagnostic about clonus. It merely represents an increase in reflex excitability and may be present in a very tense patient, one who has been straining his muscles (e.g. after defaecation), or one who has had a fright (e.g. the ankle clonus that most car drivers have experienced in their right foot after an alarming experience). Under these circumstances it rarely becomes well sustained, but as a physical sign it is only of great significance together with other signs of an upper motor neurone lesion. However, even in their absence the presence of clonus on one side only may give a hint of a pyramidal system lesion on that side.

Lesions producing increased tone

Here the results of experimentation differ from the traditions of clinical experience, but providing one is aware of the limitations of one's knowledge, for practical purposes it is wise to retain the view that a lesion of the pyramidal system produces spasticity, increased tendon reflexes, absent abdominal reflexes and extensor plantars, for long experience has proven its value in locational diagnosis.

Increase in tone is produced by any destructive lesion of the upper motor neurone. This includes cerebral thromboses, haemorrhages, tumours, degenerative diseases, inflammatory lesions and injuries; spinal cord tumours, compressions, injuries and degenerative diseases. Note however that immediately after a gross lesion of the cortico-spinal tracts tone may be lost, only to become increased after several days.

The plastic type of rigidity occurs in Parkinsonism, particularly the post-encephalitic type; in some rare instances of basal nuclear neoplasms; and in catatonia.

Cog-wheel rigidity occurs in the varieties of Parkinsonism, including arteriosclerotic degeneration of the extrapyramidal system, but it does also occur after high dosage of reserpine or chlorpromazine and its derivatives and after carbon monoxide poisoning.

Difficulties

A few moments spent in a gentle, friendly, even light-hearted manner, in establishing rapport, will save many struggling with that failure of relaxation which defeats the estimation of tone. Re-examination, when the patient knows it will not be unpleasant, may completely alter one's impression.

It is very difficult to assess minor degrees of hypotonicity. Other features, such as diminution of reflexes, have to be found before pathological conclusions can be drawn from limbs which are merely limp.

Joint changes or muscle contractures may give false impressions of increased tone which emphasises the importance of feeling the muscles themselves and examining the joints for evidence of local disease.

Another *impression* of increased tone arises when there is gross loss of postural sensibility. While the examiner is trying passively to move the limb the patient appears to be fighting against him. This is an important sign, rarely described (see p. 148).

Myotonia

This is a state in which muscle contraction continues beyond the period of time required for a particular movement to be made. It is best seen in the face and hand muscles. Ask the patient to screw up his eyes, or show his teeth, and then to 'let go'. There is delay in relaxation so that the patient appears to have not understood the instruction.

Ask him to grip the fingers, and then suddenly release his hold. This will result in flexion of the wrist, adduction and opposition of the thumb and incomplete extension of the fingers. He has to drag his hand away. Repeating the movement several times may overcome the myotonia, so look carefully the first time.

Percussing the tongue has already been mentioned (p. 95), but percussion of the thenar eminence results in slow adduction of the thumb and dimpling of the muscle, while percussion of other muscles may produce dimpling at first, followed by a raised lump to the side of the dimple. Merely a lump on hard percussion may occur as a result of myoedema in normal individuals.

MYOTONIC STATES

The two most common conditions are:
(*a*) *Dystrophic myotonica (myotonic dystrophy)* in which there is wasting of the sternomastoids and quadriceps, dystrophic features in other muscles (which may outweigh the myotonia), baldness, cataracts, testicular atrophy and steady progression.
(*b*) *Myotonia congenita.* The myotonia is present from early years, it less frequently affects the face, there are no dystrophic features and there is a much more benign course. Characteristically, as the patient moves away from a stationary position, the myotonia freezes him in his tracks for a moment after which he is able to move briskly and normally.

In *paramyotonia congenita* exposure to cold causes marked myotonia in the exposed muscles. There may also be intermittent muscle paralysis, and there may be a closer relationship to periodic paralysis than to the other myotonic disorders.

An injection of ACTH will usually cause true myotonia to diminish for a few hours and can be used to support the diagnosis. Procaine amide has a similar effect but acts for longer periods.

Chapter 17
Muscle Power

Because muscles work in combination with other muscles, and testing of movements may mean testing several muscles, it is easy to be vague, both in testing, and describing the results of testing, a patient's strength. This remark applies to neurologists as well as to other physicians. To avoid this the examiner must discipline himself to ask the following questions at each stage:

(*a*) What muscle, or muscle group, am I about to test?
(*b*) Is the limb in the right position for that muscle *alone* to be tested?
(*c*) What is the segmental nerve supply of that muscle?
(*d*) Which peripheral nerve supplies it?

Once positioning is correct the patient must be told clearly the movement he is to make, possibly illustrating it for him first. The test of power can then be carried out in two ways:

(*a*) The patient first completes the movement and then tries to maintain the muscle in full contraction while the examiner tries to overcome it.

(*b*) The examiner resists the movement throughout the whole of the patient's attempt to carry it out. This is more difficult for the patient and may detect earlier degrees of weakness. It is also a method some patients fail to understand and a false impression of weakness, or lack of co-operation, may be gained.

Steady exertion is required by both patient and examiner. Sudden movements serve only to confuse. Application of great force is unnecessary, and indeed, in hypertonic muscles undesirable, for very painful cramps may easily be produced.

While these tests are being carried out, further questions must be asked:

(*a*) Is this muscle as strong as might be expected, bearing in mind the build and age of both patient and examiner?

(*b*) Is it as strong as the same muscle on the other side?

(*c*) What is the degree of weakness, if any? (See below.)

(*d*) Is the weakness constant or variable? Does it improve on rest or on encouragement?

(*e*) Is there any painful condition (e.g. injury), or mechanical defect (e.g. ankylosis of a joint, or contracture of an antagonist) which hinders the movement.

(*f*) Are the actions the patient is known to be able to carry out compatible with any apparent weakness demonstrated? (e.g. has the patient, whose hands on formal examination are apparently almost paralysed, just undressed himself? How often one sees this in medico-legal cases!)

QUANTITATIVE ASSESSMENT OF WEAKNESS

The assessment of power may differ strikingly in the record of one examiner from that of another. For this reason many classifications of degrees of weakness have been suggested. None has been ideal, but the use of the scheme supported by the Medical Research Council at least ensures some degree of uniformity. Power is recorded by numbers ranging from the normal of 5 to complete paralysis represented by 0. It is worth remembering that even a very poorly developed individual is usually able to resist an examiner's attempt to overcome the power of a fully contracted muscle.

5 = Normal power.
4 = The muscle, though able to make its full normal movement, is overcome by resistance.
3 = The muscle is able to make its normal movement against gravity, but not against additional resistance.
2 = The muscle can only make its normal movement when the limb is so positioned that gravity is eliminated.
1 = There is a visible or palpable flicker of contraction, but no resultant movement of limb or joint.
0 = Total paralysis.

Routine tests of muscle groups

It is customary to direct attention first to major *groups* of muscles. These are the flexors and extensors of the neck; the adductors, abductors, and rotators of the shoulder; the flexors and extensors of the elbow, wrist and fingers; the grip; the abdominal muscles; the extensors of the spine; the flexors and extensors of hip and knee; the dorsiflexors and plantar flexors of the feet; and the flexors and extensors of the toes, especially the great toe.

Any weakness discovered is then more carefully analysed by carrying out the appropriate tests for *individual* muscles concerned in making the defective movement. It is here that the positioning of the limb is of such great importance.

Testing individual muscles

Full details of the actions of individual muscles are given in the text books of anatomy and the reader is particularly recommended to the late R. D. Lockhart's *Living Anatomy*. The following pages deal with those muscles that are commonly of help in neurological diagnosis. The illustrations are intended to show the movement required to bring a muscle into action rather than to demonstrate a particularly prominent muscle belly. Normal individuals, without outstanding muscular development, have been photographed.

The movements recommended should be carefully followed, for many patients learn tricks to overcome disability, which may cause confusion if the purest action of a muscle is not tested. Segmental supply is subject to individual variation, and indeed is not necessarily universally agreed; simplification has therefore been attempted by giving the segmental supply most frequently found to be relevant in clinical practice.

MUSCLES OF THE HEAD AND NECK

The *facial muscles, jaw muscles, sternomastoids and trapezii* are dealt with under the appropriate cranial nerve.

MUSCLES OF THE SHOULDER GIRDLE AND SCAPULA

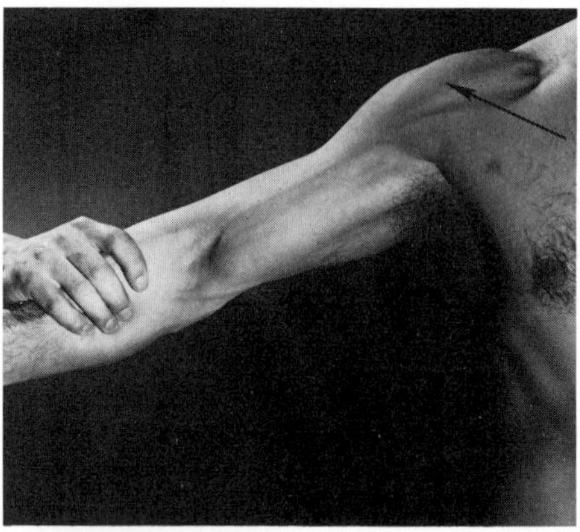

Fig. 24.
Muscle **Deltoid**
Main segmental nerve supply **C5**
Peripheral nerve **Circumflex**
Test The patient holds his arm abducted to 60° against the examiner's resistance.

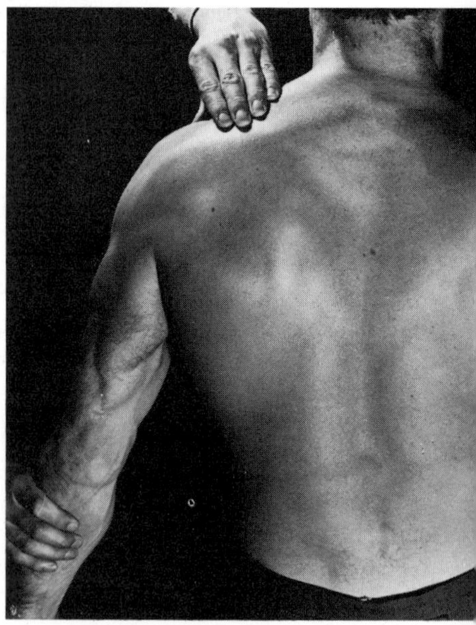

Fig. 25.
Muscle **Supraspinatus**
Main segmental supply **C5**
Peripheral nerve **Suprascapular**
Test The patient tries to initiate abduction of the arm from the side against resistance.

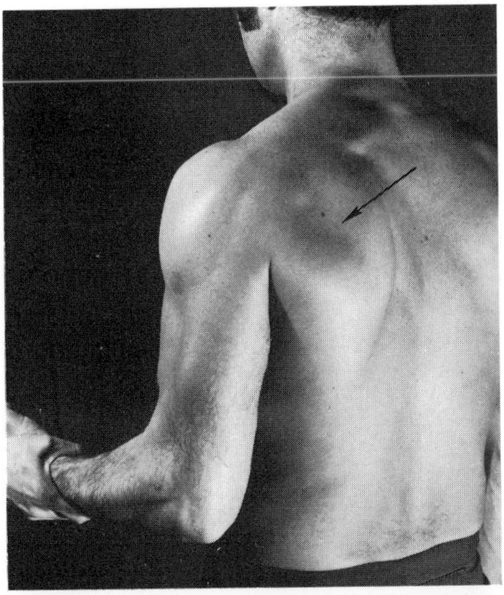

Fig. 26.
Muscle **Infraspinatus**
Main segmental supply **C5**
Peripheral nerve **Suprascapular**
Test The patient flexes his elbow, holds the elbow to his side, and then attempts to turn the forearm backwards against resistance.

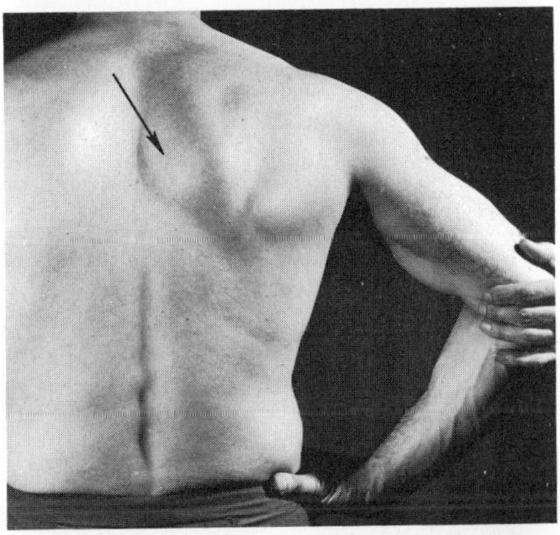

Fig. 27.
Muscle **Rhomboids**
Main segmental supply **C5**
Peripheral nerve **Nerve to rhomboids**
Test Hand on hip, the patient tries to force his elbow backwards.

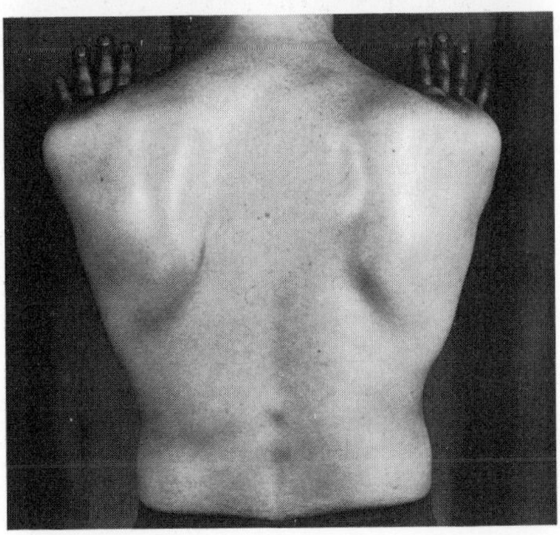

Fig. 28.
Muscle **Serratus Anterior**
Main segmental supply **C5, 6, 7**
Peripheral nerve **Nerve to serratus anterior**
Test The patient pushes his arms forwards against firm obstruction (compare this with Fig. 23).

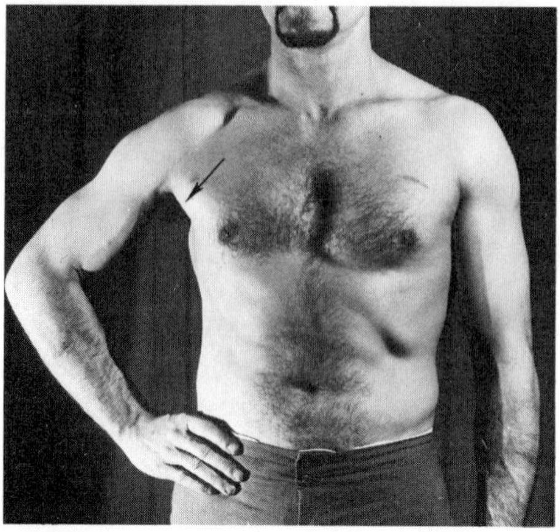

Fig. 29.
Muscle **Pectoralis major**
Main segmental supply **C6, 7, 8**
Peripheral nerve **Lateral and medial pectoral nerves**
Test Placing the hand on the hip and pressing inwards the sternocostal part of the muscle can be seen and felt to contract. Raising the arm forwards above 90° and attempting to adduct it against resistance brings the clavicular portion into action.

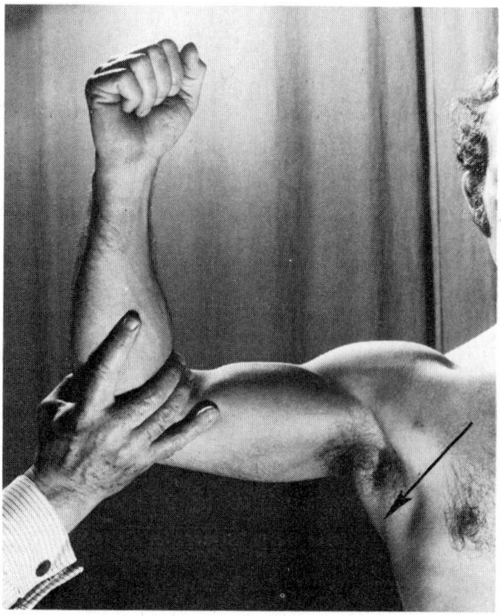

Fig. 30.
Muscle **Latissimus dorsi**
Main segmental supply **C7**
Peripheral nerve **Nerve to latissimus dorsi**
Tests (a) While palpating the muscles, ask the patient to cough.
(b) Resist the patient's attempt to adduct the arm when abducted to above 90°.

MUSCLES OF THE ELBOW JOINT

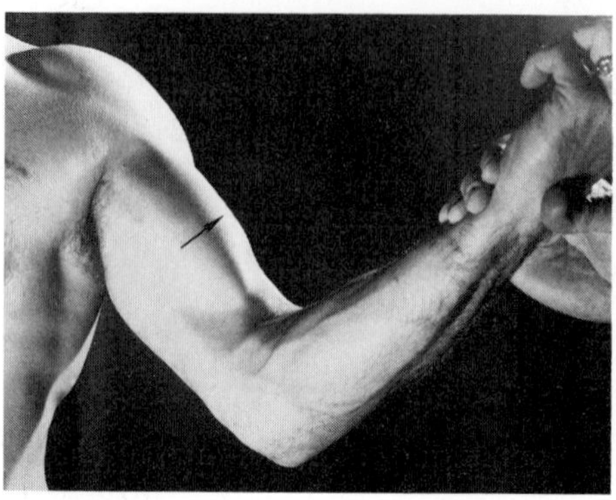

Fig. 31.
Muscle **Biceps**
Main segmental supply **C5**
Peripheral nerve **Musculocutaneous**
Test The patient flexes his elbow against resistance, the forearm being supinated.

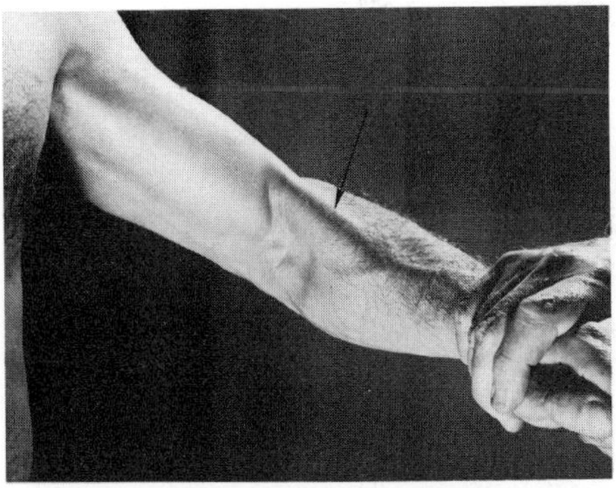

Fig. 32.
Muscle **Brachio-radialis**
Main segmental supply **C5, 6**
Peripheral nerve **Radial**
Test The patient pronates the forearm and draws the thumb towards the nose against resistance.

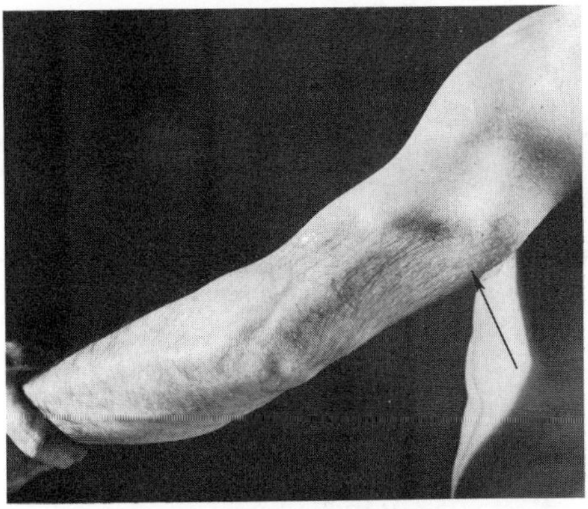

Fig. 33.
Muscle **Triceps**
Main segmental supply **C7**
Peripheral nerve **Radial**
Test The patient attempts to extend the elbow against resistance.

MUSCLES OF THE FOREARM AND WRIST JOINT

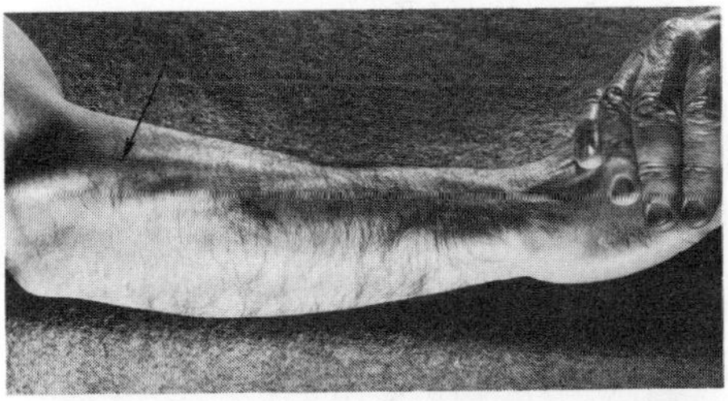

Fig. 34.
Muscle **Extensor carpi radialis longus**
Main segmental supply **C6, 7**
Peripheral nerve **Radial**
Test The patient holds the fingers partially extended and dorsiflexes the wrist towards the radial side against resistance.

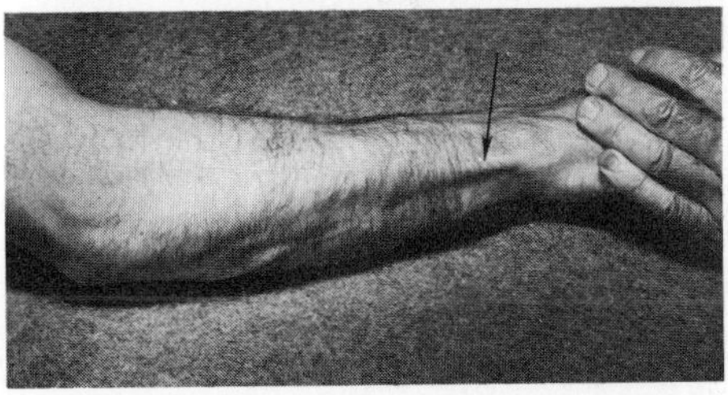

Fig. 35.
Muscle **Extensor carpi ulnaris**
Main segmental supply **C7**
Peripheral nerve **Radial**
Test As Fig. 34, but dorsiflexion must be towards the ulnar side.

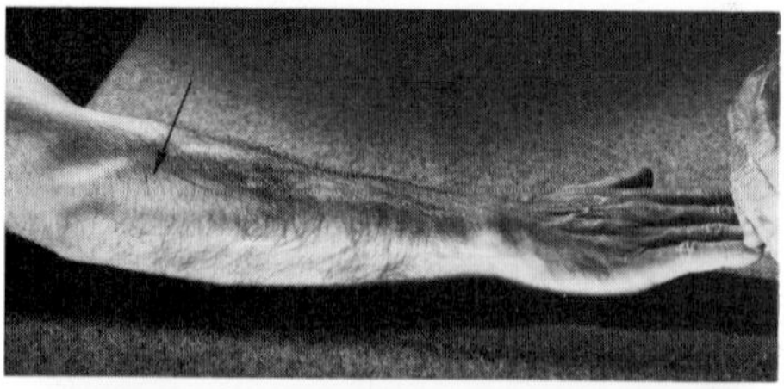

Fig. 36.
Muscle **Extensor digitorum**
Main segmental supply **C7**
Peripheral nerve **Radial**
Test The examiner attempts to flex the patient's extended fingers at the metacarpo-phalangeal joints.

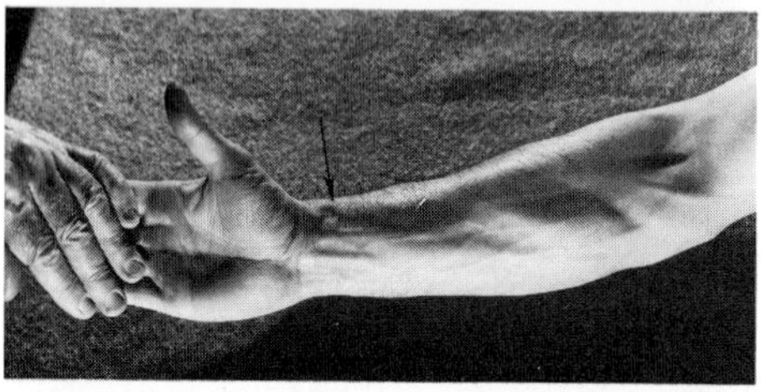

Fig. 37.
Muscle **Flexor carpi radialis**
Main segmental supply **C6, 7**
Peripheral nerve **Median**
Test The examiner resists the patient's attempts to flex the wrist towards the radial side. **Palmaris longus** is also shown.

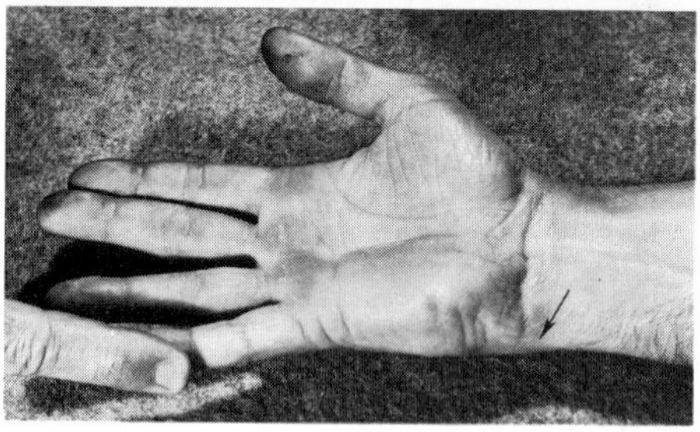

Fig. 38.
Muscle **Flexor carpi ulnaris**
Main segmental supply **C8**
Peripheral nerve **Ulnar**
Test This muscle is best seen while testing the abductor digiti minimi, where it fixes its point of origin.

MUSCLES OF THE THUMB

Note. Abduction of the thumb is the movement which brings the thumb to a right angle with the palm.

Extension of the thumb draws the thumb away in the same plane as the palm.

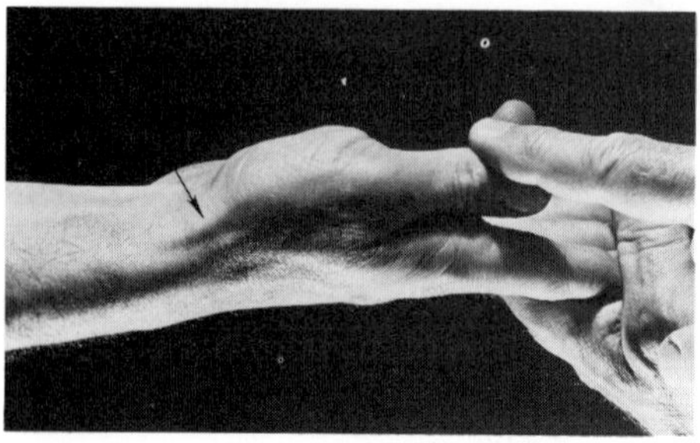

Fig. 39.
Muscle **Abductor pollicis longus**
Main segmental supply **C8**
Peripheral nerve **Radial**
Test The patient attempts to maintain his thumb in abduction against the examiner's resistance.

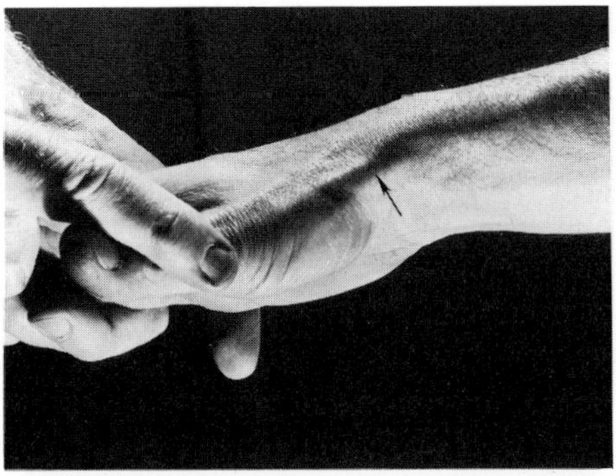

Fig. 40.
Muscle **Extensor pollicis brevis**
Main segmental supply **C8**
Peripheral nerve **Radial**
Test The patient attempts to extend the thumb while the examiner attempts to flex it at the metacarpophalangeal joint.

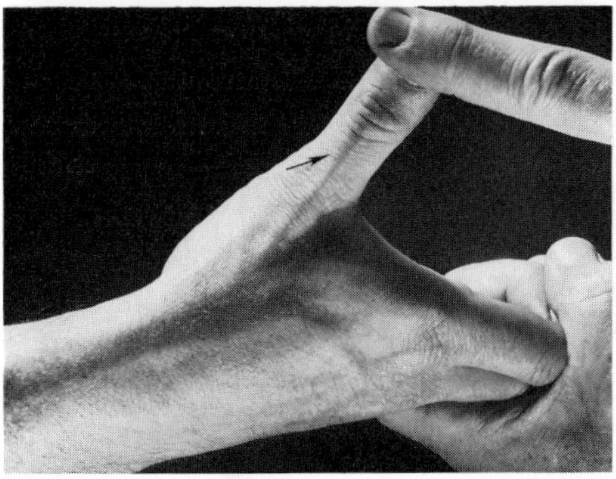

Fig. 41.
Muscle **Extensor pollicis longus**
Main segmented supply **C8**
Peripheral nerve **Radial**
Test The patient attempts to extend the thumb while the examiner attempts to flex it at the interphalangeal joint.

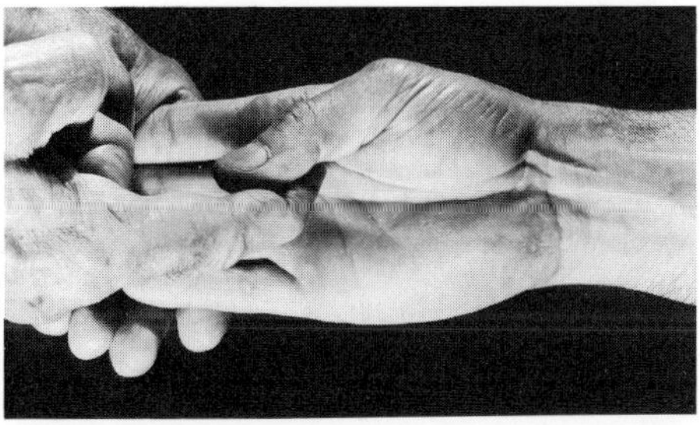

Fig. 42.
Muscle **Opponens pollicis**
Main segmental supply **T1**
Peripheral nerve **Median**
Test The patient attempts to touch the little finger with the thumb. Preserved in ulnar nerve lesions when the rest of the hand appears very wasted.

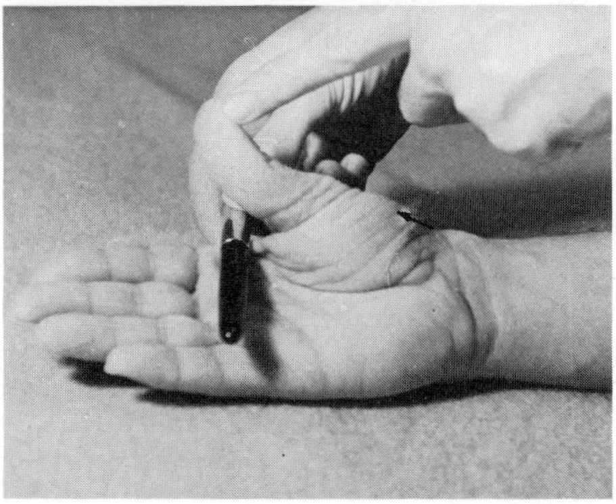

Fig. 43.
Muscle **Abductor pollicis brevis**
Main segmented supply **T1**
Peripheral nerve **Median**
Test First place some object between the thumb and the base of the forefinger to prevent full adduction; then the patient attempts to raise the edge of the thumb vertically above the starting point, against resistance. This is an important muscle, being the first to show weakness in the common carpal tunnel syndrome.

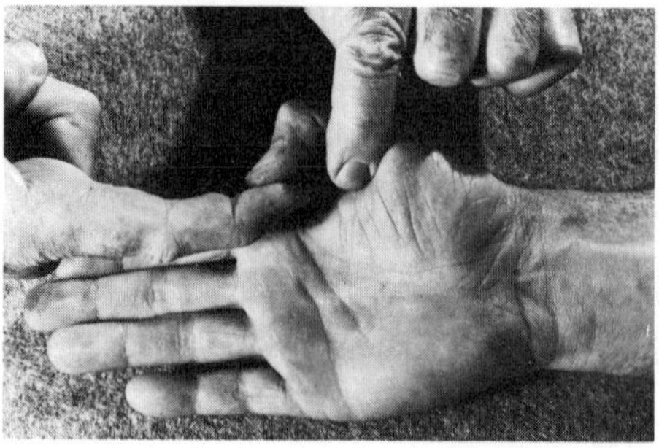

Fig. 44.
Muscle **Flexor pollicis longus**
Main segmental supply **C8**
Peripheral nerve **Median**
Test Attempt to extend the distal phalanx of the thumb against the patient's resistance. It is wise to hold the proximal phalanx.

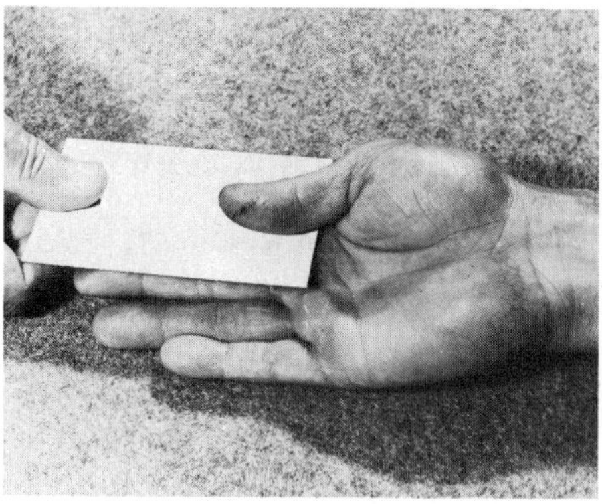

Fig. 45.
Muscle **Adductor pollicis**
Main segmental supply **T1**
Peripheral nerve **Ulnar**
Test The patient attempts to hold a piece of paper between the thumb and the palmar aspect of the forefinger.

MUSCLES OF THE HAND AND FINGERS

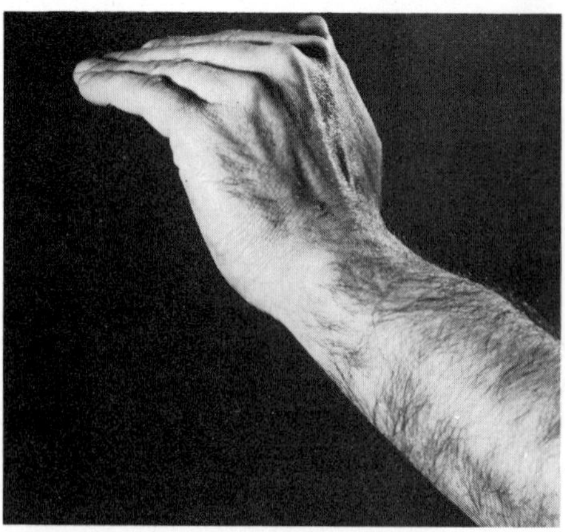

Fig. 46 (a) and (b).
Muscles **Lumbricals and interossei**
Main segmented supply **C8, T1**
Peripheral nerves **Median (lumbricals I and II); ulnar (interossei, lumbricals III and IV)**
Test (a) The patient tries to flex the extended fingers at the metacarpophalangeal joints (lumbricals).

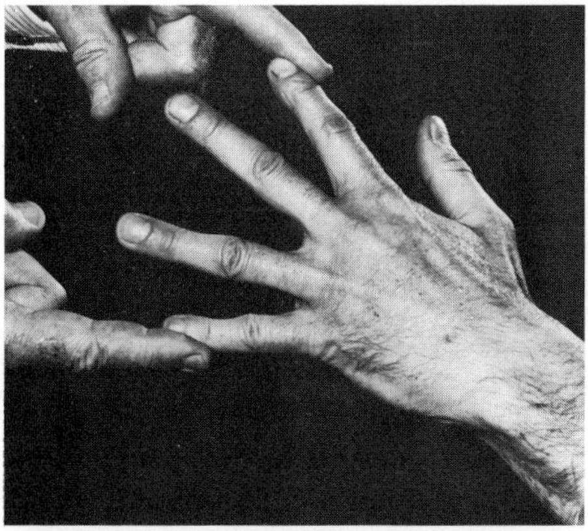

(b) Next he attempts to keep the fingers abducted against resistance (interossei).

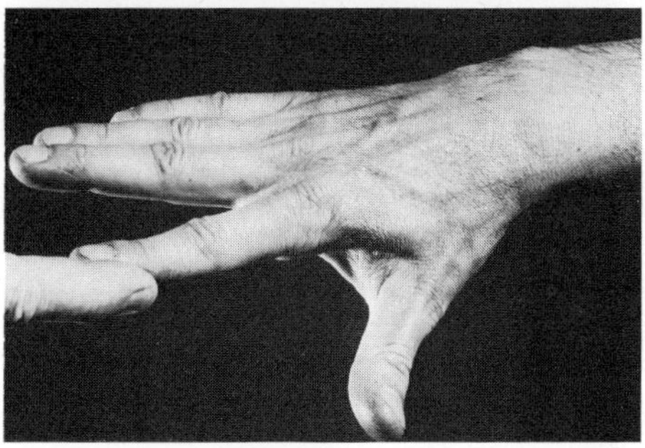

Fig. 47.
Muscles (a) **1st dorsal interosseus**
(b) **1st palmar interosseus**
Main segmental supply **T1**
Peripheral nerve **Ulnar**
Test Place the hand flat on a table. The patient then tries (a) to abduct and (b) to adduct the forefinger against resistance. (a) is illustrated. This test can be applied to other fingers, but the muscles are not easily visible.

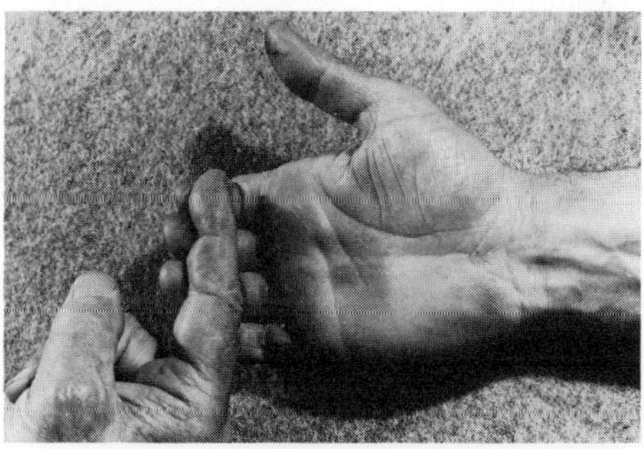

Fig. 48.
Muscle **Flexor digitorum sublimis**
Main segmental supply **C8**
Peripheral nerve **Median**
Test The patient flexes the fingers at the proximal interphalangeal joint against resistance from the examiner's fingers placed on the middle phalanx.

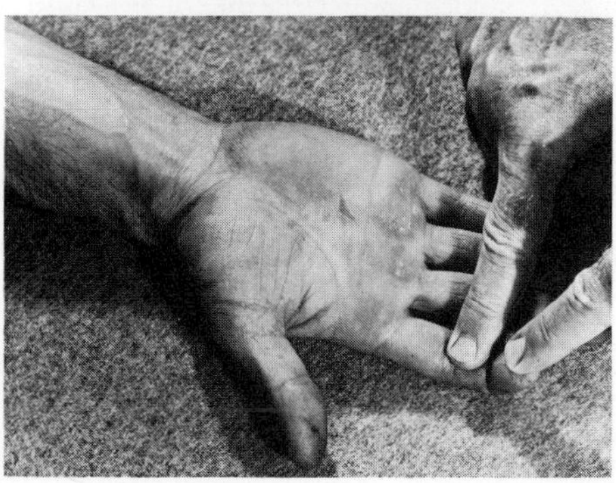

Fig. 49.
Muscle **Flexor digitorum profundus**
Main segmental supply **C8**
Peripheral nerves **Median (I and II); ulnar (III and IV)**
Test The patient flexes the terminal phalanx of the fingers against resistance, the middle phalanx being supported.

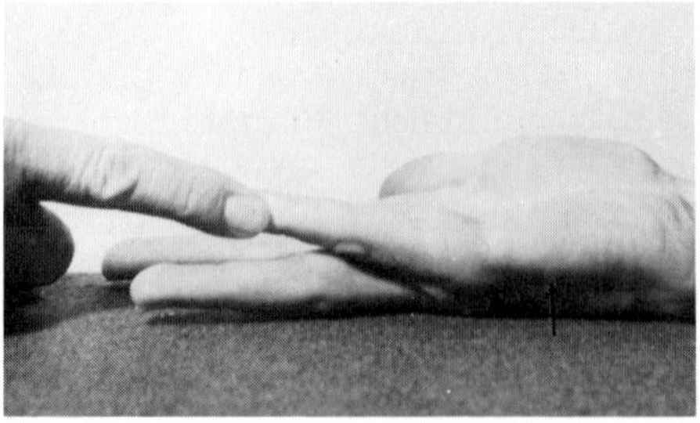

Fig. 50.
Muscle **Abductor digiti minimi**
Main segmental supply **T1**
Peripheral nerve **Ulnar**
Test The back of the hand is placed on the table and the little finger abducted against resistance (see also Fig. 38). Often the only sign of an ulnar lesion.

MUSCLES OF THE TRUNK

(Illustrations of these muscles are not helpful)

Muscles **Extensors of the spine**
Main segmental supply **All segments**
Peripheral nerves **Posterior rami of spinal nerves**
Test The patient lies on his face and then attempts to raise his shoulders off the bed.

Muscles **Intercostals**
Main segmental supply **T1–T12**
Peripheral nerves **Intercostal nerves**
Test A difficult test. Observe the movements of the ribs on expiration and inspiration and the movements of the muscles in the intercostal spaces.

Muscles **Abdominal muscles**
Main segmental supply **T5–L1**
Peripheral nerves **Intercostal, ilio-inguinal, iliohypogastric nerves**
Test The patient lies on his back and attempts to raise the head against light resistance. Watch the movement of the umbilicus.

MUSCLES OF THE HIP GIRDLE

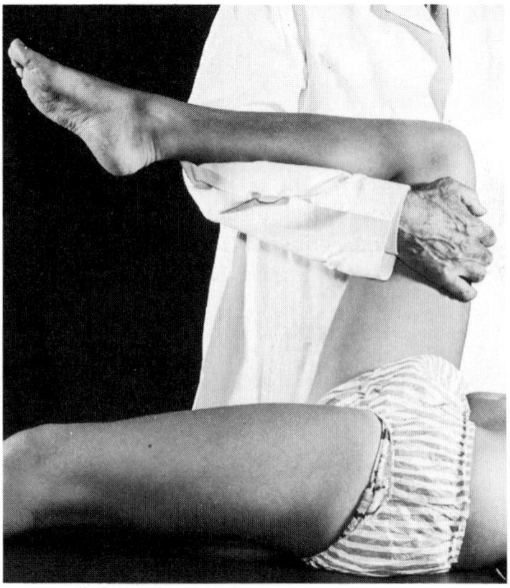

Fig. 51.
Muscle **Ilio-psoas**
Main segmental supply **L1, 2, 3**
Peripheral nerve **Femoral**
Test The patient lies on his back and attempts to flex his thigh against resistance. Similarly, with the hip fully flexed, he resists attempts to extend it.

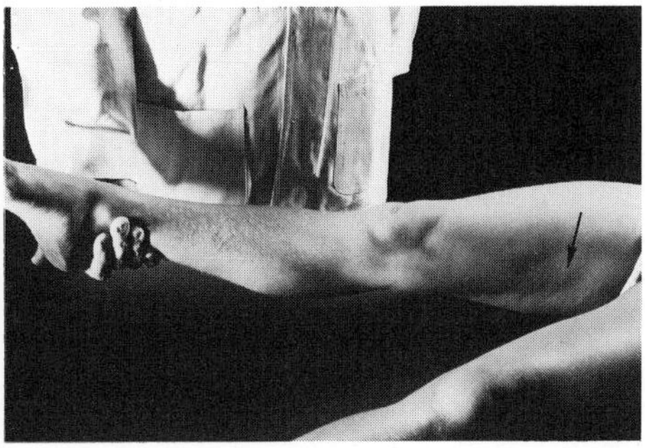

Fig. 52.
Muscle **Adductor femoris**
Main segmental supply **L5, S1**
Peripheral nerve **Obturator**
Test The patient attempts to adduct the leg against resistance.

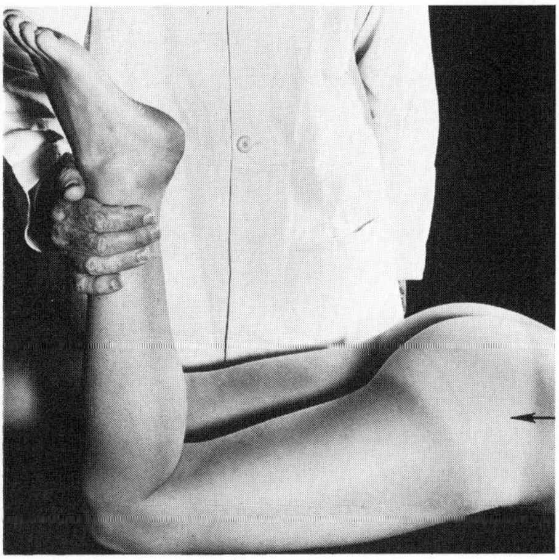

Fig. 53.
Muscles **Gluteus medius and minimus**
Main segmental supply **L2, 3**
Peripheral nerve **Superior gluteal**
Test The patient, lying on his face, flexes the knee and then forces the foot outwards against resistance. These muscles also abduct the extended leg.

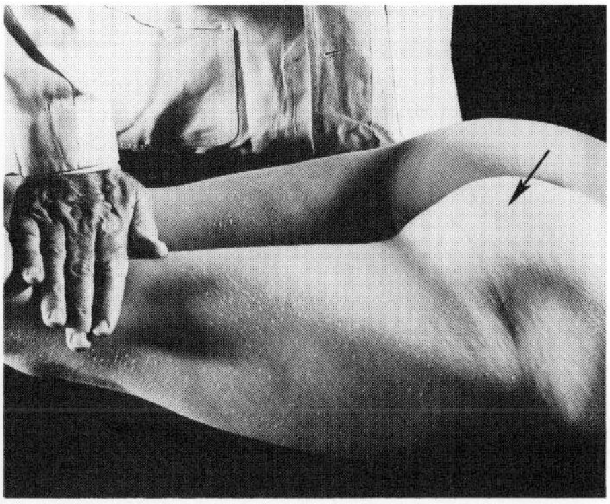

Fig. 54.
Muscle **Gluteus maximus**
Main segmental supply **L5, S1**
Peripheral nerve **Inferior gluteal**
Test The patient, still lying on his face, should tighten the buttocks so that each can be palpated and compared; he must then try to raise the thigh against resistance. Important in cauda equina and conus medullaris lesions.

MUSCLES OF THE THIGH AND KNEES

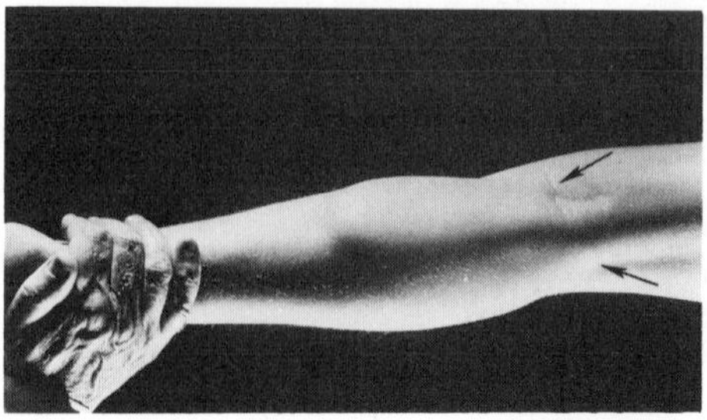

Fig. 55.
Muscles **Hamstrings (biceps, semitendinosus, semimembranosus)**
Main segmental supply **L4, 5, S1, 2**
Peripheral nerve **Sciatic**
Test The patient, lying on his face, attempts to flex the knee against resistance. The biceps is seen laterally, the semitendinosus medially.

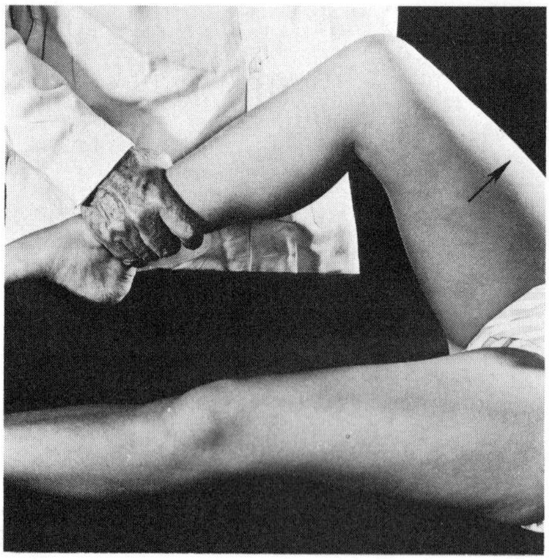

Fig. 56.
Muscle **Quadriceps femoris**
Main segmental supply **L3, 4**
Peripheral nerve **Femoral**
Test The patient, lying on his back, attempts to extend the knee against resistance.

MUSCLES OF THE LOWER LEG AND ANKLE

Note. The sciatic nerve divides into the medial and lateral popliteal nerves. The lateral popliteal further divides into anterior tibial and musculo-cutaneous branches.

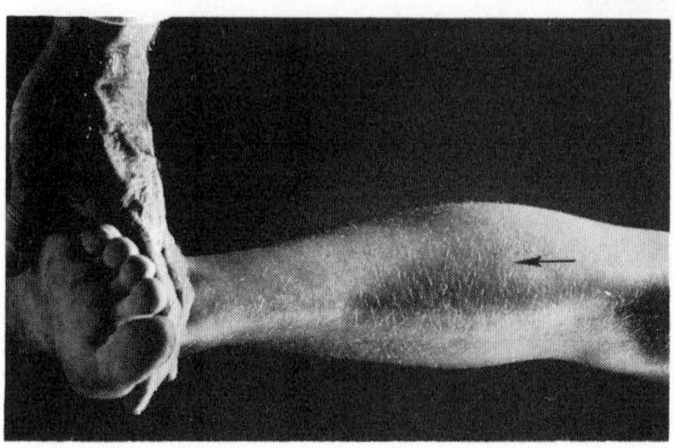

Fig. 57.
Muscle **Tibialis anticus**
Main segmental supply **L4, 5**
Peripheral nerve **Anterior tibial**
Test The patient dorsiflexes his foot against the resistance of the examiner's hand placed across the dorsum of the foot.

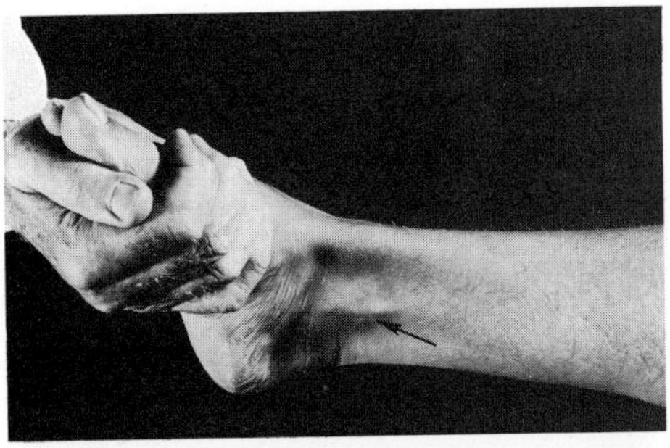

Fig. 58.
Muscle **Tibialis posticus**
Main segmental supply **L4**
Peripheral nerve **Medial popliteal**
Test The patient plantar-flexes the foot slightly and then tries to invert it against resistance.

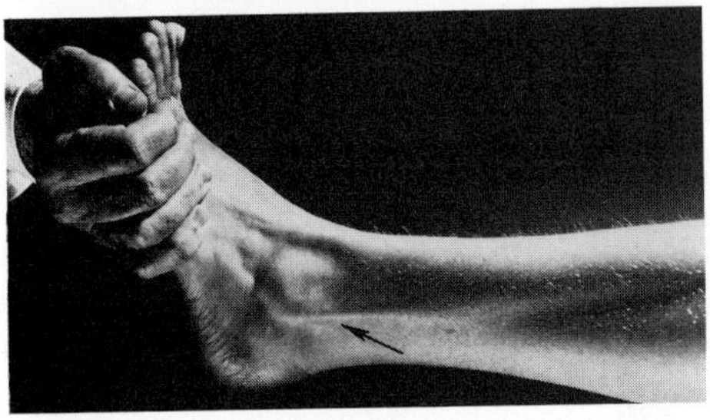

Fig. 59.
Muscle **Peronei**
Main segmental supply **L5, S1**
Peripheral nerve **Musculocutaneous (principally)**
Test The patient everts the foot against resistance. Isolated weakness may be the earliest sign of peroneal muscular atrophy.

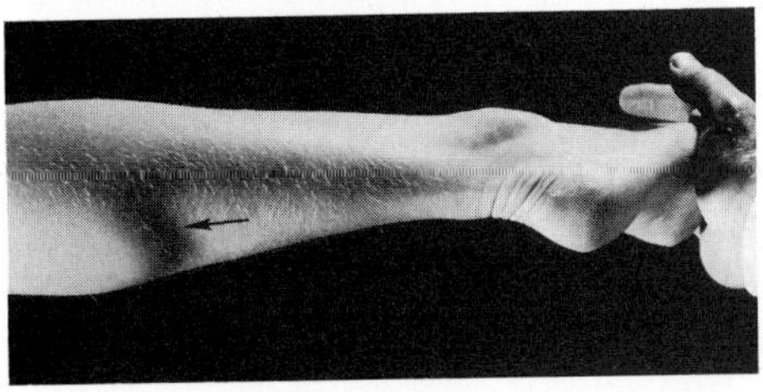

Fig. 60.
Muscle **Gastrocnemius**
Main segmental supply **S1**
Peripheral nerve **Medial popliteal**
Test The patient plantar-flexes the foot against resistance.

MUSCLES OF THE FOOT AND GREAT TOE

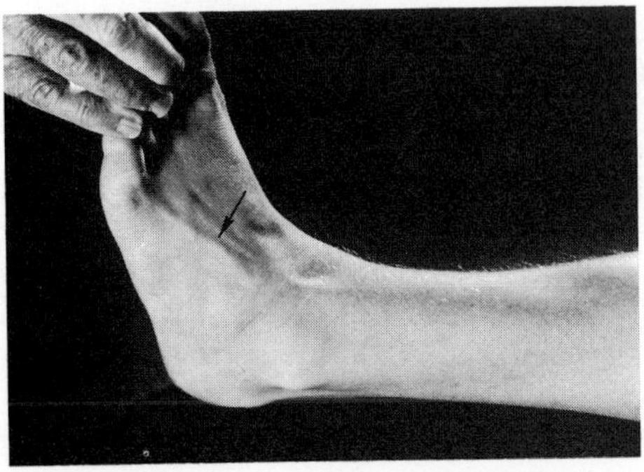

Fig. 61.
Muscle **Extensor digitorum longus**
Main segmental supply **L5**
Peripheral nerve **Anterior tibial**
Test The patient dorsiflexes the toes against resistance.

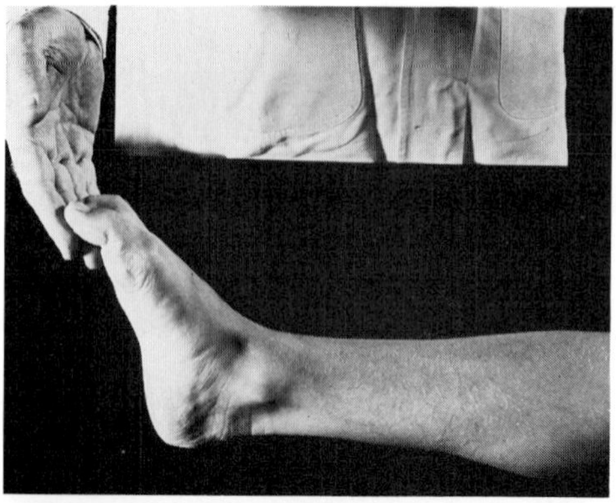

Fig. 62.
Muscle **Flexor digitorum longus**
Main segmental supply **S1, 2**
Peripheral nerve **Medical popliteal**
Test The patient flexes the terminal phalanges against resistance.

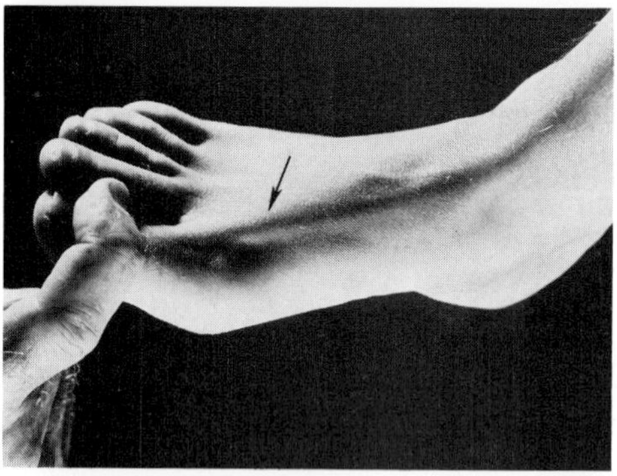

Fig. 63.
Muscle **Extensor hallucis longus**
Main segmental supply **L5, S1**
Peripheral nerve **Anterior tibial**
Test The patient attempts to dorsiflex the great toe against resistance.

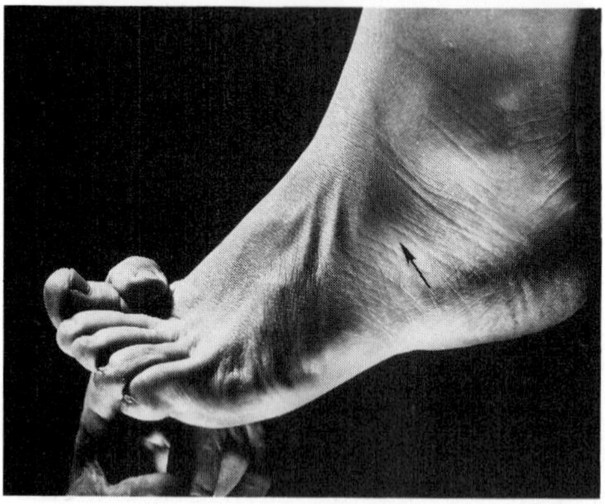

Fig. 64.
Muscle **Extensor digitorum brevis**
Main segmental supply **S1**
Peripheral nerve **Anterior tibial**
Test The patient dorsiflexes the great toe against resistance.

Types of muscular weakness

To repeat the same statement for each group or muscle in turn would be pointless, but there are certain general principles which help to distinguish different types of weakness.

WEAKNESS DUE TO PYRAMIDAL TRACT LESIONS

This tends to be a weakness that is incomplete except in the acute stages, or in the presence of a grossly destructive lesion. It affects particular movements rather than particular muscles, and is most marked in the abductors and extensors of the upper limb, and the flexors of the lower limb. Normally it is associated with increase of tone and exaggerated reflexes. Distribution is more distal than proximal, particularly in the upper limbs, where hand movements are affected earliest.

WEAKNESS DUE TO EXTRAPYRAMIDAL LESIONS

This is more of a hindrance to movement due to equal resistance from agonists and antagonists, than to true loss of muscle power. It is generalised throughout the limb and associated with rigidity and often with resultant suppression of the reflexes.

WEAKNESS DUE TO LOWER MOTOR NEURONE LESIONS

This is usually very marked, but except in extensive polyneuropathies, is limited to the muscles having that segmental supply. If of any standing it is associated with marked wasting and loss of those tendon reflexes in which the affected muscles play a part. A lesion at anterior horn or anterior root level picks out those muscles whose sole or maximal supply is from that segment, and these muscles may show fasciculation. At peripheral nerve level it affects all the muscles supplied by that nerve. In a polyneuritis, this type of weakness is often maximal peripherally in the arms and legs, and usually symmetrical.

WEAKNESS DUE TO MUSCULAR LESIONS

This can range from weakness of one muscle, such as after a local injury, to weakness of every muscle, such as in some cases of polymyositis. This type of weakness is either very localised, or very widespread but patchy. The muscles affected correspond neither to the supply of a particular spinal segment or a particular peripheral nerve. There is often individual muscle wasting, pseudohypertrophy, or tenderness. The related reflexes are lost.

Myasthenia

Though this word strictly speaking merely means muscular weakness, by custom it has come to mean that type of muscle weakness seen in myasthenia gravis, where the degree of weakness varies from hour to hour, increases as the muscle is repeatedly used, even to the extent of total paralysis, and yet recovers to its previous condition after a very short period of rest. This phenomenon, though capable of affecting any muscle in the body, is most commonly seen in the eyelids, the external ocular muscles, the facial muscles, the muscles of the tongue, throat and larynx, the muscles of the back, of the shoulder girdle and of the hand. Any of these should be tested for myasthenia either by repetition of a given action, such as maintaining

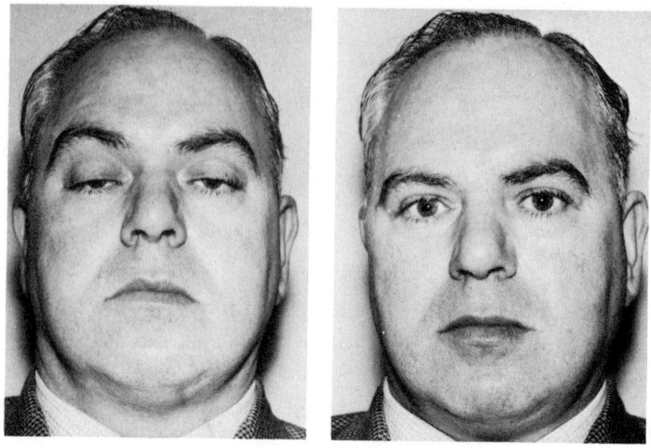

(a) (b)

Fig. 65. Effects of edrophonium chloride (Tensilon) on myasthenia gravis. (a) Before injection, (b) 60 seconds after injection.

(a) (b) (c)

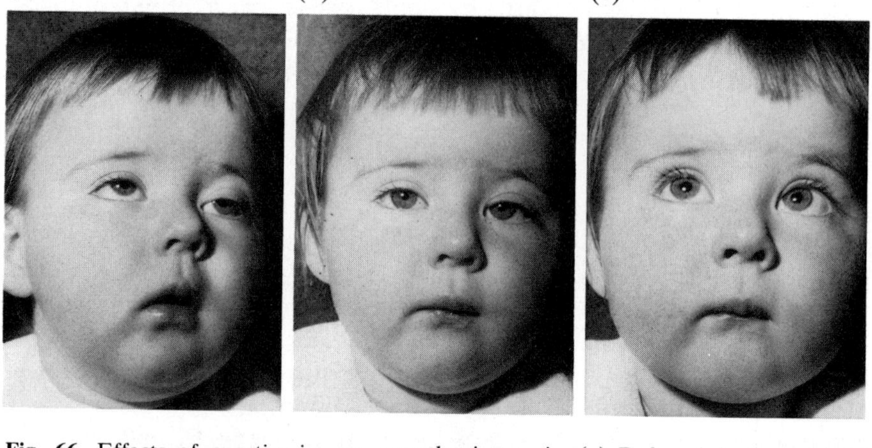

Fig. 66. Effects of neostigmine on myasthenia gravis. (a) Before injection, (b) 10 minutes after injection, (c) 30 minutes after injection. These photographs are intended also as a reminder that this disease can affect the very young.

upward deviation of the eyes for testing the eyelids, counting successively up to 100 for the bulbar muscles, or repeatedly sitting up and lying down for the back muscles.

The diagnosis can be confirmed by the intravenous injection of 10 mg of edrophonium chloride (Tensilon) when power returns within 1 minute (Fig. 65), the effect usually lasting only about 5 minutes, though in some patients it may persist longer. Eye muscle weakness responds less completely than limb muscles. An injection subcutaneously of 2.5 mg of neostigmine (Fig. 66a–c) is another striking test, when almost maximum power may be restored, but taking up to 45 minutes to do so. The effect may last 4 hours or longer. 0.6 mg of atropine should be included to minimise bowel discomfort. After either of these injections fasciculation may be seen in unaffected muscle, but if it occurs throughout all muscles, myasthenia gravis becomes unlikely. Not impossible however, if only the eye muscles are weak. In myasthenic syndromes associated with carcinoma (Eaton–Lambert syndrome) muscle strength is said to increase with repetition, and there is no dramatic response to Tensilon. Partial improvement may still be seen with neostigmine.

Cholinergic crises

An important word of caution. In patients known to have myasthenia gravis who are needing increasing dosage of anticholinesterases, increasing weakness may be a warning sign of impending cholinergic crisis, rather than worsening myasthenia. Always be on the alert for pallor, sweating, constricted pupils, hypersalivation and bradycardia. A very cautious test dose of intravenous edrophonium, using only small amounts (e.g. 1 mg) at a time will improve the situation in myasthenia and worsen it in cholinergic crises. Simply increasing the dosage of neostigmine or similar drugs may produce respiratory failure.

Hysterical weakness

This type of weakness corresponds to no set pattern of nerve supply. The antagonists to the muscle being tested are in action at the same time and this produces tremor. The power exerted by the patient is proportional to that exerted by the examiner, so that all degrees of strength produce the same failure of movement, but that failure varies from moment to moment. The grip varies. Dorsiflexion of the foot is suddenly 'let go'. By constant encouragement, the situation can sometimes be changed from one of almost total weakness to one of normal power. By watching the patient he can be seen at other times to be carrying out actions which would be impossible if the degree of weakness just shown on examination were genuinely present, and it is important to have reports from relatives and nursing staff on the degree of disability. A patient whose elbow flexion or extension can be prevented by pressure from the dorsal surface of the examiner's little finger would not be able to dress and undress if such weakness were real.

Chapter 18
Posture, Stance, Spinal Movement and Gait

The best time to observe the stance and gait is when the patient does not realise that he is being examined, for on formal testing the average person assumes a most unnatural mode both of standing and of walking. Watch the patient's movements closely on entering the room, and even more closely as he leaves. Simulated limps and other defects are frequently forgotten at the time of departure. Observations through a window of gait when leaving the building may be revealing. In the ward a casual visit may often be more informative in this respect than a set ward-round.

POSTURE AND STANCE

Formal testing is usually postponed to the end of the examination. The patient, if well enough, is asked to stand up and the position he naturally adopts is noted. Then ask him to bring both feet close together, the heels and toes touching. Watch the ease with which he does this and how well the position is maintained. Now ask him to close his eyes, assuring him that he will not be allowed to fall if he feels unsteady (and being ready to fulfil this promise). Remember that many people feel a slight sense of instability in these circumstances, and that this increases with age. Ask the patient to turn round and note whether this movement disturbs his equilibrium. The opportunity can then be taken to examine the back and spine.

THE BACK

Note the presence of kyphosis, scoliosis or abnormal lordosis, and then ask the patient to bend forwards to touch his toes. Again, note the line of the spinous processes, the conversion of the lumbar lordosis to a smooth curve, and the ease with which each part of the spine flexes. He should then flex the spine laterally in both directions. Palpate and lightly percuss the spinous processes and the para-spinal muscles.

If a muscular dystrophy or weakness of the back muscles is suspected, the patient should be told to squat down on his haunches, and to stand up again.

If he can do this he should then be asked first to lie flat on his back and then to get up on to his feet again. Most normal people will flex their hips and knees, raise their shoulders, place their hands behind them and push themselves forwards on to their feet, and so regain the upright position, possibly turning on to one side to gain better leverage.

Abnormalities of posture, stance and spinal movement

There are many conditions other than neurological disease which alter the patient's posture. These cannot be dealt with here and mention will merely be made of those abnormalities which fairly frequently bear relationship to nervous disease, with an indication of the disorders which may be suspected.

AKINESIA

This physical sign, seen principally in Parkinsonism, and quite different from rigidity, has become of immense importance to recognise, because it is this that is rapidly relieved by the various preparations containing l-DOPA. It consists of an absence or intense slowing of the initiation of voluntary movements of limbs and trunk, and of the many natural little movements which characterise human behaviour. It results in immobility of expression and of posture, great difficulty in changing posture, turning over in bed, etc., and inability to make rapid changes in movement of any sort. Best seen simply by observing the patient's usual behaviour rather than by set tests.

A STOOPED POSITION

This is common with age, excessive height, poor muscular development, some psychotic states, and in patients who have for years been under the control of overbearing relatives.

In severe Parkinsonism, the stoop affects mainly the upper spine, the head and neck being held forwards and the arms flexed at the side or in front of the body (see Fig. 2).

In some cases of motor neurone disease, myasthenia gravis, or carcinomatous myasthenia the neck muscles are so weak that the head falls forward, and the patient can only look ahead by turning his eyes upwards.

KYPHOSCOLIOSIS

A kyphotic spine does not necessarily give the impression of stooping, but in ankylosing spondylitis the stoop may be extreme.

Scoliosis is common in Friedreich's ataxia, muscular dystrophies, syringomyelia and von Recklinghausen's disease.

Gross kyphoscoliosis is capable of so distorting the theca as to cause cord compression and paraplegia.

In lumbar disc disease, a scoliosis tends to be convex to the side of the lesion, may be maximal at the affected level, and is greatly increased by bending forwards. If a congenital hemivertebra is present there is extreme scoliosis on forward flexion. This may be of no significance, but in the lumbar region it is sometimes accompanied by disc disease.

EXCESSIVE LORDOSIS

This occurs in muscular dystrophies, in some cases of generalised myasthenia gravis and in congenital hip disease. It may also be a normal racial characteristic.

A RIGID SPINE

On forward flexion the lumbar spine remains quite straight when there is paravertebral muscle spasm resulting from lumbar spine or disc disease. Flexion towards the side of the disc lesion increases the pain. In ankylosing spondylitis the whole spine moves as one and flexion occurs at the hip joints. Many patients who have been wearing spinal supports, cervical or lumbar, for a long time, develop a state of rigidity of their spinal movements which can be found even when there is very little wrong with the spine.

A TENDER SPINE

Local bony tumours and infections (such as accompany extradural spinal abscesses) cause localised tenderness on percussion. Some spinous processes, however, are always tender. Patients who constantly flinch when the paraspinal muscles are palpated, but are otherwise well, rarely have organic disease.

Abnormalities of equilibrium

Complete inability to remain upright is seen with lesions of the cerebellar vermis and in gross hypertension associated with basilar artery atheroma, and may be out of all proportion to any ataxia found while the patient was recumbent. It may also be a hysterical manifestation. In this case, the posture is bizarre and varies. It is at its worst when examined and yet, while dressing, the patient may be capable of standing and pulling his shirt over his head without falling. Other hysterical symptoms are usually present.

Falling to one side is seen in vestibular and cerebellar hemisphere lesions.

Falling backwards is seen in elderly patients with basilar atherosclerosis; in lesions involving the cerebellar vermis; and in foramen magnum lesions associated with descent of the cerebellar tonsils—such as basilar invagination and the Arnold–Chiari deformity. Such patients may be able to remain standing until they look upwards; others may find their legs becoming suddenly useless on coughing or sneezing.

ROMBERGISM

The patient sways from the heels, slightly when the eyes are open, but very markedly when the eyes are closed, to the extent that he will either fall, or separate his legs to achieve a broader base.

It is characteristic of proprioceptive deficiency and is found particularly in posterior cord compression at a high level, sensory polyneuropathies, sub-acute combined degeneration of the spinal cord, and tabes dorsalis. Some degree of swaying is not uncommon with advancing age, and in psychoneurosis. In the latter, distracting the patient's attention may stop it. It is common in vertebro-basilar disease.

SQUATTING AND STANDING UP

Weakness of the proximal leg and para-spinal muscles makes it impossible to rise from squatting. This is particularly seen in muscular dystrophies, but also in some cases of myasthenia gravis, polymyositis, and chronic polyneuropathies.

On attempting to stand up from lying flat, such patients will first turn on their face, draw their legs forwards toward their arms, place their hands on the lower part of their legs, and push themselves upright by placing the hands at successively higher levels on the legs. This is usually termed 'climbing up the legs' and is most obviously seen in children.

GAIT

First impressions, both visual and auditory, of a patient's gait are often of more help than formal testing (see Chap. 4).

At the end of the clinical examination the patient if well enough should be made to walk in a straight line for at least 10 yards (9 metres), then turn and walk back to the starting point.

Note the posture of the body while walking, the position and movement of the arms, the relative ease and smoothness of movement of the legs, the distance between the feet both in forwards and lateral directions, the regularity of the movement, the ability to maintain a straight course, the ease of turning and, finally, of stopping.

Abnormalities of gait

DRAGGING THE FEET

The patient who drags one foot usually has an upper motor neurone lesion of that leg. If this is part of a marked hemiparesis, he will throw the whole leg outwards from the hip, producing the movement called circumduction, leaning towards the opposite side with the arm flexed across the body, but often also abducting and circumducting it. This is common following hemiplegia of any cause.

In bilateral upper motor neurone lesions, both feet drag, but there is also an adductor spasm causing the legs to cross each other and each foot to trip up the other. The patient may appear to be walking on his toes (due to calf muscle contracture), and may seem almost to jump rapidly from the toes of one foot to the other. The scissors gait is most commonly seen in cerebral diplegia, in hereditary spastic paraplegia and in advanced cervical spondylosis. The more mobile a patient is despite this apparently crippling gait, the longer the lesion has been present.

HIGH-STEPPING GAITS

The patient raises the foot too high to overcome a foot drop; the toe hits the ground first, but the patient is not ataxic. This type of gait occurs unilaterally in root or peripheral nerve lesions causing anterior tibial muscle paralysis, and bilaterally in polyneuropathies and peroneal muscular atrophy. In the latter condition this gait may be very marked but apparently disable the patient very little.

A similar gait is found when, as a result of loss of position sense, the patient does not know where his foot is. The heel tends to strike the floor first, but the gait is irregular and ill-controlled, the legs move in all directions, with accompanying reeling from side to side on a broad base. The abnormality is increased in the dark and walking may be impossible if the patient closes his eyes. This is classically seen in tabes dorsalis, but as this is now an uncommon disease in many countries, it is more common in compressive lesions of the posterior columns and in carcinomatous neuropathy.

A SHUFFLING GAIT

Movement in a series of small, flat-footed shuffles occurs either due to the rigidity of extrapyramidal disease, or the combined rigidity, instability and loss of confidence of the cerebral arteriosclerotic. The Parkinsonian moves more quickly, stoops forwards with the hips and knees flexed, the steps becoming quicker as the movement progresses. There may be difficulty in stopping, and a slight push may cause rapid forward movement ('propulsion'). Sudden changes of direction cannot be made. The patient may become rooted to the spot. Such patients may have to go round several times in a revolving door before they are able to extricate themselves.

The arteriosclerotic stands upright, or leans backwards, takes tiny steps (marche aux petits pas), toes splayed outwards, legs wide apart, staring fixedly at some point straight ahead, and often pausing every few moments in the course of his movement.

AN ATAXIC GAIT

The gait of cerebellar ataxia is of two types. In one, the patient swings the legs unnecessarily and irregularly, and tends to reel in several sideways steps towards the side of the responsible lesion. The other is an ataxia of the trunk. The patient is grossly unstable, reels in any direction, including backwards, and may need the support of two people. This is seen in midline posterior fossa lesions, including tumours of the vermis and foramen magnum anomalies with descent of the tonsils (cerebellar ectopia).

The titubant ataxia of multiple sclerosis combines all these features, together with vertical oscillation of the head, trunk and arm, the arm oscillating on its stick as it moves it forwards and sideways to give additional support. It is hardly ever seen in any other condition.

A WADDLING GAIT

The pelvis is rotated through an abnormally large arc, accompanied by compensatory movements of the upper trunk and associated with marked lordosis. This accompanies congenital dislocation of the hips, but is also seen in muscular dystrophy. The rest of the physical examination will make differentiation easy. A similar gait has been seen in vitamin D deficiency.

HYSTERICAL GAITS

These are bizarre, correspond to none of the above features, vary from moment to moment, and from examination to examination, are minimised when the patient does not know he is being watched, do not cause injury, can be altered by suggestion, and are of a degree which would be accompanied by other signs of, for instance, cerebellar disease, if the process had reached a stage advanced enough to produce this type of gait. *The main danger is that of thinking that the midline cerebellar dysequilibrium is of hysterical origin.*

THE GAIT IN CHOREA

In Sydenham's and arteriosclerotic chorea one is not so impressed by the gait as by the movements of arm, neck and face which accompany walking. In Huntington's chorea, however, the patient walks wide-based, lordotic, lurching from heel to heel, with variable steps, starting and stopping, and marked by associated vigorous movements of fingers and wrist. This type of gait is often thought hysterical. In the dyskinesia of *l*-DOPA overdosage bizarre movements resembling those of Huntington's chorea may be seen in the limbs, trunk and neck while walking. In the dystonias of pre- or perinatal origin the patient may walk on the outsides of their feet, though they may be able to evert them normally on the bed.

Minor abnormalities

In order to detect minor abnormalities of gait, especially the ataxias, the patient should be made to walk heel-to-toe along a straight line. It should be noted whether he tends to reel off consistently in any particular direction. He should then be made to walk round a chair first in one direction and then the other. The patient with a right cerebellar lesion will stagger to the right and when walking with a chair on his right will tend to bump into it. On reversing the procedure, he will deviate outwards from it. These tests can be made even harder by asking the patient to close his eyes.

He should also attempt to hop on one foot. This is not possible on the side of a cerebellar lesion, but its performance will also be defective on the side of a pyramidal lesion, being slowed rather than unsteady.

There are probably few parts of the examination in which it is more important to correlate the findings with the patient's age and to temper diagnostic enthusiasm with kindness and consideration.

Chapter 19
Involuntary Movements

Analysis of involuntary movement requires intelligent use of the eyes, supplemented by a few instructions aimed at increasing, decreasing, or altering the character of the abnormality. Many movements such as shivering or startled jumping are not voluntarily produced, yet do not represent any disease process. At times, however, such phenomena may become so exaggerated as to pose problems in differential diagnosis, and for this reason alone, observations must be made at different times and under environmental conditions.

If any involuntary movement is detected at any stage in the examination, it is important to learn certain facts about it:

(*a*) What parts of the body are affected?
(*b*) Is it constant, or spasmodic in occurrence?
(*c*) Is it present only at rest, only on movement, or both?
(*d*) Does voluntary movement increase or suppress it?
(*e*) Is it altered by any particular position of the trunk or limbs?
(*f*) Is it affected by environment, temperature, or emotion?
(*g*) Is it altered by eye closure?
(*h*) Does it disappear in sleep?
(*i*) If the patient is aware of it, can he describe its onset?
(*j*) Is it present when the patient doesn't know he is being observed?

Many of these points can be observed while talking to the patient. During the formal examination, spend some time in careful observation of the whole body and then give specific instructions to bring out the behaviour of the movements more clearly.

Ask the patient first to hold his hands out in front of him, to retain them there with his eyes closed, and then to hold them above his head, palms forward. He should then grasp the examiner's hand, carry out the finger–nose test, pick up a small object such as a pin, do up or undo buttons, and make other voluntary movements requiring some degree of skill both with the affected and unaffected limbs, watching all the time the influence of the activities on the abnormality. He should then sit up, stand up and walk. Information should be added from the nursing staff or relatives as to the situation during sleep.

The quality of peripheral tremor can be emphasised by placing a piece of paper on the outstretched fingers.

As many similar movements can only be differentiated by correlating them with other physical signs, a final decision regarding their nature must await completion of the neurological examination.

EPILEPSY AND CONVULSIVE MOVEMENTS

Grand-mal epilepsy

A generalised attack characteristically is of sudden or rapid onset with loss of consciousness, rigidity of the limbs (maintained for a variable period), turning of the head and eyes, and followed by clonic jerking of face, neck, arms or legs, with cyanosis, teeth clenching, tongue biting, frothing at the mouth and incontinence. The rigidity then relaxes, the jerking dies away with a few slower jerks, and the patient goes into a post-epileptic coma, with stertorous breathing, its duration varying from a few moments to several hours. An attack may stop short at any stage.

Focal or partial epilepsy affects one side or one part of the body only, without necessarily any loss of consciousness. If the same part undergoes epileptic twitching for hours or days the condition is called *epilepsia partialis continua.*

'Salaam attacks' or infantile spasms. The arms are thrust upwards and forwards, the trunk at first extended and then flexed, the movement being followed by a cry. An EEG abnormality termed 'hypsarrhythmia' accompanies this form of infantile spasm (p. 000).

Petit-mal epilepsy

Motor manifestations are not necessarily a feature of a petit-mal attack. It may consist of no more than a few seconds of loss of attention. However, this loss of awareness may be accompanied by slight twitching of the eyelids, head nodding, a little jerking of the hands, and maybe a few repetitive words. The important features of the untreated case are the great frequency of the attacks, their very short duration, and the ease by which they can be stimulated by overbreathing.

Myoclonic jerks

These are sudden shock-like contractions of muscles which may occur singly or twice or three times in rapid succession, usually but not invariably affecting the flexors of the upper limbs and the extensors of the lower limbs; varying in degree from a contraction insufficient to move a joint to one so violent as to throw the patient to the ground. They may be provoked by touching or by sudden noise. The commonest form occurs just as a person falls to sleep.

The legs are usually affected, but the jerks may be more widespread and can interfere with sleep. These are, however, of quite benign significance. The commonest epileptic form usually starts in adolescents, affects the upper limbs and occurs just after waking in the morning or shortly after rising. They may herald a grand-mal attack or remain the only epileptic feature, but can be provoked by over-breathing, sometimes simply by eye closure, and often by photic stimulation. Myoclonus may also be seen in a number of degenerative and infective diseases of the brain and even of the spinal cord, and is not of localising value.

A special type of myoclonic jerk is seen in subacute sclerosing panencephalopathy (inclusion body encephalitis), and affects both trunk and limbs. It is slower than other jerks and the sudden movement is followed by a coarse tremor, during which the limb moves slowly upwards for a few inches. There are, in association, episodes of loss of tone of the neck, limbs and trunk.

Opisthotonus

Opisthotonus is a state of extreme hyperextension of the neck and spine, varying from arching of the spine to a state of rigidity so great that only heels and vertex touch the bed. It may be permanent or episodic, may be precipitated by noise or interference.

Maintained opisthotonus is seen in extreme meningeal irritation, usually in small children, or in extreme extrapyramidal rigidity, such as in the late stages of subacute encephalitis. If spasmodic, it occurs in tetanus, in the so-called brain stem fits due to pressure from posterior fossa neoplasms, occasionally in pontine haemorrhage secondary to tentorial pressure coning, and has been seen in brain stem encephalitis. It can be an hysterical manifestation.

CHOREAS AND DYSTONIAS

Chorea

This condition varies both in degree and on different occasions from the severe form where the limbs are flung about in rapid movements, no two in succession being the same, often described as semi-purposive, but really having no purpose at all, accompanied by respiratory irregularity and rapid protrusion and retraction of the tongue, with 'flapping' of its tip; to minor degrees where the movements may be slight, but being brought out by voluntary movement and disorganising it, may be mistaken for a cerebellar ataxia. The limbs are hypotonic, yet the reflexes are usually retained. The joints can be hyperextended, and bizarre postures of the fingers and wrists are adopted, and if the arms are held above the head with palms forwards, this position cannot be maintained. The movements are minimal at rest and in quiet surroundings, and maximal when the patient is frightened or embarrassed. The patients rarely injure themselves or anyone else, but may frequently drop or knock things over.

It is essential to look particularly for (*a*) the flapping of the tongue, (*b*) the respiratory irregularity, (*c*) hypotonia and hyperextensibility, (*d*) the inability to hold the hands above the head with palms extended, and, of course, (*e*) any cardiac lesion.

Similar movements occur in several varieties of chorea:

(*a*) *Sydenham's chorea* (usually children, often with cardiac abnormality and a positive anti-streptolysin titre).

(*b*) *Huntington's chorea* (patients in middle life, without hypotonicity, no cardiac lesion, progressive dementia, and a family history).

(*c*) *Chorea of pregnancy* (usually a first pregnancy).

(*d*) *Chorea in patients on oral contraceptives.*

(*e*) *Senile or arteriosclerotic choreas* (in the later age groups, often of sudden onset, and with evidence of degenerative vascular disease).

(*f*) *Chorea in primary polycythaemia.*

(*g*) *Hereditary chorea without dementia* (now a recognised entity with dominant transmission, not always 'benign').

Athetosis

In contrast to chorea, this is a slow writhing movement, best seen at wrists, fingers and ankles. The fingers writhe, the wrists flex, the forearm and arm rotate inwards, abduct, and then rotate outwards in abduction. The foot is inverted. The impression is one almost of voluntary movement, and except in severe cases, most marked in a limb not at that moment being examined. The movements are absent during sleep, little altered by eye closure, increased by voluntary movement, and interfering with it. Respiratory rhythm is normal; there is no tongue flap, but similar movements of face and tongue may occur, especially when athetosis is bilateral.

Choreo-athetosis

This is a combination of the above. The movements have both slow and quick elements, and either may predominate. It is rather characteristic that, just as one is about to diagnose, say, athetosis, a movement typically choreic appears, and vice versa. The respiratory rhythm and tongue movements are abnormal. The movements are very apparent on voluntary effort and straining with one limb will increase the movements greatly in the others. No cardiac lesion is present.

Both athetosis and choreo-athetosis occur in a variety of lesions of the corpus striatum distinguishable only by histology. They are most commonly the result of lesions at birth or in the neonatal period, and may also follow an infantile hemiplegia. Mental retardation may often be much less than the impression given by the bizarre movements.

Dyskinesias

Dyskinesia is a generic term to describe all the above involuntary movements, but its special importance nowadays is the frequency with which it is seen in patients receiving *l*-DOPA treatment for Parkinsonism. The choreic element is less rapid than in other choreas, the athetoid element of lesser amplitude. Indeed the movements, though so obvious, are often preferred by the patient to the previous akinesia. The movements may be absent from a limb previously treated stereotactically. Lowering the *l*-DOPA dosage will reduce or stop the movements at first, and they tend to occur only at the time of peak action of the drug. Later, the dyskinesias increase in duration and can occur throughout the day. Orofacial movements are most prominent.

Hemiballismus

This is the most dramatic of all involuntary movements. Usually affecting the proximal joints of one arm, there are wild, rapid, flinging movements of wide radius, occurring constantly, or with short periods of freedom, sufficiently violent to injure the patient and others. They are not altered by eye closure, are absent during sleep, but prevent sleep because of their violence, and may be accompanied by increased tone and reflexes in the affected limb. This condition is often of sudden onset, is totally disabling and exhausting, but may lessen under observation. It is due to a lesion in the vicinity of the sub-thalamic nucleus interrupting its immediate connections, usually vascular in origin, though occasionally due to metastatic or primary neoplastic infiltration. It may sometimes follow stereotaxic operations for Parkinsonism, and may require a larger lesion to cure it.

Dystonia musculorum deformans

In this state, the patient's trunk and limbs undergo very forcible, wide amplitude, writhing movements, mainly at the proximal joints, with quicker, smaller movements super-added. Marked hypertrophy of the dystonic muscles may develop. In the advanced state the patient is frequently brought into a clinic strapped into his chair. The slower movements consist of arching of the back and neck, strong rotation of the neck and arms into positions of extreme distortion which are held at their maximum for 5–10 seconds. The more rapid movements are seen at the beginning and end of each slow movement, especially the neck turning. There is usually grimacing, grunting and protrusion of the tongue. All features are greatly increased by nervousness, are absent during total relaxation and sleep, and become progressively worse as repeated attempts at voluntary movement fail. Such patients may be able to feed themselves at home, and yet in the outpatient department may be unable to grasp the examiner's hand. Intelligence may again be much higher than the superficial appearance suggests.

This condition is almost invariably due either to anoxia at birth, birth trauma, infantile encephalitis, or, very rarely, to encephalitis in later life.

INVOLUNTARY MOVEMENTS OF THE FACE AND NECK

Almost any of the movements described may involve the face and neck, but in certain conditions the abnormality is limited to this part of the body.

Facial tics

Many bizarre facial movements are probably not due to organic disease and are synonymously called habit spasm. However, the total lack of firm data about idiopathic tics as a whole precludes dogmatic insistence that they are psychogenic or organic. Generally tics are stereotyped, repetitive movements which are easily produced voluntarily, such as blinking, screwing up the face, pursing the lips. They are present when under observation, sometimes absent when concentrating on something else, common in childhood, increased by nervousness, and though they may remain stereotyped for months or years, singly or occasionally, multiple tics may persist or even evolve throughout life. Voluntary suppression is possible for a while, but increasing inner tension ultimately causes their return, with associated momentary relief from tension. Though commonest in the face, such movements frequently involve the shoulder girdle, causing shrugging movements, retraction of the neck, and, at times, contraction of individual muscles such as the platysma, the pectorals, or even one-half of the abdominal muscles. The whole muscle is always in action and the movement is in every respect similar to voluntary contractions of those muscles. A rare disorder, the syndrome of Gilles de la Tourette, is characterised by multiple persistent tics often accompanied by inarticulate cries or barks or compulsive utterance of obscenities.

Hemifacial spasm (facial clonic spasm)

In this condition, the muscles in one part of the face go into spasmodic contraction, drawing the mouth towards that side, with a series of fine twitches after it is drawn up. The muscles round the eye are similarly involved. Each spasm starts suddenly and stops suddenly, is very embarrassing, made worse by nervousness, stopped by concentration or by sleep, is always the same in type if not in degree, and after some years may be accompanied by facial weakness. The aetiology is uncertain, but irritation of the facial nerve by an aberrant arterial loop, aneurysm or acoustic neuroma can be responsible.

A somewhat similar twitching is seen long after a facial palsy, but the facial muscles show contracture already, the spasm is initiated by voluntary movement even though very slight, and fasciculation is often present at rest.

Focal facial fits may simulate facial spasm, but the contractions are much slower and coarser and, though the onset may be similar, they do not cease suddenly, but through a series of lessening twitches, and, of course, are frequently accompanied by other manifestations of a grand-mal attack.

Facial myokimia

This differs from myokimia in the orbicularis muscles being of sudden onset, affecting the whole of one side of the face by undulating flickering waves of contraction on a background of constant contraction. It may occur bilaterally, is of self-limiting course, and has been seen in vascular lesions of the stem, multiple sclerosis, and pontine gliomata. Short runs of lesser degree affecting only a small portion of the facial musculature are not very uncommon and have the same benign significance as periorbital myokimia.

Peri-oral tremor

A constant, coarse tremor of the orbicularis oris and chin is seen in general paralysis of the insane, and may be the only site of the tremor.

Spasmodic torticollis

This consists of forced turning of the head to one side, or even backwards, with elevation of the chin and dropping of the occiput. There may be a long sustained spasm, a series of rapid spasms, or short-lived spasms with intervals of normality, often accompanied by grimacing, overaction of the platysma, cracking noises from the neck and considerable pain. It is made worse by nervousness and embarrassment, and relieved by total rest. In long-standing cases there is hypertrophy of the sterno-mastoid. How often torticollis is due to an organic lesion is uncertain for such lesions are but rarely demonstrated. It may be part of, or the first sign of, generalised dystonia. It undoubtedly is often of psychogenic origin with clear psychopathology and other psychogenic history and symptoms. (This statement will be hotly denied by many, who have swung too far towards the organic theory for all and every case, though quite unable to produce any consistent neuropathological or neurochemical evidence to support them.)

Facial dystonia and tardive dyskinesia

Bizarre grimacing of the face, associated with intermittent protrusion of an apparently hypertrophied tongue, occurs certainly in generalised dystonic states, but also as an isolated phenomenon. This may be seen in some varieties of Huntington's chorea, and in the Gilles de la Tourette syndrome, where involuntary noises or utterances may occur. Tardive dyskinesia is a similar phenomenon not uncommon after prolonged heavy dosage of phenothiazine-type drugs especially in females. It is seen more commonly with increasing age and in patients in institutions. A dyskinesia of the face may be isolated from generalised dyskinesia and occur during treatment of Parkinsonism by *l*-DOPA being relieved by lowering the dose, but possibly recurring on progressively smaller dosage.

Titubation

This is a vertical oscillation of the head, present when the head is maintained in an upright position, and therefore seen when the patient sits or stands, and disappears on his lying down. It is indicative of disease of the cerebellar connections, and is most commonly seen in multiple sclerosis. It differs from the isolated head nodding forming part of the torticollis spectrum, and is always accompanied by marked signs of other neurological disease, although there is an idiopathic variety associated with so-called essential tremor.

TREMORS

In these paragraphs the words 'fine' and 'coarse' frequently appear. A fine tremor is intended as one visible only on close inspection, and best brought out by balancing a piece of paper on the patient's fingers. A coarse tremor is one which is very obvious, needs no special measures to see it, but still produces a movement of a few millimetres only. The term 'very coarse' is applied to those which move the fingers or limb through an appreciable distance.

Nervousness

This is the most common tremor. It is rapid, varying from fine to coarse, affecting mainly the fingers, but capable of spreading to the whole arm or body. It is present at rest, increased by any voluntary movement which the patient fears he may not do correctly or quickly enough (such as the finger–nose test, or undressing), not increased during automatic movement, made worse by speaking sharply to the patient, reducing towards the end of the examination as he realises that it is not a very alarming experience, and often absent on a second examination for the same reason. A 'physiological' tremor is present whenever a muscle contracts (due to subtetanic contractions of motor units). This is not visible, but becomes so when 'enhanced' by B-adrenergic stimulation of the segmental stretch reflex. The frequency is fast, 10–15 Hz, and this is the tremor of nervousness.

The anxiety state

A similar tremor, more marked, coarser and more persistent, though also greatly influenced by emotion. It also is an exaggerated 'physiological' tremor. It differs in being accompanied by dilated pupils, tachycardia, cold, clammy, sweating extremities, and not varying to the same degree on repeated examination.

Thyrotoxicosis

This is a fine rapid tremor, present constantly, greatly influenced by emotion, and accompanied by sweating and tachycardia, *but the extremities are very warm,* there is lid retraction, possibly exophthalmos, and loss of weight.

Alcoholism

A variable tremor, often very coarse, capable of affecting the whole limb and trunk (as in acute alcoholic tremulousness). Nearly half of a given population of chronic alcoholics, *not* in withdrawal, show a tremor. The tremor is postural, between about 6 and 10.5 Hz and shows no relationship to the person's age or the duration of excessive drinking. It is present constantly, not greatly influenced by emotion or voluntary movement, but may be sufficiently severe to interfere with fine movement. There is usually a good response to β-blockers. If the examiner's palm is pressed against the patient's outstretched fingers, a curious impression is transmitted of clicking between the bones at the interphalangeal joints, a feature rarely found in any other type of tremor. It may remain long after withdrawal from alcohol. This is probably the basis of Quinquad's sign where the patient holds his fingers flexed at the metacarpophalangeal joints and extended at the interphalangeal joints, while the examiner presses his palm against the finger tips. A worm-like sensation is transmitted from the proximal joints. Tremor on acute withdrawal is of two varieties. One is less than 8 Hz in frequency, similar to essential tremor. A second type is of frequency greater than 8 Hz.

Other toxic tremors

Almost any drug taken in excess over a prolonged period may give rise to a tremor which resembles alcoholic tremor. Inorganic mercury compounds are particularly liable to produce coarse tremor, but are rarely a problem in these days. Addiction to stimulant drugs, including some of those used as anti-depressants are now more commonly responsible than industrial toxins. The tremor caused by *withdrawal* from alcohol and opiates is an 'enhanced physiological' tremor again. Lithium, nicotine and *l*-DOPA are further examples of agents that can induce this form of tremor. Toluene abuse ('solvent encephalopathy') is a recent problem, producing an acute illness with coma, ataxia, behavioural disturbance and convulsions. Withdrawal from such 'glue-sniffing' can provoke tremor, and an intention tremor occurs during intoxication along with other 'cerebellar' signs.

Essential heredo-familial tremor

This is a coarse tremor, constantly present, influenced by emotion, worrying to the patient, sometimes disabling, present throughout life usually, but not necessarily, with a definite history of similar tremor in the family. The characteristic feature is that though the tremor is very marked when the hands are held outstretched, if the patient is asked to pick up a pin the tremor will stop just at the moment of grasping it, so that fine movement is little affected. One calls essential tremor a *postural-action* tremor in that instance, but it can only be purely *intentional*. The frequency is about 8 Hz.

Parkinsonian tremor

A rhythmical 4–8 Hz tremor varying from the simple movement of one thumb to a state in which so gross is the shaking of the whole limb and body that the tremor can be heard as well as seen as the extremities thump the chair or floor. In the earliest stages, the movement is seen in the tip of the thumb as a flexion–extension movement. The next stage occurs when the thumb comes into opposition with the forefinger, which itself produces a flexion tremor at the first interphalangeal joint. As the tremor advances, the fingers are moved *en masse,* rather than individually, and the flexed position becomes permanent at rest. The tremor is absent in total relaxation, or in sleep, and often immediately after waking. It is increased by emotion, and is present at rest providing some form of posture is being maintained and usually suppressed by the initiation of voluntary movements. It will return as soon as that movement becomes maintained or a new position taken up. It may be accompanied by cog-wheel rigidity at the wrist and fingers and slowing of each movement. Masking of the face may be obvious even when the thumb alone is involved. Occasional patients with Parkinson's disease show an exaggeration of the tremor with movement. In other words, there are features of 'essential' tremor. *l*-DOPA is responsible for raising adrenalin levels when decarboxylated systemically, and so superimposes an enhanced physiological tremor. However, there are more intriguing associations, because it is a fact that more patients with Parkinson's disease have had pre-existing 'essential' tremor than chance alone would predict. Considering that heredity plays *no* important part in Parkinson's disease, but 50% of people with essential tremor have a family history, this is a very interesting association!

Tremor in collagen disease

This is a coarse, side-to-side, irregular tremor of the digits, each moving independently and out of step with its neighbour, in a manner which a normal person is incapable of imitating. It is increased by attempts to maintain posture, and by emotion, and completely disappears on total relaxation. It is seen in the collagenoses, in polyarteritis nodosa particularly, and in severe rheumatoid arthritis with accompanying rheumatoid polyneuropathy, which is itself probably due to an arteritis.

Intention tremor

A coarse tremor (4–6 Hz) characterised by the difference between its absence at rest or on the initiation of voluntary movement, and its development as the moving limb approaches its object. It then usually appears as a side-to-side oscillation (e.g. in the finger–nose test), which in advanced cases may be so gross as to move the limb over a distance of more than a foot, so preventing any object from ever being reached and in this case is utterly disabling. In mild degree it appears as a few oscillations, best shown as the finger is maintained on the nose for a few moments after reaching it.

It indicates a lesion of the cerebellar connections, and is seen most clearly and consistently in multiple sclerosis.

Red nucleus tremor

This tremor, usually unilateral as in Benedikt's syndrome, is slow, coarse, and rhythmical, present at rest and also throughout a voluntary movement and by virtue of its site of origin, usually associated with ataxia on that side. Rubral tremor, so-called, is really a severe cerebellar tremor with the responsible lesion more likely in the superior cerebellar peduncles. (The frequency is 2.5–4.0 Hz.)

Tremor in Wilson's disease

Characteristically, on holding the hands outstretched, this tremor is seen as an irregular, vertical, flapping movement at the wrist, with large amplitude movements from the shoulder, asymmetrically on the two sides. It is grossly increased by further voluntary movement, and may then become a wild, inco-ordinate, choreic flinging of the arm in all directions. It is absent on total relaxation, so that the patient may be able to conceal it, but it appears as soon as any attempt is made to maintain posture. The youth of the patient, the family history, increasing dementia, and, of course, the pathognomonic Kayser–Fleischer ring, confirm the diagnosis, evidence of liver disease usually being present only at a late stage.

'The liver flap'

This is a similar wing-flapping tremor at the wrists, which is seen in patients with advanced liver disease. Its particular importance is that its appearance is often a warning of impending hepatic coma. The other features of Wilson's disease are absent.

Asterixis

Very similar to the liver flap, this consists of a sudden loss of posture in arms held outwards with wrists dorsiflexed. The drop may be followed by a compensatory jerk, so that objects may be thrown around. It is seen in severe chronic respiratory insufficiency and is of grave prognosis. It can be regarded as a form of 'negative' myoclonus.

Pseudo-athetosis or 'searching movements'

This is an important physical sign, and is seen when a patient lies with his eyes closed and his hands either held outstretched in front of him, or resting on a flat surface such as a bed table. Slow wandering movements occur of the fingers, accompanied by flexion at the metacarpophalangeal joints so that the palm is drawn away from a flat surface. As this happens the fingers gradually close, the wrist flexes, and there is internal rotation of the pronated forearm. In many ways the movements resemble athetosis, but it is suppressed when the patient watches his hand, and he is usually unaware of its occurrence. *It is always accompanied by gross loss of postural sensibility.* Occasionally the toes, or even the legs, may show similar involuntary movements. When such a limb is moved passively the examiner gains the impression (incorrectly) that the patient is resisting him voluntarily. Any lesion causing very severe loss of position sense may produce this phenomenon. When tabes dorsalis was a common cause for loss of position sense these movements were called 'tabetic athetosis' but nowadays it is most common in those cases of cervical spondylosis where the spinal canal is very narrow, so that backward displacement of the cord results in compression of its posterior aspect. In this condition it may affect only the arms, but it is also seen in carcinomatous sensory neuropathy where it may affect arms and legs equally. It occurs with cerebellar ectopia at foramen magnum level and very occasionally, unilaterally, in parietal lobe lesions. It can occur, but it is rare, in multiple sclerosis, and here it may remit completely.

MOVEMENTS LIMITED TO THE MUSCLES

If there is tremor, the muscles of that limb will show this movement. It is, therefore, essential to look at the limbs as a whole when any abnormal movement is noted in one of its muscles. There are, however, certain movements confined to the muscles.

Fasciculation

This term, by common clinical usage, is applied to an irregular, nonrhythmical contraction of muscle fascicles, sometimes fine, sometimes coarse, most easily seen in the larger muscles such as deltoid or calves, and present at rest, stopping during, but increased after, voluntary movement, stimulated by smacking or warming the muscle, but usually not felt by the patient. It varies greatly in degree and may be so coarse and gross as to be visible through the clothes, when the whole muscle seems alive and like a bag of worms. Fasciculation is a better word than fibrillation, which is too fine a movement to be seen, though it can be measured on the electromyograph. It indicates degeneration of the anterior horn cell, or irritation of the anterior root, when the fasciculation is very coarse, and repetitive in muscles having the same root supply. The finer fasciculation is seen classically in motor neurone disease, where it normally is associated with wasting, but exaggerated reflexes, and is almost diagnostic of this disease when affecting the tongue and accompanied by an exaggerated jaw jerk. It may also be seen in the tongue in syringobulbia, but the jaw jerk is then absent. It occurs also in muscles recovering from poliomyelitis; in calves after lumbar disc lesions or laminectomies which have caused much arachnoiditis; in a very coarse form in cases of collagen disease, and as a transient state in presumed infective or allergic lesions, such as myositis. If seen in wasted muscles with absent reflexes, thyrotoxic myopathy, syphilitic amyotrophy, and peroneal muscular atrophy must be considered. Widespread fasciculation can be produced in non-myasthenic individuals by an injection of 2.5 mg of neostigmine, sometimes after edrophonium (Tensilon), and in the unaffected muscles in some myasthenics. In pathological states a much smaller dose will greatly increase any fasciculation already present. (See Chap. 39 for electromyographic definition.)

Myokimia

This, the most common involuntary movement of the muscles, is seen in two forms.

(*a*) As a fine, very rapid rippling of muscle fibres persisting *in the same group of fibres* for minutes at a time, most commonly in the orbicularis oculis and easily felt by both patient and observer. If a fold of the skin below the eye is held between the thumb and forefinger a sensation is experienced similar to touching a purring kitten. It is usually a manifestation of fatigue, but is common in psychoneurosis.

(*b*) The second type is a much coarser contraction of bundles of muscle fibres, again both visible and palpable, and though usually not moving a limb, if near enough to a joint is strong enough to do so. This is common in the outer aspect of the thigh or upper arm, but occurs in any muscle, including the pectorals and intercostals. It is not due to organic disease, but is common in fatigue and neurasthenic states. It can be stopped by temporarily obliterating the circulation to the limb and is not increased by prostigmine. (See also *Facial Myokimia,* p. 143).

Shivering

This is quite frequently seen in the muscles of patients who are cold or nervous, without the rest of the limb or body being involved. It may, therefore, be mistaken for fasciculation. Its rapid, regular movement of the whole muscle, its appearance in a series of bursts, and its cure by warmth and correcting the other simple causative factors, distinguishes it from more serious conditions.

Clonus

It is possible for individual muscle bundles to go into clonus without any active measure having been taken to elicit it and without movement of the limb as a whole. It is entirely regular, occurs only in a hypertonic limb with exaggerated reflexes, is present when that muscle is in some degree of tension, and is stopped immediately by altering the position of the limb so that the muscle is in relaxation.

Do not assume that abnormal movements are of psychogenic origin if they disappear when not under direct observation. Most involuntary movements are least obvious on complete relaxation, a state rarely achieved during physical examination.

Part IV
The Sensory System

Chapter 20
Basic Principles for Examination of Sensation

There is probably nothing more frustrating and fatiguing than the detailed examination of sensation, particularly in a patient who is so unreliable that answers are too variable to be of value, or in one so determined to report minor differences that the end result is equally confusing. It is often wise to carry out sensory examination in several stages, testing different parts of the body, or different modalities, on different occasions.

Whichever modality is being examined, try to form a mental picture both of the pathway that that particular sensation follows from the site of stimulation to appreciation in consciousness, and the relationship of that pathway to neighbouring nervous structures.

This entails a little anatomical knowledge, but though there are many varieties of sensation, long practice has taught the value of studying those forms whose tests are simple and whose anatomical pathways are well established.

It is also important to bear in mind that sensory loss is of far greater importance in some conditions than in others—e.g. in suspected syringomyelia, or in searching for the level of a lesion causing a paraplegia, or in delineating a peripheral nerve lesion, exact assessment is vital. In a hemiplegia, however, the *detailed* analysis of superficial sensory loss rarely adds much information of value.

The modalities of sensation to be tested

(*a*) Pain; light touch; and temperature. These are the exteroceptive sensations derived from sources outside the body.

(*b*) Sense of position; passive movement; vibration; and deep pain. These are the proprioceptive sensations derived from the body itself.

(*c*) Stereognosis; graphaesthesia; and two-point discrimination. These are the combined and cortical sensations.

Visceral or interoceptive sensation is a fourth group, but is rarely examined as a clinical bedside routine. In fact the word 'interoceptive' is unknown to most examiners.

Essential features of the sensory pathways

In the following paragraphs, a very complex subject is over-simplified in order to state briefly some anatomical facts that form the basis for the localisation of lesions producing sensory disturbances.

(*a*) *All forms of sensation* must travel via a peripheral nerve and a sensory root to the spinal cord, or for cranial nerves, the brain stem. A nerve or root lesion will, therefore, cause loss of all forms of sensation from the area which it supplies.

(*b*) *Fibres serving pain and temperature sensation* enter the postero-lateral aspect of the spinal cord, travel upwards a few segments and then cross to the opposite antero-lateral spino-thalamic tract. A superficial cord lesion will cause loss of these sensations on the opposite side of the body, or a central cord lesion on both sides but over a limited area. This tract ascends to the brain stem, where it lies lateral to the median fillet, and is joined by the quinto-thalamic tract (p. 65) in the pons. These fibres pass dorsal to the red nucleus and end in the ventro-lateral nucleus of the thalamus. A lesion here will cause loss of sensation throughout the whole of the opposite side of the body. It is, however, now thought that many pain fibres end in the reticular formation of the brain stem. From the thalamus, sensory impulses pass through the posterior limb of the internal capsule and the thalamo-parietal radiations to the post-Rolandic cortex, but lesions at cortical level cause little disturbance of pain and temperature.

(*c*) *Fibres carrying the sense of light touch* ascend the posterior columns of the spinal cord on the same side as they enter, as far as the nuclei gracilis and cuneatus, and further fibres then cross the midline to ascend the brain stem in the median fillet, where they are joined by touch fibres from the face. They then pass to the thalamus and on to the post-Rolandic cortex. Other elements of touch, however, on entering the cord, ascend several segments, and then relay across the midline to follow the course of the spino-thalamic tract in its anterior portion. It is for this reason that some cord lesions, especially central lesions, affect pain and temperature but not light touch.

(*d*) *The fibres carrying sense of position, of passive movement, and of vibration* ascend the cord in the posterior columns on the same side, as far as the nuclei gracilis and cuneatus, than synapse, decussate, and form the median fillet, continuing as described above. A posteriorly situated cord lesion will cause loss of these sensations below the lesion on the same side—this applies also to (*e*).

(*e*) *Stereognostic and discriminative sensations* follow the same pathway as proprioceptive sensation, but they should not be considered as separate tracts, for stereognosis depends on the sense of touch and position, and two-point discrimination on the sense of touch.

(*f*) *Facial sensation* is described in Chap. 9.

Arrangement of the sensory fibres

In the posterior columns, fibres from the lower part of the body are displaced medially as more fibres enter. *In the spino-thalamic tract*, fibres from the lower part of the body are displaced to lie superficially to those from the upper part. *In the thalamus*, fibres from the lower part of the body lie laterally to those from the trunk and arms, fibres from the face lying most medially of all. *In the sensory cortex*, fibres from the lower limbs terminate near the superior longitudinal fissure, and those from the face in the lower part of the post-Rolandic gyrus. The hand and mouth occupy a very much larger area in relation to size than other parts of the body.

Sensory dermatomes

A visual image must constantly be borne in mind of the spinal segmental supply to each area under stimulation, the shape and extent of the sensory dermatome in which it lies, and which of the peripheral nerves supplies it.

Avoid testing at the fringes of these dermatomes for considerable overlap occurs. Unfortunately, such patterns can only be learnt by heart and, though not necessarily the same in different text books, the accompanying diagrams give a practical workable scheme (Fig. 67).

Doctors, more than most, use mnemonics to help memory. In this context it is better to memorise certain key facts, and this applies to the following notes regarding sensory dermatomes, because if some facts are indelibly imprinted on one's mind, the others can be deduced.

(*a*) The patient is always considered to be standing with the palms of the hands facing forwards.
(*b*) C1 gives no supply to the skin, the occiput being supplied by C2.
(*c*) C5 supplies the outer aspect of the shoulder tip.
(*d*) C7 (the longest cervical spinous process) supplies the middle finger (the longest finger).
(*e*) T3 dermatome lies in the axilla.
(*f*) T8, T10, T12 supply the rib margin, the umbilicus and the pubis respectively.
(*g*) L3 dermatome lies at the knee. L5 runs diagonally from the outer aspect of the tibia to the inner aspect of the foot.
(*h*) S1 includes the little toe.
(*i*) S3, 4, 5 are in concentric rings round the anus.

Skin areas supplied by peripheral nerves are more difficult to remember (Fig. 67). Fortunately, though any nerve may be damaged, comparatively few are injured or diseased with any degree of frequency. These are the Vth cranial nerve, the circumflex branch of the axillary nerve (Fig. 68, Chap. 24), the radial, median and ulnar nerves (Fig. 69, Chap. 24), the femoral nerve, the lateral cutaneous nerve of the thigh, the sciatic nerve and its branches, the external popliteal and the anterior tibial nerves (Fig. 68, Chap. 24).

The purposes of all sensory tests

(*a*) To demonstrate clearly and consistently the limits of any areas of abnormal sensation.

(*b*) To determine which modalities are involved within those limits.

(*c*) To compare the findings with known patterns of abnormal sensation.

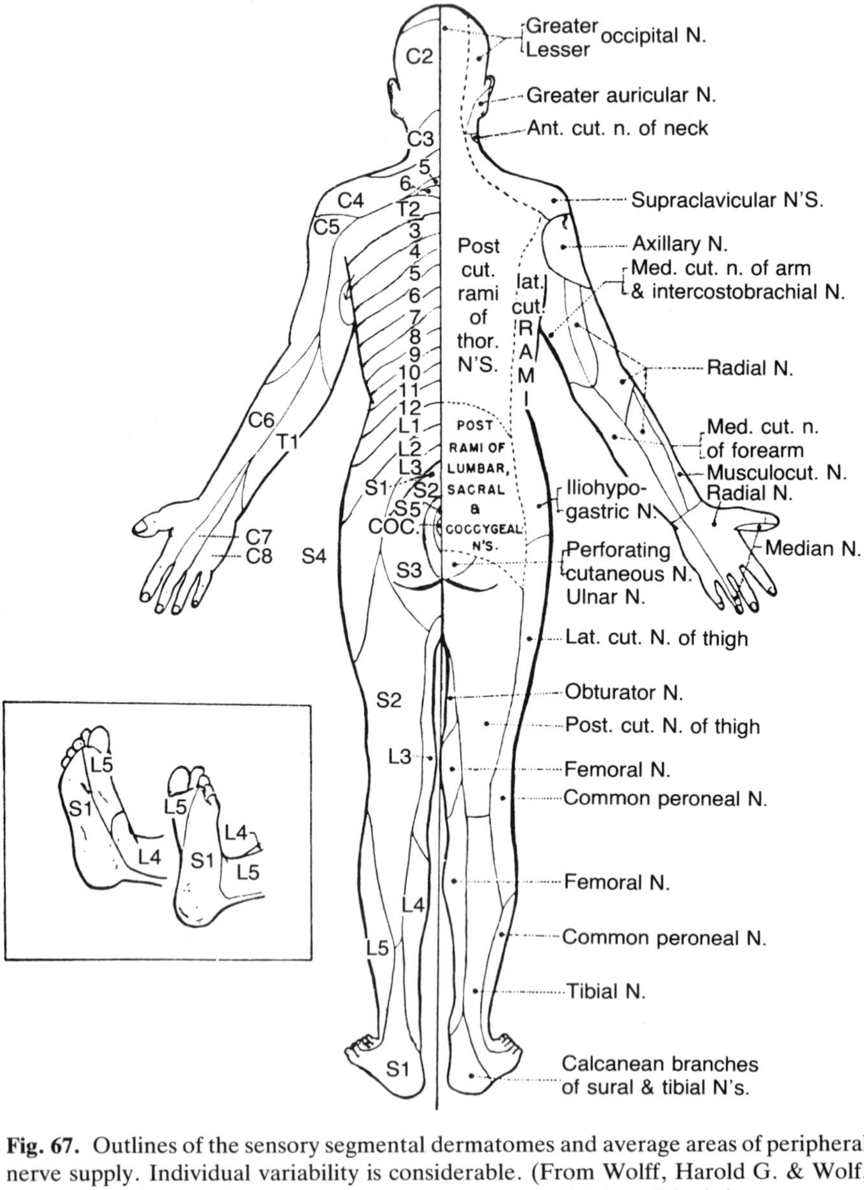

Fig. 67. Outlines of the sensory segmental dermatomes and average areas of peripheral nerve supply. Individual variability is considerable. (From Wolff, Harold G. & Wolf, Stewart (1958) *Pain*. Courtesy of Charles C. Thomas, Publisher, Illinois.)

The more experienced one becomes, the more one learns to recognise the type of case in which sensory impairment is a vital diagnostic feature and must be minutely examined; and conversely the case in which, even if present, its importance is minimal and barely justifies a tedious analysis. The less experienced must complete the examination, but must also ask himself 'is this apparent sensory impairment relevant to the diagnostic problem, or might it be a red herring drawn across the path by too minute attention to detail?' For instance, in a spastic hyper-reflex paraparesis, spending a lot of time over a very vague and inconsistent sensory level, may be completely

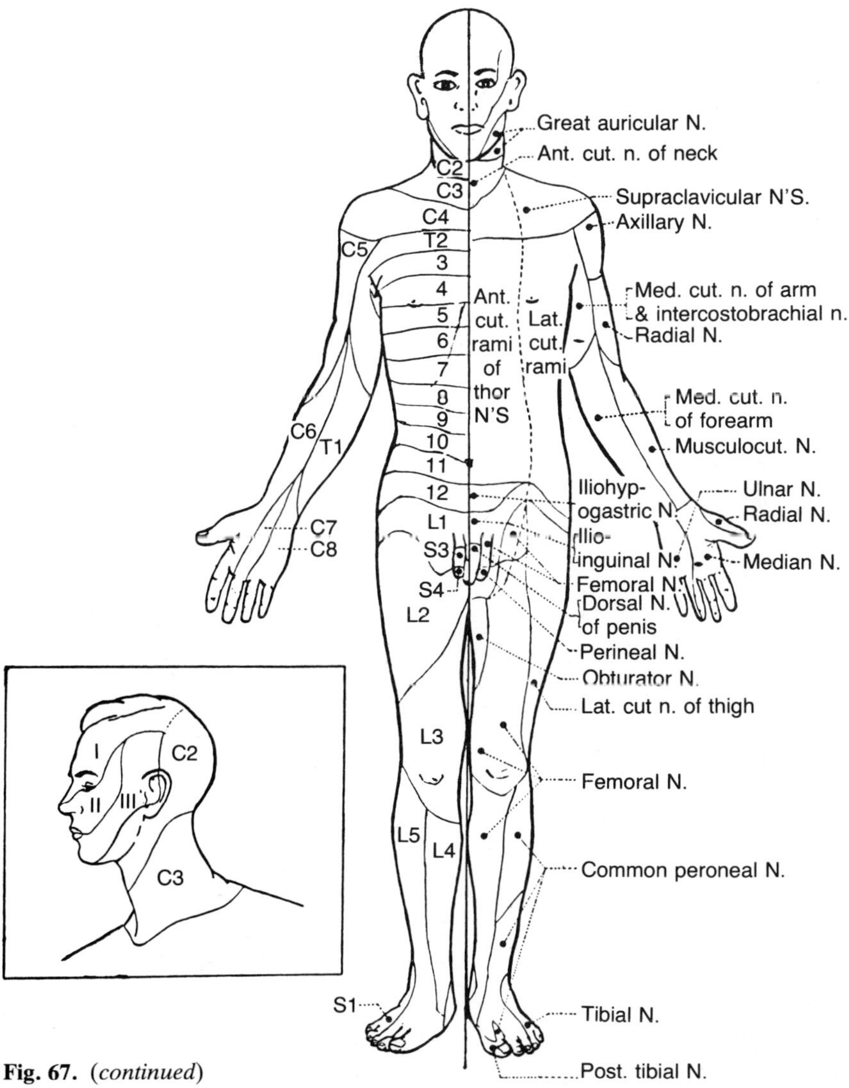

Fig. 67. (*continued*)

wasteful if one has not appreciated that the jaw jerk is grossly exaggerated so that the lesion must therefore be above the mid brain stem, and spinal sensory levels are irrelevant.

In the following chapter, each modality of sensation is considered in turn and advice is given on the methods of testing most likely to produce the clear consistent results without which this part of the examination is pointless.

Chapter 21
Pain, Touch and Temperature

PAIN

Modern investigative procedures have to a large extent supplanted the very detailed sensory testing considered so important in years gone by. But such procedures are not necessarily available to the first person who examines a patient. All sensory tests are open to faulty observation, by both patient and examiner. To try and produce uniform or graduated stimuli while testing pain, numerous pieces of apparatus have been suggested, but in practice, the simplest remains the best, and a *sharp* pin with a rounded head will serve most purposes.

Preliminary screening

First choose a part of the patient's body which, from the history, is expected to be normal and touch him precisely, but not too firmly several times with the point of the pin. Ask him (*a*) if he can feel anything, (*b*) what it is that he can feel. If he says that he can feel a point ask (*c*) if it is sharp or blunt. Remember that a single prick may not always register pain.

Having established that he recognises the stimulus, compare quickly the appreciation of the sensation in a number of areas, including the face, the shoulders, the inner and outer aspects of the lower forearms, the thumb and little finger, the upper and lower chest and abdomen, the front of the thighs, the lateral and medial aspects of the lower legs, the dorsum of the feet, the little toe, and the buttocks. Bearing in mind the *aide-mémoire* in the previous chapter, this will give a very good general idea of the overall pattern of sensory defect.

From the history, attention may have been drawn to areas likely to be abnormal. The next stage, therefore, whether the preliminary screening revealed any abnormality or not, is to test these areas particularly and in the same way.

More detailed analysis

If possible, it is wise to postpone closer analysis to a later examination. One should now go at once to the area previously roughly defined as abnormal, and, moving the pin from the centre of this area, ask the patient to say immediately the sensation changes and to describe the type of change. Mark this point and change the direction of the pin, *always moving from impaired sensation to normal sensation*, for the change is easier to detect. Do not stimulate too rapidly or the slowly reacting patient may still be referring to the last prick but one. Avoid asking 'Is it sharp?' and 'Is this sharper than that?', for a nervous patient may agree with something he does not really mean. A patient may also truthfully answer 'Can you feel that?' by saying 'Yes' even though no pain is produced. It is quite sensible to ask if there is any difference between different areas, and then what the difference is.

TOUCH

Practically all the previous remarks apply equally to the examination of light touch. Again many methods are used, but a small piece of cotton wool answers most needs, does not cause sufficient pressure to stimulate deep sensibility, and produces a sensation familiar to the patient. After similar preliminary screening, tell the patient to shut his eyes and to say 'Yes' each time he feels anything. The cotton wool is shaped to a point and the skin is then touched lightly, but not too lightly, testing again in dermatome areas, and mapping out abnormalities more clearly later by the methods already described.

TEMPERATURE

For preliminary screening, the patient can compare the temperature of a cold object such as a tuning fork in the main sensory areas of the body. After this, use test tubes containing hot water (110°F or 43°C), and cold water (45°F or 7°C). Extremes of heat and cold should not be used, for these stimulate pain fibres, but the temperatures must be maintained throughout testing.

The same principles again apply. The patient has the eyes closed, is first asked what he can feel, whether there is any difference when the other tube is used, and what that difference is.

A note on sensory levels

In the cord, the spinal segments are not necessarily at the level of the vertebra bearing the same number. In the highest cervical region they do correspond; in the low cervical region there is one segment difference, i.e. C8 spinal segment is opposite C7 vertebra. In upper thoracic regions the difference is of two segments, in mid-thoracic, three, and the lumbar and sacral segments are all opposite T11–L1 vertebrae.

In cord lesions there may be a clear-cut upper level of sensory abnormality, defined by a zone of hyperaesthesia. Remember always to test for a lower level also, for 'sacral sparing' is common.

When testing for a sensory level by moving the pin from lower to higher spinal segments, there is a danger of error. If one passes from one skin area to an adjacent area supplied by a much higher spinal segment, at the point of segmental change the patient thinks there has been a sudden increase in the intensity of the stimulus. This is easily shown on the chest, where T3/4 and C4 are adjacent, around the upper arm (T2–C5), and the thigh (S2–L2). Unless one is aware of it, a false impression may be gained of an abnormal sensory level. Try it on yourself—it is quite normal, and has been called 'the summation of sensory stimuli'.

Difficulties and fallacies

These are all 'subjective' tests; one is at the patient's mercy to some extent and it is difficult to give strictly comparable stimuli. No apparatus has found permanent favour over those described above, but care, concentration and patience are essential qualities for both examiner and patient.

Remember that the pulp of the fingers is relatively insensitive to pin-prick, but very sensitive to touch. Stimulate with the pin just proximal to the nail.

Simulation of sensory impairment is usually fairly easy to detect. The sensory loss does not correspond to known anatomical patterns; it is often confined to the *whole* of one limb; variability of margins and suggestibility are frequent; and the disability that such a severe sensory loss would produce is not apparent. Turning the patient over and repeating the tests may reverse the side affected. A sudden, painful stimulation in the analgesic area while talking about something else may produce a definite reaction, if only muscle contraction, a blink, or dilatation of the pupils, yet it is enough to show that the stimulus has been appreciated. When testing touch, the well-tried method of asking the patient, whose eyes are closed, to say 'Yes' each time he feels a touch, and 'No' each time he does not, still works in a high proportion of the less alert members of the community.

Abnormal sensory patterns are described in Chap. 24.

Chapter 22
The Proprioceptive Sensations

POSITION SENSE AND SENSE OF PASSIVE MOVEMENT

These two closely related sensations are examined together. Where most people refer to tests of position sense, or joint sense, they are usually, in fact, referring to the sense of passive movement.

Position sense

The patient's eyes should be closed throughout the examination.
(*a*) Place the patient's arm in a particular position, then move it away and ask him first to replace it himself, and then to place the opposite limb in a similar position.
(*b*) Ask him to touch the forefinger of one hand with the forefinger of the other, and make it harder by moving his finger to different positions.
(*c*) Let him try adopting similar positions with his legs, and later ask him to raise one leg to touch his own outstretched hand with his big toe.
(*d*) Ask him to place his forefinger accurately on the tip of his nose, and his heel accurately on his knee (see Chap. 26).

Sense of passive movement

The patient's eyes must still be closed. The digit (thumb, finger, or big toe) is held firmly and moved up and down, while the patient is asked if he can feel any movement. If so, he should be told that he is going to be asked whether his thumb (or toe) has been moved upwards or downwards. Move the digit widely in the appropriate directions so that he understands which movement he is to call 'up' and which 'down'. *This apparently elementary instruction is very necessary.*

Hold the sides of the digit between the finger and thumb, so that uneven pressure above or below does not reveal the direction of the movement, and make a clear and precise movement in one or other direction. Repeat the test several times, avoiding alternate movements, and if any error is made, the test should be continued until at least six successive correct responses are given, or until one is satisfied that the defect is constant.

If digit movement could not be detected in the first place, the same test is carried out at the wrist, elbow and knee.

If one suspects a very minor defect, the test can be varied by asking the patient to say 'Now' at the moment he first feels the toe moving. The movement is then made slowly, but precisely, and a remarkably slight degree of displacement is normally detected immediately. Defects of the sense of passive movement may be so gross that the patient has no knowledge of wide displacement at shoulder or hip.

Subjective awareness of posterior column deficit. It is common for a patient with posterior column defect to complain of a 'numbness' in the affected limb—a numbness which cannot be demonstrated objectively as loss of touch, pain or temperature.

Difficulties and fallacies

The most frequent difficulties are of one's own making, when the test becomes so automatic that the patient is expected to know exactly what he has to do without preliminary explanation. Waggling the toe vigorously and then suddenly moving it in one direction may be satisfactory with an intelligent and co-operative patient, but merely confuses the less alert, his responses, and the physician. The movement should always be clear and precise.

Some patients blissfully lapse into a rhythmical, alternate repetition of 'up' and 'down.' If one draws the patient's attention to this by saying firmly 'Now, think hard, I am not just going to move it up and down, up and down,' a simple measure such as this, surprisingly enough, will almost invariably overcome the difficulty, and it is rarely necessary to record the findings as 'too unreliable to be of value.' However, the patient who consistently and with unerring accuracy places his finger one inch to one side of his nose during the finger nose test is unlikely to have a genuine postural loss, especially if he does the same thing when the eyes are open.

A patient who briskly and invariably gives an answer opposite to the actual movement made need not necessarily be simulating a non-existent fault. He may quite genuinely have misunderstood the directions—hence the importance of the preliminary demonstration, which may need to be repeated.

VIBRATION SENSE

A tuning fork (128 C° or 256 C^{1}) of well-maintained vibration is shown to the patient and then placed on his clavicle to allow him to identify the sensation of vibration. He then closes his eyes, the fork is struck* and placed on bony

*It is a wise neurologist who strikes his fork on his percussion hammer or other resilient material, for constant striking on his own knee is capable of producing effusion in the joint. The senior author can testify to this!

points, starting peripherally at the internal malleolus and the lower end of the radius. If there is gross deficiency here it can then be placed on the tibial tuberosity and the elbow, the anterior superior iliac spine and the clavicle or the ribs. *Placing it in turn on the spinous processes of the vertebrae and moving upwards until it is appreciated may, on rare occasions, give the only clear sensory level of a posteriorly situated spinal tumour.*

The patient is first asked if he can feel the vibration. Do not say 'Can you feel that?' because he probably will, in fact, be able to feel the fork. Then ask him to say immediately the vibration stops. The fork is stopped by touching it and the speed with which he recognises this is noted. The two sides are now compared, first by asking if the degree of vibration feels the same, and then by comparing the promptness with which he notes the cessation of vibration. Next allow the fork to run down by itself, asking the patient to say when he can feel it no longer. Move it then quickly to the other limb, where normally vibration will still be detectable for 3–5 seconds. In minor degrees of abnormality, it is not detected when transferred from normal to abnormal side, and persists longer than usual when moved from abnormal to normal side.

Difficulties and fallacies

Always test the vibration of a strange fork first; it may be barely perceptible.

A bony point must be used. On soft tissue it may be quite imperceptible. In fat people it may be difficult to find any bony points, but in oedematous legs, the oedema can be compressed away before starting.

Unless the test is clearly explained, many patients think it is the sound that they are meant to detect and they may well hear that when *vibration* sense is lost. Do not confuse the issue by using the word 'humming'.

In increasing age, vibration sense diminishes steadily and over the age of 65 some deficit at the ankles is common. In diabetes it is reduced at a much earlier age, even in the absence of other signs of a polyneuropathy.

MUSCLE SENSITIVITY

To assess the degree of discomfort produced, the thumbs are firmly pressed into the muscles of the forearm and calves. Normally, by the time one has to strain the hand muscles a little, the patient will complain of discomfort. If the muscles are abnormally tender, there will be obvious distress under lighter pressure and the pain will continue for a few seconds after release. In states of diminished sensitivity, the patient will allow all possible force to be exerted without complaint. Squeezing the tendo achilles between the finger and thumb will allow diminished deep sensation to be assessed.

Increased muscle tenderness is found in 'infective' polyneuritis, subacute combined degeneration of the spinal cord, myositis and in some psychogenic states. Diminished tenderness occurs in tabes dorsalis, syringomyelia, carcinomatous neuropathy and in lesions of the posterior roots and root entry zones of the spinal cord.

Chapter 23
Stereognosis, Discriminative Sense and Graphaesthesia

STEREOGNOSIS

This is the ability to recognise an object purely from the feel of its shape and size. Test objects must be familiar, easily identifiable and large enough for a weak hand to feel. The patient should close his eyes and the object is placed first into the hand suspected of abnormality, and he is asked to identify it. If he fails, or takes a long time to decide, it should then be placed in the other hand and comparison made both of the accuracy and speed of response.

Abnormalities

It will usually be obvious at once whether the patient recognises the object or not. If stereognosis is defective the normal skilled movements of exploring an unknown object are absent. The hand moves as a whole instead of as a series of small joints. Often it is evident that the patient is not aware that anything has been placed in the hand and may perhaps allow it to fall out, and yet go on apparently trying to feel it.

Stereognosis is defective if touch and position sense are defective and may, therefore, be defective in severe lesions of the sensory pathway at any point. Its particular value in localisation arises when, though other forms of sensation are normal or only slightly affected, yet there is astereognosis. The lesion responsible then lies in the parietal lobe.

Difficulties and fallacies

A very weak hand may be unable to make the movements required to feel the object properly. In this case, the patient's fingers must be held closed over it.

A hand which is partly paralysed, oedematous, or deformed by some process such as rheumatoid arthritis, may be unable to close over a small object and may give a false impression unless a large enough object is used.

As stated above, severe loss of sensation will include astereognosis, so that a parietal lobe lesion must not be automatically diagnosed. Stereognostic sensation travels in the posterior columns, which means a cord lesion can produce it. It is a finding that must be taken in conjunction with the rest of the examination.

TWO-POINT DISCRIMINATION

This is the ability to detect that a stimulus consists of two blunt points when they are simultaneously applied. Explain the test to the patient first, and illustrate the sensation for him by touching his finger with the two points widely separated. He must then close his eyes and the pulp of the finger is touched firmly with either one point or two, starting with them far apart, and approximating them until he begins to make errors. The threshold is thus determined and the other hand can be compared. The same test can be carried out on the feet, preferably stimulating the dorsum of the foot. Avoid areas of calloused skin both on hands and feet.

The normal ability to distinguish the two points from one varies in different parts of the body. On the fingers it should be possible at less than 5 mm separation, but on the dorsum of the foot, separation of even 5 cm may be required and still be normal.

Two-point discrimination depends on the integrity of light touch, but if this is only slightly deficient or normal, and no signs of severe posterior column disease are present, then impairment of two-point discrimination indicates a parietal lobe lesion.

Difficulties and fallacies

Many dealers and hospitals supply a pair of compasses for this test. These are useless unless the points have been well blunted, for one must not stimulate pain fibres.

The usual cause of faulty interpretation, however, comes as a result of forgetting how different the discriminative threshold is in different parts of the body, and expecting the foot to be as sensitive as the hand.

GRAPHAESTHESIA

This is the ability to recognise letters or numbers written on the skin with a blunt point. The patient closes his eyes and letters or numerals are traced out on the palm of the hand or the anterior aspect of the forearm, thigh or lower leg. Clear figures such as 8, 4, and 5 should be used first and, if correct, the more difficult 6, 9, and 3 can be used as finer tests.

If peripheral sensation is lost, graphaesthesia will be absent, but if peripheral sensation is normal, the absence of graphaesthesia is then a sign of a parietal cortical lesion.

LOCALISATION OF TOUCH

The patient closes his eyes and then is touched on some point of the body with examiner's finger or a pin. He is asked to indicate the point touched with his own forefinger. The significance of the test is the same as for graphaesthesia and two-point discrimination.

Other sensory abnormalities associated with parietal lobe disease are described in Chap. 30.

Chapter 24
Common Patterns of Abnormal Sensation

No two patients are exactly the same. Their size, their faces, their eyes and the colour of their skin varies, and one might expect their neuroanatomy to vary similarly. It is however quite extraordinary how constant, within only a slight range, are the signs on the body of a lesion of the sensory pathways. This of course is of utmost value to that fundamental initial stage in diagnosis—the location of the lesion. In addition, this reproducibility is vital in detecting a sensory abnormality that is genuine, for sensation is after all a purely subjective phenomenon and alleged sensory loss is common, but anatomical knowledge is not!

The most common patterns of sensory abnormality are now illustrated, remembering that though anatomical pathways may not vary, lesions do vary greatly, so that the intensity of sensory abnormality may range from total loss to very slight reduction, or even hypersensitivity, and it is in these latter cases that great experience is needed for judgement of the significance of any abnormality that may be found.

Total unilateral loss of all forms of sensation (Fig. 68a).
This indicates an extensive lesion of the thalamus or its immediate neighbourhood. If all forms of sensation are truly lost, there must be gross disability. For instance, total postural loss is incompatible with normal use of a limb, and if this is claimed, and the limb used normally, the sensory loss must be non-organic.

One must however be wary of the late result of a long-standing thalamic lesion (such as a vascular episode) when motor function may have returned, but sensory diminution, not total loss, may remain.

Unilateral loss confined to all exteroceptive sensation
This can be caused by a partial lesion of the thalamus, or a lesion laterally situated in the upper brain stem. Associated signs, such as motor impairment in thalamic lesions, or cranial nerve palsies, or perhaps red nuclear tremor if in the midbrain, are likely.

When no other signs are present this also is often a hysterical sign, but the sensory impairment then usually stops exactly at the midline or some way over it, instead of a short distance from it.

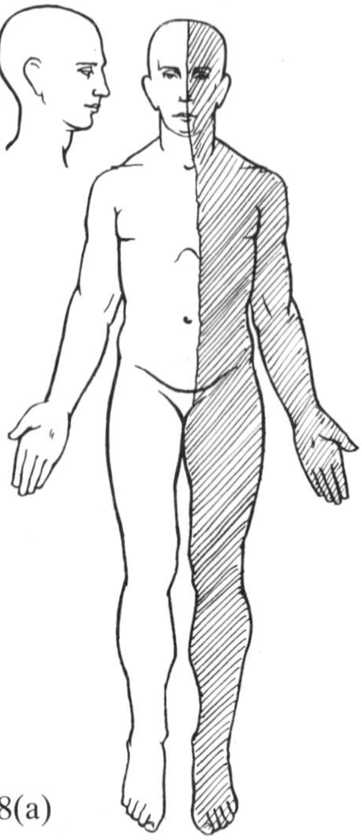

68(a)

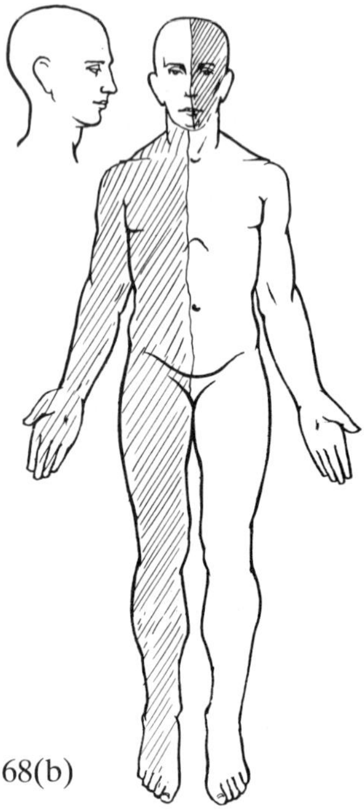

68(b)

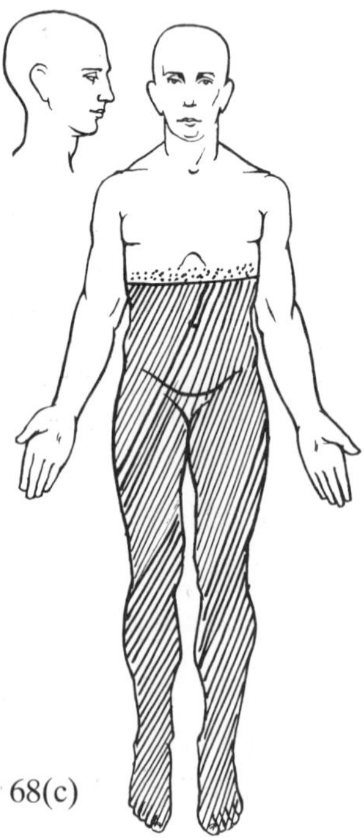

68(c)

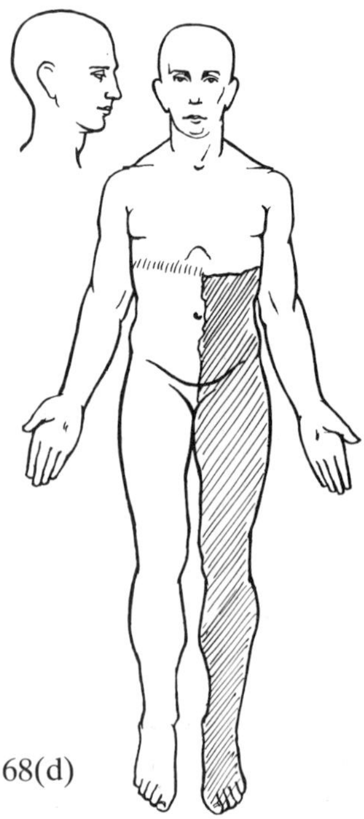

68(d)

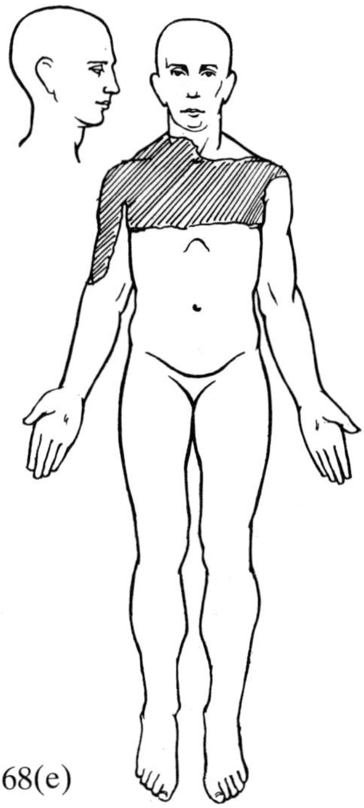

68(e)

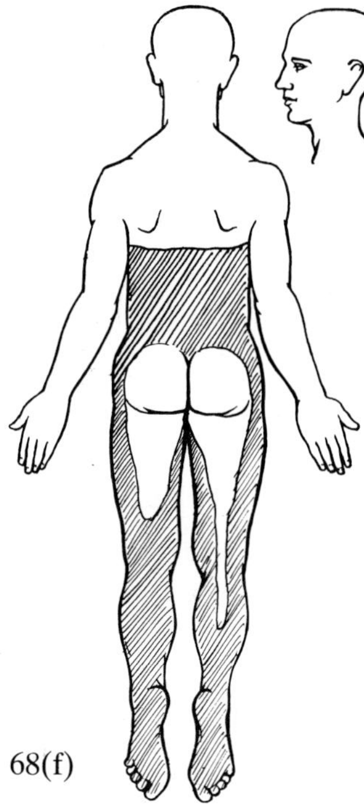

68(f)

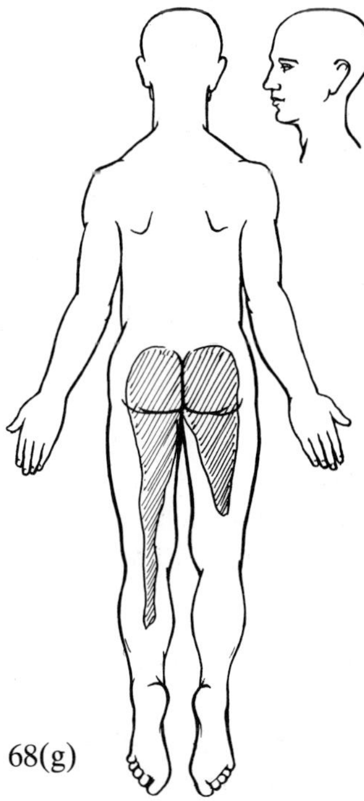

68(g)

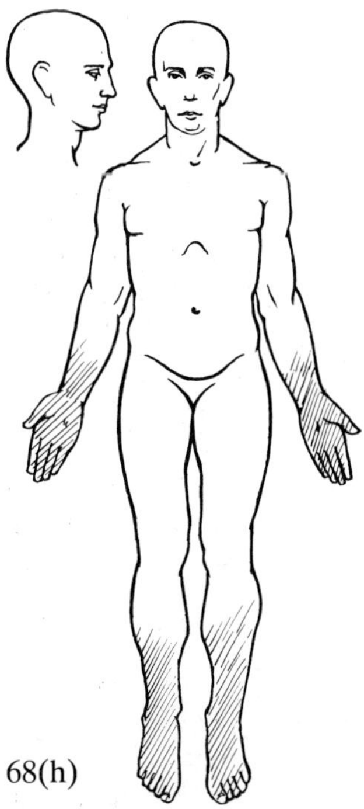

68(h)

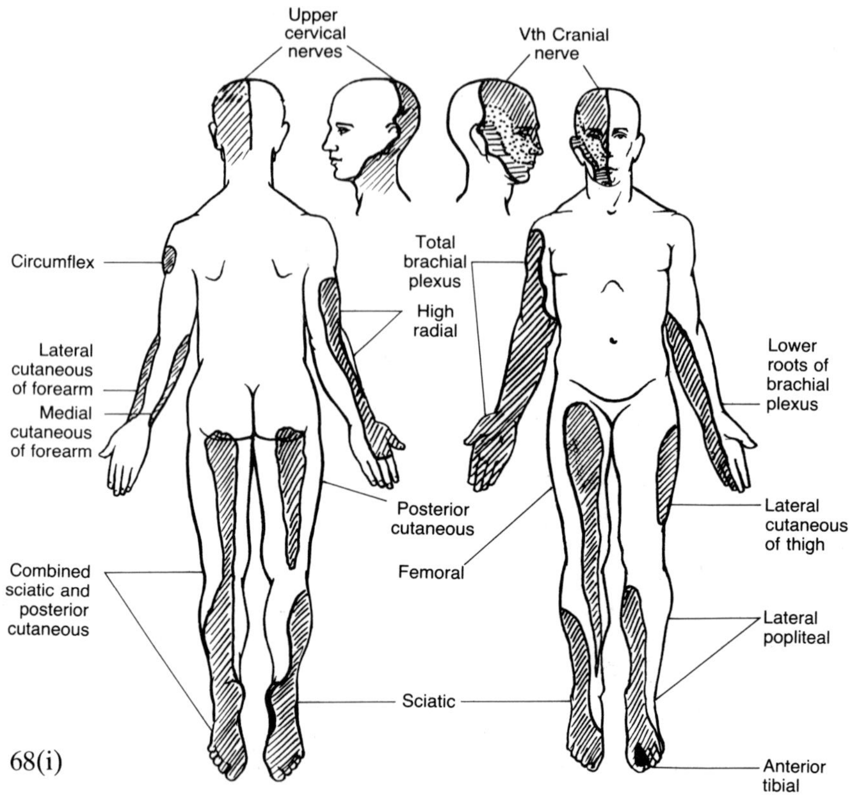

68(i)

Fig. 68. (a) Total hemianalgesia —thalamic, or upper brain stem lesion. (b) Lateral medullary lesion (usually vertebral artery deficiency). (c) Transverse lesion of the cord. (d) Brown-Séquard lesion—hemisection of the cord. (e) Cuirasse analgesia—central cord lesion. (f) Sacral sparing—cord compression, often extrinsic. (g) Saddle analgesia—cauda equina or conus medullaris lesion. (h) Glove and stocking analgesia—polyneuritis; hysteria. (i) Average areas of sensory loss resulting from the more common peripheral nerve lesions. Variation is considerable and in incomplete lesions the area involved may be greatly reduced.

Unilateral loss confined to all proprioceptive sensation

This can be caused by a partial lesion of the thalamus, or a lesion medially situated in the upper brain stem. A very uncommon finding and grossly disabling.

Unilateral loss of position sense and cortical sensation, with disturbance of light touch and the quality of pain

This indicates a parietal lobe lesion between the thalamus and the cortex. As the lesion becomes more superficial, so it would have to be increasingly large to affect all the diverging fibres. Superficial lesions, therefore, tend to affect one localised area only. Responses are characteristically variable from one moment to the next.

Unilateral hyperalgesia and hyperaesthesia

This commonly follows partial lesions of the thalamus. Usually of vascular origin and often associated with thalamic pain.

Loss of pain and temperature on one side of the face and the opposite side of the body (Fig. 68b)

This indicates a lesion of the medulla affecting the descending root of the Vth nerve, and the ascending spino-thalamic tract from the rest of the body.

This 'lateral medullary syndrome' used to be thought due to thrombosis of the posterior inferior cerebellar artery, but is now known to be due to vertebral artery deficiency and particularly likely to occur if there is, as occurs not too infrequently, a major difference between the size of the two vertebral arteries.

Bilateral loss of all forms of sensation below a definite level (Fig. 68c)

This indicates a gross lesion of the spinal cord. The upper level of the lesion may be indicated by a zone of hyperaesthesia and it is the upper level of this that should be taken as showing the highest spinal segment affected. Note this segment is not necessarily at the same level as the equivalent vertebra (see Chap. 21, p. 160).

If the upper level is vague and there is no zone of hyperaesthesia, the actual level of the lesions may be many segments higher than the sensory level suggests. See note on sacral sparing below.

If pain and temperature only are affected it will be the anterior aspect only of the cord that is involved.

Unilateral loss of pain and temperature sensation below a definite level (Fig. 68d)

This indicates a partial unilateral lesion of the spinal cord. The *Brown-Séquard syndrome* of hemisection of the cord consists of ipsilateral motor and proprioceptive impairment and contralateral loss of pain and temperature, while at the highest level on the side of the lesion there is a thin band of analgesia representing involvement of the root entry zone. It is more common, however, for compression, injury or demyelination to produce incomplete examples of this syndrome.

Impairment of pain and temperature sensation over several segments with normal sensation above and below (Fig. 68e)

This indicates an intrinsic lesion of the cord, placed near its centre and so involving the crossing fibres. If more posteriorly than anteriorly, proprioceptive sense may be lost over a similarly limited area. A common lesion in syringomyelia and intrinsic cord tumours. Loss of sensation over *many* segments (e.g. T6–S2) with normal sacral sensation is, however, common in extrinsic cord compression also (Fig. 68f).

Loss of sensation of 'saddle' type (Fig. 68g)
This is the description given to impairment of sensation over the lowest sacral segments. If affecting all forms of sensation, accompanied by loss of leg reflexes and sphincter control, it indicates a major lesion of the cauda equina. If touch is preserved, the lesion is in or near the conus medullaris, in which case the plantar reflexes may be extensor and the knee jerks may be retained.

Glove and stocking anaesthesia (Fig. 68h)
Peripheral loss of sensation affecting both hands and both feet is common in polyneuritis of any cause. In such cases there is normally impairment of reflexes as well, and this type of sensory defect with no other signs or symptoms, or with symptoms relating to some totally different part of the body, is often hysterical.

Loss of all forms of sensation over a clearly defined area in one part of the body only (Fig. 68i, Fig. 69)
This could be due to a lesion of a sensory root, or of a peripheral nerve. To differentiate, comparison must be made with the known sensory dermatomes and peripheral nerve distributions (Fig. 67). Few peripheral nerve lesions are purely sensory, while pure posterior root lesions will be.

Quite apart from common disorders such as diabetes, polyneuropathies, and one must include multiple isolated peripheral nerve lesions (mononeuritis multiplex), are seen in the collagen diseases, especially, as regards the latter, in polyarteritis nodosa, but these days they must also be carefully looked for in patients on one of the many cytotoxic preparations, for they may represent an early toxic manifestation.

Loss of vibration sense alone
If affecting the lower limbs, this is common in intrinsic cord lesions such as those produced by multiple sclerosis and syringomyelia, and has led some to suggest that vibration sensation has a different pathway from other proprioceptive sensations. Impairment is common in old age.

Loss of position and vibration sense alone
This indicates a lesion of the posterior columns which is often difficult to

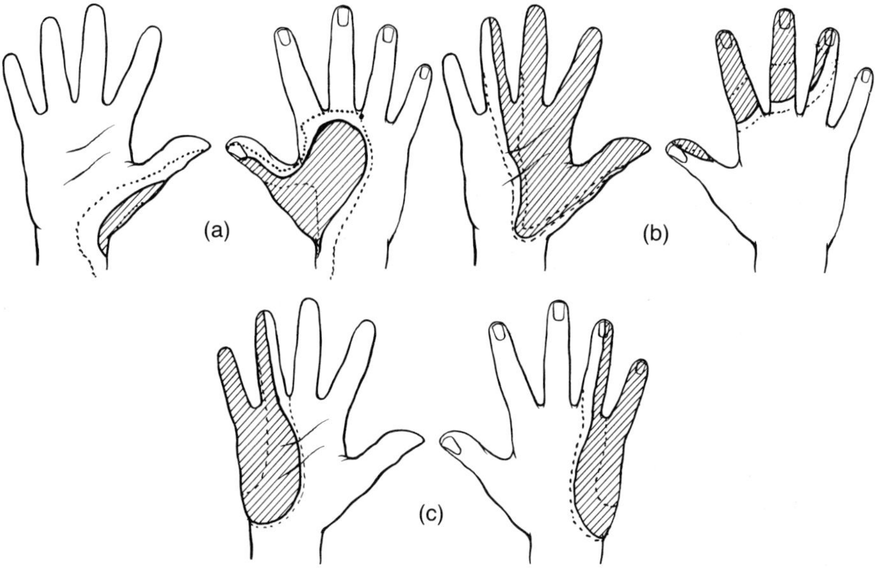

Fig. 69. Area supply of (a) radial, (b) median, (c) ulnar nerves. In each the heavy line represents the average areas of loss to touch and the dotted lines the degrees of variation which are common. Pain is often lost over less than the smaller area of supply.

localise. It is common in tabes dorsalis, sub-acute combined degeneration, Friedreich's ataxia, carcinomatous neuropathy and certain toxic states such as those due to organic mercurial compounds.

If lost only below a definite level, there may be compression of the posterior part of the cord. If the arms are affected to a much greater extent than the legs, and asymmetrically, the lesion may be due to a combination of cervical spondylosis and a very narrow vertebral canal; or to foramen magnum lesions, especially with tonsillar prolapse (see also page 135).

Miscellaneous features

Patchy areas of loss of sensation below a certain level are common in intrinsic lesions of the spinal cord secondary to such conditions as cervical spondylosis. They are also found during recovery from a Brown-Séquard lesion. Patches of sensory loss irregularly scattered throughout the body occur in chronic polyneuritides, and in leprosy. Patches on the face, the forearms, the lower legs and bands of abnormality on the trunk occur in tabes. Except in defining a mononeuritis multiplex, the exact charting of very vague patches of sensory loss rarely gives clinical information of a value comparable to the time taken to complete the task. It is the overall picture and pattern that needs to be assessed.

Areas of hypersensitivity, if corresponding to the segmental dermatomes, indicate lesions of the posterior root or the root entry zone of the cord. If these areas correspond with the distribution of the peripheral nerve, they usually mean an incomplete or recovering lesion of the nerve. Very transient, very localised areas of hyperaesthesia are not uncommon in normal people; their aetiology is uncertain but they do not represent a disease process.

Part V
The Motor-Sensory Links

Chapter 25
The Reflexes

Any reflex action requires a stimulus, a sensory pathway, a link with a motor unit, a motor neurone, and, finally, a contractile or other effector element. Any breach in this arc results in an absent reflex. Most reflex arcs are also influenced by higher centres, and where there is a breach in the pathways from these centres, the behaviour of the reflex is fundamentally changed.

Purpose of the examination

No matter which reflex is being examined, one must determine:

(*a*) Whether the reflex is present or absent.

(*b*) If present, whether it is normal, or showing signs that influences from higher centres are defective.

(*c*) If absent, whether the arc is breached on the motor or sensory side.

(*d*) Whether any abnormalities are unilateral, bilateral, affecting all reflexes, or whether a definite level can be detected in the nervous system at which abnormalities first appear, for reflex 'levels' may be as helpful as sensory levels.

THE TENDON REFLEXES

Any skeletal muscle will contract reflexly when suddenly stretched, the tendons merely being convenient structures with which to produce this stretching. Certain muscles are, however, easy of access and by long experience their normal and abnormal responses have been defined.

For clarity of results there are certain requisites:

(*a*) A good percussion hammer (p. 5).

(*b*) An examiner with flexible wrists who allows the weight of the hammer to decide the strength of the blow.

(*c*) A patient who is warm, comfortable and relaxed.

(*d*) A muscle placed in the optimum position, slightly on stretch, but with plenty of room for contraction.

(*e*) A constant mental picture of the segmental and peripheral nerve supply of each muscle as its reflex is being tested.

The jaw jerk

This is described under the Vth cranial nerve (see Chap. 9). It represents one of the most helpful in finding a 'level' of reflex abnormality.

THE UPPER LIMBS

If possible the patient should at first be partially propped up, the elbows slightly flexed, the hands lying loosely across the abdomen, the fingers just not touching (see illustrations). In this position, the biceps and supinator jerks can be tested.

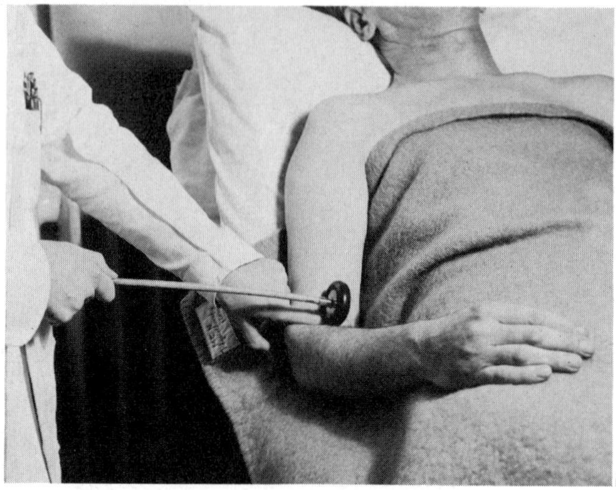

Fig. 70. The biceps jerk.

The biceps jerk (Fig. 70)
Technique. Press the forefinger gently on the biceps tendon in the antecubital fossa and then strike the finger with the hammer.
Normal result. Flexion of the elbow and visible contraction of the biceps muscle.
Segmental innervation. **C5** *Peripheral nerve.* **Musculo-cutaneous**

The supinator jerk (Fig. 71)
Technique. Strike the lower end of the radius about 2 inches above the wrist. Watch the movement of the forearm and fingers.
Normal result. Contraction of the brachio-radialis and flexion of the elbow. The biceps often contracts as well and slight flexion of the fingers may occur (see p. 188 for the 'inverted supinator reflex).
Segmental innervation. **C5–6** *Peripheral nerve.* **Radial**

The triceps jerk (Fig. 72)
Technique. By holding the patient's hand, draw the arm across the trunk and allow it to lie loosely in the new position. Then strike the triceps tendon 5 cm (2 inches) above the elbow. If there is no response, repeat two or three times either side of the original point.

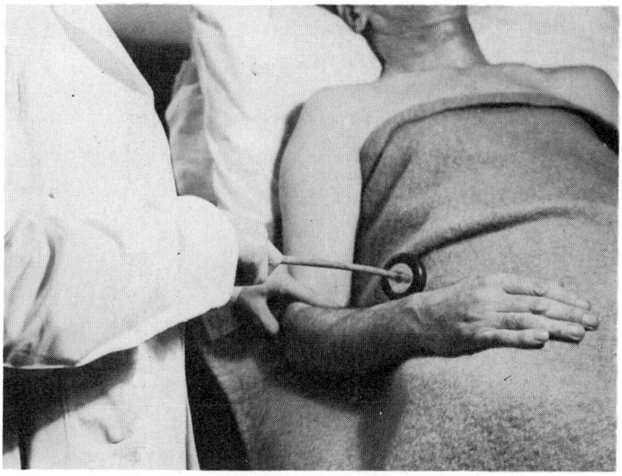

Fig. 71. The supinator jerk.

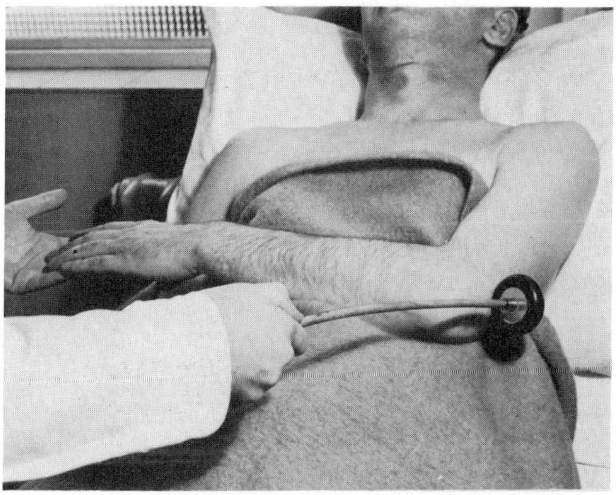

Fig. 72. The triceps jerk.

Normal result. Extension of the elbow and visible contraction of the triceps.
Segmental innervation **C6–7** *Peripheral nerve.* **Radial**

The pectoral reflexes
Technique. Place the tips of the fingers on the pectoral muscle as it forms the anterior margin of the axilla and strike the fingers.
Normal result. Adduction of the arm and visible contraction of the pectoralis major.
Segmental innervation. **C5–T1** *Peripheral nerves.* **Lateral and medial pectoral**

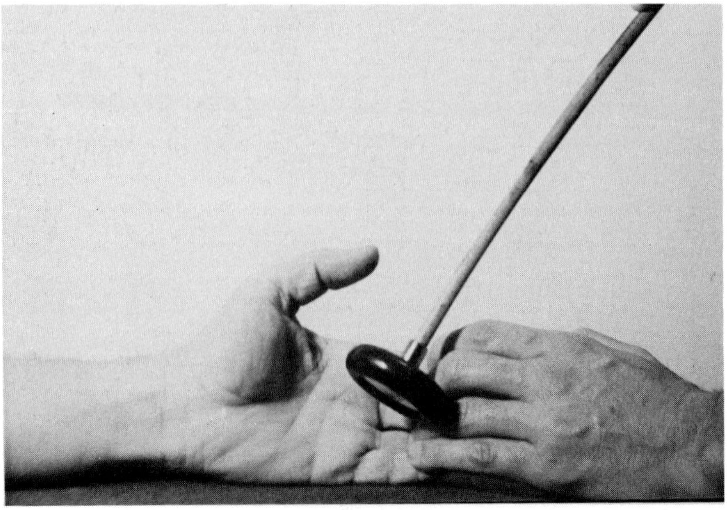

Fig. 73. The finger flexion reflex

The finger flexion reflex (Fig. 73)
Technique. Allow the patient's hand to rest palm upwards, the fingers slightly flexed. The examiner gently interlocks his fingers with the patient's and strikes them with the hammer.
Normal result. Slight flexion of all fingers and of the interphalangeal joint of the thumb.
Segmental innervation. **C6–T1** *Peripheral nerve.* **Median**

THE LOWER LIMBS

The patient should lie in the same position as described for the upper limbs, but care should be taken to see that the legs do not extend beyond the foot of the couch which in most hospitals appear to have been constructed for medieval man.

The knee jerk (Fig. 74)
Technique. The eye should not be too high above the patient's knees, and so if the bed is too low the examiner may have to kneel. To compare the two sides, the left arm (for a right-handed examiner) is placed under both knees in order to flex them together. If the patient holds the legs rigidly, instruct him to lie back and let his heels fall on the bed. This often produces complete relaxation. The patella tendon can then be struck lightly on each side, increasing the strength if there is no response. A light tap is best for comparing the two sides. Watch the movements of the lower leg and of the quadriceps muscle.

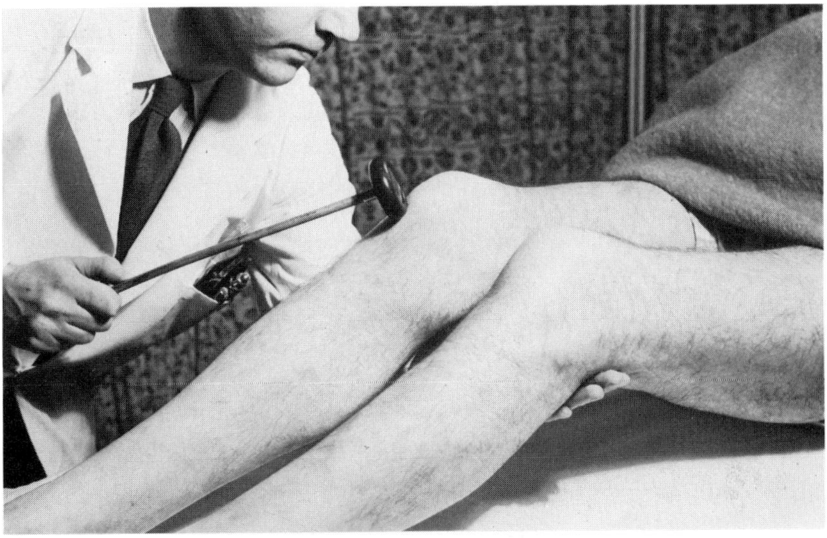

Fig. 74. The knee jerk.

Normal result. Extension of the knee and visible contraction of the quadriceps.
Segmental innervation. **L3–4** *Peripheral nerve.* **Femoral**

Alternative methods
Place the finger just above the patella and, while the legs are extended, strike it in a peripheral direction. The quadriceps contracts and the patella will be pulled upwards. This method detects slight differences between the two sides and can be used when the lower leg has been amputated, or the patella removed.

Another well-known method is to seat the patient on the edge of the couch so that the legs are dangling. This may produce a reflex in unrelaxed patients, but often the rigidity persists. It will, however, clearly show the pendular character of the reflexes in cerebellar disease.

The ankle jerk (Fig. 75)
Technique. This reflex appears to present technical difficulties, and is frequently recorded as absent when correct technique produces a perfectly normal response. The patient's leg should be externally rotated and slightly flexed at the knee. The back of the examiner's left hand should then be placed along the sole of the patient's foot, slightly dorsiflexing the foot (Fig. 75a).

For the left leg, the palm of the left hand is used, the examiner moving to the other side of the bed (Fig. 75b). The achilles tendon is then struck and

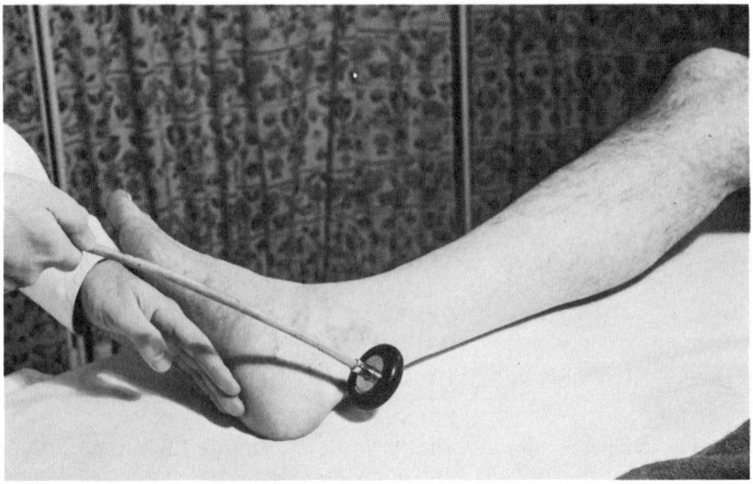

(a)

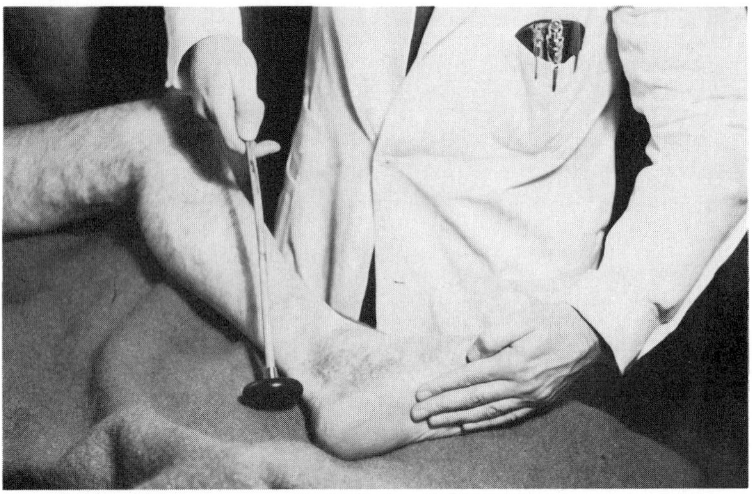

(b)

Fig. 75. The ankle jerk.

both the movement of the foot and the contraction of the calf muscles are watched.

Normal result. Plantar flexion of the foot and contraction of the gastrocnemius.

Segmental innervation. **S1** *Peripheral nerve.* **Medial popliteal**

Alternative method

A patient who is fit enough can kneel up on a cushioned or blanketed chair, with his back to the examiner and the feet projecting over the edge. The achilles tendon can then be struck from above, and it is very easy to compare the responses on the two sides.

Examination with reinforcement

If a tendon reflex appears reduced or absent, this need not necessarily be of pathological significance. Such a situation is often found in patients involuntarily tensing themselves, and those very relaxed, such as a happy young child, and perhaps rather surprisingly very muscular individuals. If other muscles are placed under strain, it often becomes possible to obtain a normal reflex.

For the upper limbs, the patient should clench his teeth tightly, or while one arm is being examined he should clench the fist of the other.

For the lower limbs, these measures can still be used, but the well-tried method of Jendrassek is more reliable. The patient interlocks the flexed fingers of the two hands and pulls one against the other at the moment thc reflex is stimulated.

Whatever the method used, the patient must make the movement at the moment that the reflex is tested and relax afterwards.

OTHER ALLIED REFLEXES

The Hoffman reflex (Fig. 76)

The terminal phalanx of the patient's middle finger is flicked downwards between the examiner's finger and thumb. In states of hyper-reflexia, organic

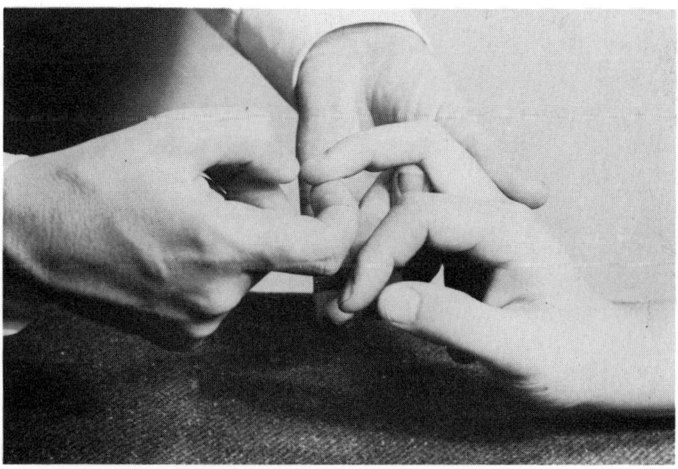

Fig. 76. Testing the Hoffman reflex.

or emotional, the tips of the other fingers flex and the thumb flexes and adducts. It is finding it on one side only that is useful for this can sometimes be an early sign of unilateral pyramidal tract disease.

Wartenberg's sign (Fig. 77)
The patient supinates his hand, slightly flexing the fingers. The examiner pronates his hand and links his similarly flexed fingers with the patient's. Both then flex their fingers further against each other's resistance. Normally, the thumb extends, though the terminal phalanx may flex slightly. In

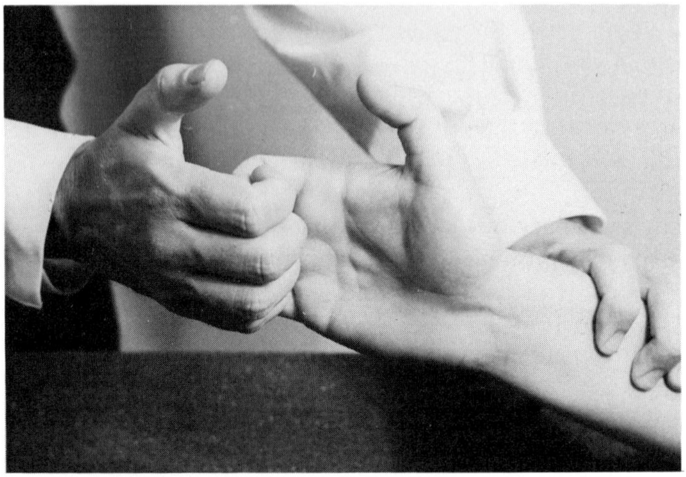

Fig. 77. Wartenberg's sign. Normal result. Note the extension of the patient's thumb.

pyramidal tract lesions the thumb adducts and flexes strongly. Unfortunately, this is not a constant sign, but if present on one side only it can indicate an early stage of pyramidal tract disease.

Rossolimo's reflex
The patient lies supine with the leg extended and the foot partially dorsiflexed. The ball of the foot is then struck with the hammer and in hypertonic states there is a brisk contraction of all toes. The same reflex can be obtained by flicking the toes in an upward direction. Its significance is the same as the finger flexion reflex in the upper limb.

Abnormalities of the tendon reflexes

Only by repeated examination of reflexes can sufficient experience be gained to judge a particular response as normal or abnormal. It is therefore very important, as in examination of the fundus, for tendon reflexes to be examined in all patients, not only those suspected of neurological disease. Gross abnormalities are easy to recognise, but when deviations from normal are slight, it is necessary to re-examine several times before a decision is reached.

EXAGGERATION

(*a*) A reflex may be *excessively brisk*, the movement being a sudden, short-lived jerk. Sometimes its amplitude may be very small and unless both limb and muscle are watched it may be thought to be reduced. This type of reflex is seen in lesions of the upper motor neurones, and in clinical practice is generally taken to be one of the manifestations of a lesion of the pyramidal system. Similar reflexes occur in agitation, fright, anxiety, and after violent exercise, but they return to normal on rest and relaxation, and there are no other features of pyramidal lesions.

(*b*) The reflex may be *excessively prolonged*. This can occur in two ways. In cerebellar lesions, particularly if there is some element of upper motor neurone disease as well, the reflex is not so much a brisk one as a large one—the amplitude being greater, the speed reduced. In certain positions of the limb it may sway back beyond its starting point and oscillate in a pendular fashion. Secondly, prolongation occurs in myxoedema. The movement is retarded, especially during relaxation, so that the impression of a slightly slow-motion film is obtained, the reflex appearing to 'hang-up' compared with a normal jerk.

(*c*) A reflex may be *clonic*.The muscle which has been stretched goes into clonic contractions until the stretch is relieved. This is most commonly seen in the knee and ankle jerks and sometimes in the finger jerk. It indicates a marked degree of reflex excitability and usually means pyramidal system disease.

REDUCTION OR ABSENCE

Reflexes appreciably reduced or absent in normal individuals become normal on reinforcement. Pathologically, reduction occurs under the following circumstances:

(*a*) When there is a breach in any part of the reflex arc, e.g. lesions of the sensory nerve (polyneuritis), the sensory root (tabes dorsalis), the anterior horn cell (poliomyelitis), the anterior root (spinal compression), the peripheral motor nerve (trauma), the terminal nerve endings (polyneuritis), or the muscle itself (myopathies, periodic paralysis). There are, of course, many other possible disorders at these various sites.

(*b*) In the state of so-called cerebral or spinal 'shock' which occurs immediately after a severe cerebral catastrophe or spinal injury. Spasticity and reflex overactivity may be delayed for hours, days or weeks. An extensor plantar response often appears long before the tendon reflexes return.

(*c*) When great rigidity, spasticity or muscle contracture more or less splint the joints so that movement cannot occur. Advanced spastic paraplegia and severe extra-pyramidal rigidity usually cause this situation, but it can be found in normal individuals completely unable to relax. In the latter, re-examination at another, less anxious, time usually produces satisfactory reflexes. An ankylosed joint may not move, but the muscle whose tendon is being tapped will show the contraction.

Two important combinations of reflex abnormality

The inverted supinator jerk

When the supinator jerk is tested, there is often a slight flexion of the fingers. This may become very obvious when all the reflexes of the upper limb are exaggerated. If, however, finger flexion is the only response, contraction of the brachioradialis and elbow flexion being absent, then the reflex is said to be 'inverted'. In practice, this is usually associated with an absent biceps jerk, and exaggeration of the finger and triceps jerks. The difference between the reflex activity of the biceps and triceps may be so marked that striking the biceps tendon produces *extension* of the elbow.

The inverted supinator reflex indicates a cord lesion at the fourth or fifth cervical level, causing a lower motor neurone lesion of C5 and an upper motor neurone lesion of reflexes innervated below this level. It is very common in cervical disc disease, syringomyelia, cervical trauma and sometimes in cervical neoplasms. It is invaluable in localising lesions responsible for a spastic paraparesis which have no sensory abnormality or clear-cut level. This applies particularly to cervical spondylosis.

Lesions of the conus medullaris

Classically the ankle jerks only are absent in lesions of the conus medullaris. In practice, as these lesions frequently extend into the conus from higher in the cord, there may however be loss of both knee and ankle jerks, but, at the same time, an extensor plantar response. This is associated with symmetrical dissociated saddle anaesthesia, spontaneous segmental sweating in the sacral segments, and loss of bladder and rectal control.

In combined upper and lower motor neurone lesions, such as occur in sub-acute combined degeneration of the spinal cord, or tabo-paresis, a similar combination of reflex changes may be found, but there is not the characteristic segmental sensory loss and loss of sphincter control.

Difficulties and fallacies

Failure of relaxation is the major difficulty in examining tendon reflexes. Re-examination is wise just before leaving the patient, for, knowing that it is all over, he will be in a greater state of relaxation than at any other time, providing the techniques used have been gentle and sympathetic.

Faulty positioning of the limb, especially for the ankle jerk, is another cause of difficulty and advice has been given at some length on this point.

Many patients make a confusing, semi-voluntary jerk of the limb shortly after the reflex has occurred. Pointing out to the patient that it is he who is doing it, that it is confusing, and bluntly asking him to stop it, seems to be effective.

Arthritic patients often fear that the test will be painful, hold themselves rigid, and jump violently when the tendon is struck. Start with a very gentle tap and gradually work up to the normal strength of stimulus.

Always watch the muscle itself as well as limb movement. When the biceps reflex is absent, on striking the tendon, the elbow may appear to flex, but a glance at the biceps itself will show no contraction at all.

The jaw jerk is often thought to be of little importance, but its value is, in fact, very great (see p. 67).

In amputees, the reflex muscular contraction may be normal, but the amount of limb to be moved is so small that there is apparently a very brisk response. In a normal patient with a below-the-knee amputation, the stump may even go into a form of clonus.

No apology is made for repeating that clonus is only a manifestation of heightened muscle tone, and it may occur in very tense or frightened individuals, after straining, or after exercise. It is, however, rarely long-sustained as in pyramidal system disease, it is usually equal on the two sides, and truly clonic reflexes are not obtained.

THE SUPERFICIAL REFLEXES

For practical purposes, only four of the many superficial reflexes are routinely tested—the abdominal reflexes, the cremasteric reflexes, the anal reflex, and the all-important plantar reflexes.

The abdominal reflexes (including the epigastric reflex)

Technique. The patient should first lie flat. Palpate the abdomen gently to assess the degree of relaxation and the sensitivity of the skin. Then explain that something is about to be drawn across the stomach, illustrating the manoeuvre on the chest. Any physician who has unexpectedly had his abdominal reflexes examined will appreciate the value of this warning.

Lightly stroke the abdomen with a pencil, key, or two-point discriminator, from without inwards, stimulating each of the four quadrants of the abdomen and the lower margins of the thoracic cage in turn.

Normal result. The muscles in the quadrant stimulated contract and the umbilicus moves in that direction.

Segmental innervation. Epigastric **T7–9**; upper abdominals **T9–11**; lower abdominals, **T11, 12** (sometimes also L1)

Abnormal responses

(*a*) *Exaggerated abdominal reflexes* occur in psychoneurosis, often in the absence of overt anxiety, and may also be brisk in simple nervousness.

(*b*) *Absent abdominal reflexes* may be due to:

1 Defects of technique, relaxation, or observation.

2 A breach of the appropriate reflex arc, due to lesions such as herpes zoster, or surgical operations which have damaged the peripheral nerves or the muscle itself.

3 Pyramidal system lesions above the upper level of segmental innervation. This is more common in spinal lesions (ipsilateral or bilateral) than in cerebral lesions (contralateral), but the reflexes are not necessarily absent in all such cases, or in one case on all occasions.

(*c*) *Easily fatigued reflexes.* In the young this may be a sign of early pyramidal disease.

(*d*) *An inverted response.* Occasionally, when the abdominal reflexes are absent on one side, stimulation on that side produces muscular contraction on the normal side, so that the umbilical deviation takes place towards the normal side.

Difficulties and fallacies

If the patient has a very fat abdomen, one scarred by enthusiastic surgeons, or exhausted by frequent pregnancies, muscular contraction may not be visible or may not occur. Slight contraction of the external oblique may still be visible, and stimulation near to the ribs and inguinal ligaments often produces a local response not visible elsewhere.

If a patient has difficulty in relaxing, it may be possible to obtain these reflexes by testing them with the patient sitting on the edge of the bed, or even standing upright.

The stimulus should be light and never unpleasant. Pins should not be used. An abdomen resembling a problem in Euclid carries the trade mark of a bad examiner.

Heavy stimulation may produce a deep abdominal reflex, which, being a tendon reflex, is often exaggerated when the superficial reflexes are absent.

A big fallacy is a belief that abdominal reflexes are rarely retained in multiple sclerosis. They are, indeed, often absent, but their presence in no way invalidates the diagnosis, and they may persist in the advanced stages of the disease.

The cremasteric reflexes

Technique. The upper inner part of the thigh is stroked in a downward and inward direction, the patient lying down or standing up. Watch the movement of the scrotum and testicle.

Normal result. The contraction of the cremasteric muscle pulls up the scrotum and testicle on the side examined.
Segmental innervation. **L1–2**

Abnormal responses

Exaggeration has no special importance. The reflex is often absent in:
(*a*) Elderly men and those who have hydroceles, or have had scrotal operations.
(*b*) Any breach of the reflex arc, including impaired sensation over the skin of the thigh.
(*c*) Pyramidal tract disease, but there is the same inconstancy of response shown by the abdominal reflexes.

The anal reflex

Technique. Lightly scratch the peri-anal skin.
Normal result. Contraction of the external sphincter.
Segmental innervation. **S4, 5**

The plantar reflex

This is the most important reflex in the body, and yet the most frequently misinterpreted.
Technique. Many methods are recommended; even more are used. If the following instructions are observed, many of the difficulties are overcome.

Start by positioning the patient so that the knee is slightly flexed, and the thigh externally rotated. The outer aspect of the foot should now rest on the couch as for testing the ankle jerk. Warn the patient that the sole of the foot will be scratched and ask him to try to let the foot remain loose. The outer aspect of the sole is then firmly stroked with a *blunt* point such as a key, the end of the percussion hammer handle, or the two-point discriminator. The stimulator should move forwards and then curve inwards towards the middle metatarso-phalangeal joint (Fig. 78). The stimulus must be firm, but not frankly painful. A pin should not be used, nor should the stimulus be a tickle, for this produces abnormal responses in normal individuals. Do the stimulation slowly and allow yourself time to see what is happening.

Watch the first movement of the metatarso-phalangeal joint of the great toe, which in this position is immediately visible. Watch also the movement and behaviour of the other toes. The test should now be repeated with the knee in extension, and in case of doubt the knee may even be pressed downwards. In this new position, early abnormalities may be detected which disappear when the knee is flexed. The two methods serve as a check on each other.
Normal result. Normally, no matter what its shape may be, the great toe will

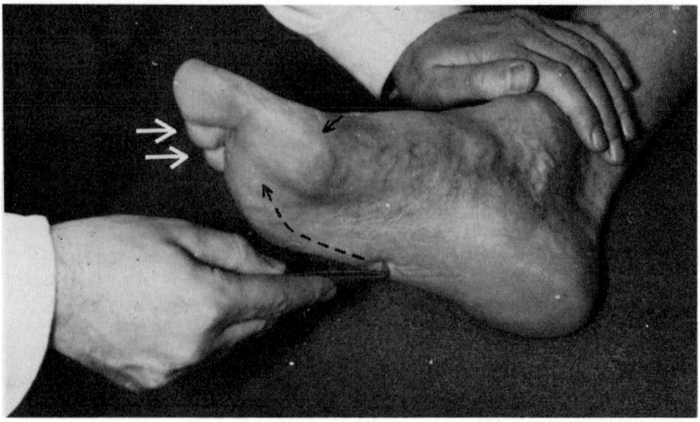

Fig. 78. The plantar reflex. The dotted line indicates the direction taken by the instrument. The arrows indicate the points to watch.

flex at the metatarso-phalangeal joint, even if the terminal joint appears to extend. At the same time, the other toes will flex and close together. The true reflex movement normally does not start when the stimulus is started, but when the instrument is about one-third of the way along the foot, or sometimes not until the end of the movement.

Abnormal responses

No response at all usually indicates that the patient is not relaxed or is very cold. Sometimes total loss of sensation interferes with the sensory side of the reflex arc, or total paralysis of the muscles makes any movement impossible.

The Babinski response

The Babinski response consists of extension of the great toe at the metatarso-phalangeal joint, and usually the interphalangeal joint as well, while the other toes open out in a fanwise manner and are dorsiflexed. The movement is usually a slow one, but may be jerky and repeated. This may particularly happen if the stimulus is ended in a quick flick. If only the great toe extends this may be a true extensor response; if the whole foot extends it is often a voluntary movement. In advanced cases the whole foot dorsiflexes, the knee and hip flex, and the contraction of the muscles responsible can be felt. In cases where the toe does not move, there may be palpable and visible contraction of the tensor fasciae latae.

The Babinski response indicates disturbance of the function of the pyramidal system, a fact on which there is both clinical and experimental agreement. It does not necessarily mean a structural lesion of the pyramidal tract and may, for instance, be found in coma from almost any cause. In advanced pyramidal disease this response may be obtained from stimulating over a wide area, even as high as the thigh.

Difficulties and fallacies

The main difficulties arise from failure of relaxation, and from voluntary movements made as a result of the unpleasant sensation. The preliminary warning and avoiding the use of traumatic stimuli are the first steps in overcoming this problem.

Some patients, however, are truly unable to tolerate the sensation. Stimulating the outer *side* of the foot, even slightly on the dorsum, causes less distress, or the stimulator may be placed on the sole and pressed inwards, then drawn slowly forwards without altering the pressure. This will often allow the response to be seen before the patient withdraws his foot. If, during the test, the patient takes a deep breath, attention is distracted enough to allow a few moments of relaxation.

In marked pes cavus, it is difficult to assess the movement of the big toe. At times the movement may be frankly extensor, but this need not be a sign of a new pathological process. The toe may be so retracted as to appear to be in the extensor position to start with and if the terminal joint only is observed a further extension may be quite misleading. Always watch the metatarso-phalangeal joint.

Deformities may prevent any movement of the big toe at all. This applies particularly to a surgically corrected hallux valgus. In such cases, the type of movement of the other toes must be observed.

Complete paralysis of the extensors of the toes may make Babinski's response impossible. This is only rarely of importance, however, for such total paralysis is likely to be of lower motor neurone origin. The contraction of the tensor fasciae latae must be observed.

The plantar response is normally extensor below the age of six months, and this may persist up to twelve months in about 75% of children. After this, however, it should be flexor.

A Babinski response is an extensor plantar response. 'Babinski flexor' is a contradiction of terms.

Several other methods of obtaining the plantar reflex have been described. The three most commonly used are:

(*a*) *The Oppenheim reflex.* A firm stroke with the finger and thumb down either side of the anterior border of the tibia, greater pressure being applied to the medial side.

(*b*) *The Gordon reflex.* A hard squeeze of the calf muscles.

(*c*) *The Chaddock reflex.* A light stroke below the external malleolus, on the outer side of the foot.

Each has the same significance as the Babinski response, but each is less reliable. These methods can, however, be applied to (*a*) patients whose soles are extremely sensitive; (*b*) some patients whose co-operation is poor; and (*c*) children, while their attention is directed elsewhere.

OTHER IMPORTANT REFLEXES

The tonic neck reflexes

A lesion situated high in the brain stem, or basal nuclei, will produce a state of *decortication*. The patient lies with flexion of the arms and extension of the legs (cf. *decerebration* where arms and legs are rigidly extended). In such a case, forced turning of the head to one side produces extension of the arm on that side, and increased flexion on the other, the limbs returning to their original positions when the neck is no longer moved.

In some cases of hemiplegia due to lesions at this level, the same movements can be seen, but only on the affected side. The value of the test is that it can be carried out on totally unco-operative and stuporose patients, and that it indicates the likely site of the responsible lesion. Vascular accidents, injuries, high brain stem tumours, and diffuse encephalitic processes most commonly produce this state.

The grasp reflex

First place the first and second fingers of one hand between the thumb and forefinger of the patient's hand and try to draw them lightly away. Then place these fingers on the palm of the patient's hand and move them peripherally towards the tips of the fingers. If a grasp reflex is present the fingers will be held tightly by the hand in the first instance, the hold increasing as the effort to draw away is increased. In the second instance, the patient's fingers will flex strongly.

This reflex is normal in babies under four months. It occurs in mental deficiency and birth injuries; in tumours and vascular accidents in the premotor cortex, particularly on the medial surface of the brain; and in lesions of the corpus callosum, probably due to neighbourhood involvement of the medial frontal lobes. It is not infrequently found in very diffuse lesions of the brain when it is difficult to say which part is responsible, so that bilateral grasp reflexes are not of great localising value.

The embarrassing situation of being unable to extract one's hand (embarrassing also to a conscious patient) can be overcome by massaging the ulnar aspect of the dorsum of the patient's hand, when the grasp will be released.

The forced groping reflex

Lightly and repeatedly touching the side of the palm results in the hand following the stimulus and perhaps attempting to grasp it. This is usually demonstrated in states of lowered consciousness and severe mental defect due to widespread cerebral lesions and is not of great localising value.

The sucking reflex
Touching the corner of the mouth produces a sucking movement of the lips and deviation of the mouth in the direction of the stimulus. This is seen in advanced and diffuse cerebral atrophic lesions, and in states of stupor from widespread encephalitic or traumatic lesions. It is normally present in infants.

THREE CLASSICAL SIGNS

Chvostek's sign
Tapping over the facial nerve or the branches of the facial nerve produces marked twitching and retraction of the corner of the mouth. This is present in tetany, and other states of muscular irritability. It may be seen to a slight degree in motor neurone disease. A similar movement occurs during regeneration of a damaged facial nerve.

Trousseau's sign
If the upper arm is compressed by a sphygmomanometer band for not more than four minutes, the hand goes into the *main d'accoucheur* position. This is an important sign of latent tetany, and can be increased and accelerated by hyperventilation.

Lhermitte's phenomenon
Forward flexion of the neck results in a burst of electric-shocklike paraesthesiae shooting into all four limbs, or down the centre of the back. Sometimes this may occur in lower limbs only, or even on one side only. It was once thought to be pathognomonic of multiple sclerosis, and is most commonly found in this disease, but it also occurs in high cervical compression from spondylosis, or cerebellar ectopia, and is also seen in the early stages of radiation myelopathy and occasionally in sub-acute combined degeneration.

The number of reflexes, named and unnamed, is legion. One textbook lists over 700. Fortunately few possess any special advantages over those described, which are easy to elicit and whose reliability has earned their place in the routine examination.

Chapter 26
Co-ordination

Co-ordinate movement requires that both motor and sensory systems should be intact, for any satisfactory voluntary effort requires:

(*a*) Efficient, smooth, adequate, but not excessive, movement of a group of muscles.

(*b*) Appropriate and smooth relaxation of the correct antagonists, together perhaps with the contraction of other muscles, such as joint fixators, to ensure the efficiency of the movement.

(*c*) Knowledge of the position of the moving part before, during, and at the end of each movement.

(*d*) Knowledge of the position of the point to which the part is to be moved, and the relationship between the two at any moment during the movement.

Co-ordinate action of the muscles is under cerebellar control, and influenced by the extrapyramidal system, but intact proprioceptive sense combined with an accurate image of one's own body and its relationship to the environment are equally essential for the movement to be completed satisfactorily. Lesions in many sites may therefore produce inco-ordination.

Purposes of the tests

To give the patient simple movements to perform which the examiner can, from past experience, compare with the normal. A certain stereotyping of tests is required, for the possible number is, of course, uncountable.

The aim of each test is to decide whether any defect demonstrated is due to:

(*a*) Cerebellar dysfunction.

(*b*) Proprioceptive deficiency.

(*c*) Some other factor, such as muscular weakness, simple lack of comprehension as to what they are supposed to do, or, and very important, perfect comprehension, but a determination to do it wrongly for a variety of reasons, none representing organic disease.

Methods of testing co-ordination

Co-ordination of ocular movements, speech and gait are dealt with in their appropriate sections.

THE UPPER LIMB

Preliminary observations

Ask the patient to hold both arms outstretched in front of him. Watch the movement, and how well the posture is maintained. Then ask him to close his eyes and continue to watch the posture.

Next, telling the patient to keep his arms up, tap each briskly and observe the displacement and return to the previous positions, both when his eyes are open and closed. Next press downwards on each in turn and suddenly release the pressure. Normally very little displacement occurs.

Abnormalities

On first raising the arms, if there is cerebellar disease the arm on the affected side will usually overshoot and have to be brought back to be parallel with the other. Frequent correction of its position has to be made so that the arm appears to bounce and often deviates towards the other. The hand may show hyperextension of the metacarpo-phalangeal joints with partial flexion of the wrist.

When the eyes are shut, these features may increase in cerebellar disease, but if the arm now begins to drift upwards and sideways (possibly outwards), this usually indicates postural deficiency.

If the arm falls slowly, this may also indicate postural deficiency, but more commonly is due to simple muscle weakness.

External rotation of the hand, bizarre posturing of the fingers, and little writhing movements of the thumb and fingers may also be seen in severe postural deficiency, as well as in dystonic states (see p. 148).

The arm is easily displaced on tapping due to (*a*) motor weakness, when it remains in the displaced position, each tap displacing it further; (*b*) cerebellar hypotonia, when it tends to return after several bounces to the previous position; and (*c*) postural deficiency, when, with the eyes closed, the arm may be grossly displaced without the patient realising it, and if told to replace it, he assumes an entirely incorrect position.

In cerebellar disease, with the eyes open or closed, after releasing pressure, the arm will fly upwards, sometimes so vigorously as to hit the patient (or the examiner) in the face. In postural deficiency, when the eyes are closed, the arm tends to remain in the new position without much rebound.

The finger–nose test

Unless illustrated clearly for them, many patients for some reason have difficulty in following the first simple instruction which is to 'point the forefinger.' They may then perform the next movement in a quite unnatural manner, making assessment very difficult.

Each arm in turn is drawn out to full abduction and the patient is told to

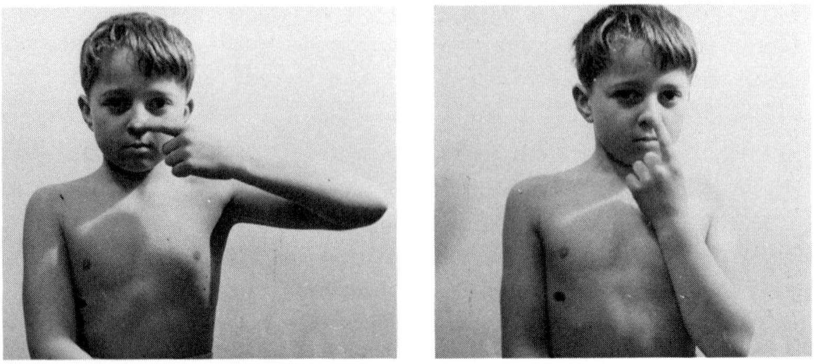

(a) (b)

Fig. 79. The finger–nose test: (a) right, (b) wrong. The arm must be held in abduction or many of the abnormalities will be concealed.

place the finger-tip on his own nose and hold it there (Fig. 79). Again, if the instruction is not clear, a surprising number of patients try to touch the examiner's nose, a gesture which causes general embarrassment. Note the ability to point the correct finger, the smoothness of the movement, the accuracy of placing and the steadiness with which the finger is held on the nose to a count of 5. Repeat the test with the eyes closed. Minor abnormalities can be emphasised if the patient touches his forefinger to the examiner's out-stretched finger and then moves it backwards and forwards from nose to finger quickly, the examiner holding his finger in a different place for each movement.

Abnormalities

In cerebellar disease the arm on the side of the lesion may first be flung wildly outwards, striking near-by objects. The finger moves to the nose in a wavering side-to-side, or up-and-down, but not a jerky fashion, at the last moment being brought on to its object fairly accurately. This is increased slightly by eye closure, and emphasised by the harder tests. In milder lesions, all that is seen is the wavering to either side of a straight line during the course of the movement, with a tendency to overshoot the object at first, towards the side of the lesion.

This wavering must not be confused with *intention tremor*, which is a side-to-side oscillation which develops as the finger approaches the nose, or occurs shortly after the finger touches the nose. It may be so wild as to make it impossible for the movement to be completed, or so slight as to consist merely of two or three oscillations while the finger is being held on the nose for a few seconds after touching it.

In postural ataxia, the movement from start to finish can be a smooth one, though it is usually hesitant, and the finger hesitates before finally touching the nose. When the eyes are closed, however, the finger is unable to find the nose and, after first touching somewhere else, is then dragged along the skin of the face towards its object. If the finger is briskly, constantly and confidently placed on the cheek a little to one side of the nose, in the same place each time, this almost without exception reflects a non-organic state, and completely without exception if it is still constantly done with the eyes open.

THE LOWER LIMB

Preliminary observations

Exactly the same principles are used as in the arms, but such fine movements cannot be expected.

The patient is told first to raise one leg to touch the examiner's outstretched hand with his big toe. A patient with normal muscle strength will be able to do this with only a little 'bounce' at the end of the movement.

Abnormalities

A patient with cerebellar disease is likely to overshoot, perhaps wildly, the leg will need several bounces before it reaches its object, and the knee may be unnecessarily flexed.

The heel–knee test

The heel must then be placed on the opposite knee. It is wise to touch the appropriate heel and knee, for otherwise some patients whose comprehension is slow flounder helplessly at a simple verbal instruction. others always perform the movement with the opposite limb, and some even attempt the discouraging manoeuvre of trying to place the heel on the knee of the same leg.

When the movement is completed the patient should be told to run the heel down the front of the shin to the top of the foot. The whole test is then repeated on the other side, and finally it is carried out again with the eyes closed.

Abnormalities

In *marked cerebellar disease* the heel overshoots the knee sideways, and develops a rotary oscillation as it approaches it, which is the equivalent of the intention tremor in the upper limb. As the heel moves down the shin it oscillates from side to side and finally shoots off the opposite foot in an uncontrolled manner.

In *mild degrees of cerebellar ataxia* the side-to-side oscillation may be the only obvious defect.

In *sensory ataxia* the heel is lifted too high in the first place and the patient raises his head to see what the relationship is of the two limbs. Deficiencies in the rest of the movement are not rhythmical, though the leg may fall off the other several times during its course. When the eyes are then closed, the patient is only able to find the knee by allowing the heel to land on some part of the thigh and then sliding it downwards.

In *combined ataxia,* elements of the two types of abnormality are present and the movement may be equally disorganised whether the eyes are open or closed. Again, in non-organic states the heel is brought down confidently and repeatedly, eyes open or closed, in exactly the same place, usually about 15 cm (6 inches) below the knee.

Dysdiadochokinesis

This is a failure efficiently to perform rapidly alternating movements.

The patient should sit with his arms flexed at the elbow, holding the forearms vertically with the palms facing inwards. He is then told to rotate the hands rapidly at the wrists. This will require both illustration and encouragement. Most people are less skilful at this with the non-dominant hand and children are less adept at it than adults.

The patient with *cerebellar disease*, however, makes a movement which is coarse, irregular and slow, with the hand dorsiflexed and the fingers extended, so that the whole palm is being shaken rather than the wrist rotated. If repeated with the fist clenched, a jerky flexion-extension of the wrist is superimposed on the attempted rotation.

In *motor weakness*, especially due to pyramidal tract lesions, the movement may be clumsier and slower on the affected side, but the particular features mentioned above are not seen.

Past-pointing tests

Past-pointing is a sign found both in cerebellar and labyrinthine disease. It must not be confused with the inaccurate placing of a position sense defect.

The patient sits opposite the examiner holding his arm forwards horizontally, so that his fingers touch the fingers of the examiner's similarly outstretched arm. He should then either lower the arm to his side, or raise it above his head, and bring it back to the original position, first with the eyes open and then when they are closed. The test should be repeated several times with each arm.

In *cerebellar disease* the arm on the side of the lesion will deviate outwards towards the side of the lesion instead of accurately regaining its original position.

In *unilateral labyrinthine disease* both arms will deviate towards the side of the lesion. This will be in the same direction as the slow component of the nystagmus, which will undoubtedly be present (q.v.).

Additional tests

These are tests which are altered in cerebellar, pyramidal and extrapyramidal disease, and, though demonstrating ataxia, are of less value in its analysis.

RAPID HAND TAPPING

Hand tapping is a good method of detecting a unilateral motor deficit, but does not fully analyse it. The back of one hand is tapped rapidly with the fingers of the other. Again, the non-dominant side is normally less skilful. In *cerebellar disease* the tap becomes a rotary stroking movement. Such dysmetria can be emphasised by telling the patient to rotate the hand while tapping so that alternate taps are carried out by the palmar and dorsal surfaces. This test can also be adapted for the feet, but the speed of tapping normally possible is much less.

TAPPING IN A CIRCLE

A circle 1 cm in diameter is drawn and the patient, given a pencil, is asked to tap out a series of dots, all within the circle. In *any* ataxia the patient will spread the dots irregularly over a wide area, outside as well as inside the circle. In *unilateral cerebellar disease* more of the dots may be found displaced to the side of the lesion.

This test is a good method of recording in the notes a deterioration or improvement in ataxia.

SPIRAL DRAWING

Ask the patient to draw a spiral. This is totally impossible in severe ataxia, tremor or chorea. It is not a specific test, but serial drawings offer a useful method of comparing improvement or deterioration.

Difficulties and fallacies

Poor performance of these tests, especially the heel–knee test, is not necessarily a sign of true ataxia. They are not easy tests to do for the first time and an agitated patient must be encouraged to take his time and to do them slowly. Remember this may be the tenth patient that afternoon you have told to put his right heel on to his left knee, but for the patient this may be the first time in 65 years that he has been given this improbable instruction.

Note the presence of any static tremor in the hands at rest, for at the end of the finger–nose test this might be mistaken for intention tremor.

Marked muscular weakness may interfere seriously with the heel–knee test, the heel repeatedly falling off the shin, but the difficulty in raising the thigh and maintaining the knee in extension will have been noted in the early stages of the test.

Pyramidal and extrapyramidal lesions slow up the performance of tests requiring rapid fine movement, but the execution of the individual stages of the movement is correct and there is not the decomposition seen in cerebellar ataxia.

Always correlate the degree of ataxia demonstrated on the couch with your observations of what movements the patient is able to perform when he does not realise he is specifically being examined. Precise co-ordinated movements may be seen which are not merely automatic, and a suspected simulated ataxia may be confirmed.

N.B. The failure to demonstrate abnormalities of co-ordination when the patient is lying in bed must never be considered to exclude cerebellar disease, for in a midline posterior fossa or cerebellar vermis lesion, or in one in which the cerebellar tonsils are displaced through the foramen magnum (e.g. in the Chiari deformity and other anomalies in this area) gross ataxia of gait may be the only physical sign, tests of co-ordination while recumbent being normal. Before this was realised many patients with gross ataxia of gait were wrongly labelled as hysterical, and even these days many still are.

Part VI
Examinations of Particular Difficulty

Chapter 27
The Unconscious Patient

'Normal consciousness' has not, so far, been satisfactorily defined, and it is easier to describe abnormalities of the conscious state. There are two aspects of the conscious state that can vary independently in different types and distribution of brain disease. One is the *content* of consciousness, the sum of mental function; the other we call the *state* or *level* of consciousness, which is the degree of *alertness* or *arousal*. So there are conditions in which the patient, though awake and responsive, is imperfectly aware of himself, his actions, and his environment. Here, the *content* is affected. Alternatively, in other states of impaired or lost consciousness we see defects of *arousal* of varying degree. Anatomically, the central reticular formation of the brain stem is the basis of *arousal*; the *content* of consciousness depends on the activities of the cerebral cortex and thalamus. Full conscious behaviour requires intact cerebral hemispheres and a normal brain stem. In both cases, an acute lesion is more likely to influence consciousness than a slowly developing one. Destructive lesions of the hemispheres, if slowly evolving, have to be extensive before consciousness is impaired. On the other hand, discharging lesions, as in epilepsy, are often small. Similarly, only relatively small, bilateral, lesions of the brain stem are required to disturb consciousness profoundly.

The purpose of the examination

(*a*) To determine the *state* or *level* of consciousness.
(*b*) To identify or exclude systemic disease known to cause disturbances of consciousness without primary disease of the brain.
(*c*) If due apparently to a neurological lesion to determine its site in the brain or brain stem. One thinks in terms of 'north or south', rostral or caudal.

The attitude towards investigation is bound to differ in units fully equipped for intracranial emergencies, and in the more general hospitals. The majority of the remarks in this chapter are based on the fact that most comatose patients are not primarily admitted to neurological or neurosurgical units, but in the final paragraphs there is an indication of the steps such units would undertake.

HISTORY

So much information can be gleaned from the history that no amount of trouble should be spared to obtained the fullest details. Relatives, friends, work-mates, police, ambulance men, or other witnesses must be searched out and questioned, making certain that the information obtained is precise, relevant, factual and not supposition, and determining whether it comes from direct knowledge or hearsay.

The points of particular importance in the history are:

(*a*) *The mode of onset.* Was the loss of consciousness abrupt as in cerebrovascular catastrophes or epileptic states; rapid, over a period of a few hours, as in some cases of intracranial haemorrhage and in toxic states, or gradual, over days, as in expanding intracranial lesions?

(*b*) *Premonitory symptoms.* Complete absence of premonitory symptoms would suggest a primary intracranial vascular accident or an epileptic attack. Previous episodes of a similar nature suggest either epilepsy, the recurrent administration of drugs, or, very rarely, the blocking of cerebrospinal fluid pathways by some intermittent obstruction to the ventricles, such as an intraventricular mass or cyst.

Headaches, with vomiting, progressive mental change, increasing weakness or unsteadiness of the limbs, would all suggest an expanding intracranial lesion.

Progressive severe loss of weight, anorexia and asthenia suggest metastatic disease, while symptoms such as a cough, dyspnoea, anorexia, melaena, lumps in the breast, past mastectomy or gastrectomy, may indicate the probable site of the primary lesion.

Any active infection in the ears, chest of sinuses, may suggest intracranial infection.

A history of severe psychological disturbance, especially depression, raises the possibility of self-administered drug intoxication.

A history of alcoholism may be obtained, but it is often very difficult to get an honest assessment, even from would-be helpful relatives.

Most important is the question of trauma, remembering that the elderly are prone to intracranial bleeding after relatively slight degrees of trauma. The cause and type of the injury must be established, its severity, the length of the interval between its occurrence and the loss of consciousness, i.e. whether immediate, or after a delay of minutes, hours, or days; if gradual or abrupt in onset; and whether there was initial recovery and then relapse.

It is also important to know if there has been any associated fracture of long bones which might have been the source of cerebral fat embolism.

EXAMINATION

Much of the examination will consist of careful observation, carried out repeatedly and perhaps over a long period of time, both in the patient's immediate vicinity and also from a position where a patient who might be feigning unconsciousness is not aware that he is under observation.

Assessment of the degree of altered consciousness

This must be decided at once, for the future examination will be largely governed by the conscious level, which should be described in detail. There are infinite gradations of altered consciousness characterised by defects of arousal, but the terms *drowsiness, stupor,* and *coma* usefully describe the three major stages which can be clinically recognised.

Drowsiness

A state resembling normal sleepiness. Stimulation rouses the patient to a state of complete wakefulness and co-operation, but he tends to sink into sleep again if stimulation ceases. Normally the full neurological examination can be carried out. This state is common in high brain stem disturbances, direct or indirect, and in drug toxicity.

Stupor

Left to himself, the patient appears to be completely unconscious, but nevertheless may be restless. On vigorous stimulation he can be roused sufficiently to resist painful stimuli, or even for short periods to respond to commands or to answer simple questions. No satisfactory co-operation is obtained and as soon as stimulation ceases the patient reverts to his original state. Bilateral cerebral hemisphere disease (anoxic, toxic or traumatic) and compression or disease of the upper brain stem may all cause stupor.

In the variety called *akinetic mutism*, the patient lies motionless and speechless but with eyes open as if awake. He is not unresponsive or resistive and his eyes may appear to gaze about him. One has the curious impression that these patients are just on the very brink of saying something, but never quite achieve it. Yet there is always an amnesia for the duration of this state. It occurs in association with lesions in the neighbourhood of the third ventricle, or sub-acute encephalopathies, and is probably a consequence of involvement of the reticular formation in the upper brain stem. It illustrates the dissociation which may occur between wakefulness and awareness.

There is another similar condition but having important differences. All movement save for blinking and vertical gaze is paralysed; but consciousness is retained. The patient is aware of himself but physically 'locked-in'. When the cause is a peripheral disorder such as acute polyneuritis (Guillain–Barré syndrome), it is not difficult to recognise that the patient is conscious. But when central processes lead to this 'de-efferented' state, coma may be readily simulated. The responsible lesion is in the ventral pons, either vascular or demyelinating. Vertical eye movements are served from the superior collicular region of the midbrain and are thus preserved in the presence of a tetraplegia and facio-bulbar paralysis.

Coma

The patient is deeply unconscious. He will respond only in the most elemental way to painful stimulation and cannot be roused to any degree of co-operation. He is usually lying immobile and incontinent. There is some justification in describing a coma which is bordering on stupor as 'light' and one in which no form, even of reflex activity exists, as 'deep'. The deeper degrees of unconsciousness are common in pontine and low brain stem lesions; pupillary, corneal and swallowing reflexes may be abolished. Three particular aspects of the behavioural response have been used in the now widely accepted 'Glasgow Coma Scale' (see Appendix D p. 350). Various grades of eye opening, verbal and motor response can be recorded on a special chart to provide consistent standard of appraisal. Such methods help to avoid the errors which often result from the imprecise use of language by the medical or nursing staff. (*Never* use the phrase 'semi-coma'.)

In addition to these three states, there are other abnormalities of awareness (content) which must be recognised though they need not necessarily be accompanied by any disturbance of *arousal*. Diffuse disturbance of the cerebral hemisphere is responsible.

Confusion and disorientation

The confused patient may be quite alert and even co-operative, but is incorrect in his comprehension and assessment of his own state or his environment. It is usual to test in three dimensions.

(*a*) *Time*. Ask his knowledge of the day, date, month, year and how long he has been in his present place.

(*b*) *Place*. Ask where he is, what room, what building, what town, what country.

(*c*) *Person*. Ask who he is, what is his work, what is his age.

Finally, ask if he knows who the doctors, or nurses, or relatives are who may be around the bedside.

Delirium

In this state the patient appears out of touch with his surroundings and is spontaneously producing evidence of his confusion and disorientation by muttering, rambling, shouting, often offensively, often continuously, with evidence of delusion and hallucination, and often with so much associated motor activity that physical exhaustion overcomes him. This is to be seen in toxic and infective states, and most strikingly in the delirium tremens of alcoholism, a condition which once seen will never be forgotten.

Catatonia

This is most frequently a symptom of a psychotic state in which the patient, otherwise entirely normal, lies mute, immobile and unresponsive. He does not follow movements; does not appear to be paying any attention to his surroundings; and will often have a plastic rigidity of the limbs, which may remain in any position in which they are placed, however bizarre that may be. Modern drug therapy has greatly reduced its frequency. Similar states may be seen in organic frontal and hypothalamic lesions, including mutism, but other neurological signs are present.

Having assessed the level of consciousness and the degree of co-operation to be expected from the patient, a general inspection of the face, skin, position and movements of the body must be carried out before passing on to examination of the cardiovascular and central nervous systems.

GENERAL OBSERVATIONS

The purpose of the following paragraphs is to indicate a train of thought set up by certain observations and they must not be taken as a suggestion that these observations give the diagnosis.

Colour and condition of the skin

Pallor and sweating occur in syncope, severe blood loss, and hypoglycaemia, but may be seen in brain stem vascular deficiency, and following some epileptic attacks.

Suffusion of the face is seen in hypertension, alcoholism and sometimes in cerebral haemorrhage.

Cyanosis of the face and neck accompanies respiratory obstruction, epilepsy, and some intracranial vascular accidents. It is, of course, a crucial sign requiring correction as a matter of urgency if possible, and should therefore, until proved otherwise, be assumed to be due to respiratory obstruction.

Cyanosis of the limbs is seen in peripheral circulatory stagnation, severe coma and collapse.

Jaundice may suggest multiple metastases, but may also indicate hepatic coma due either to primary liver disease, or to drug toxicity.

A cherry red colour is seen in carbon monoxide poisoning.

Petechiae and ecchymoses are found after a fit; in bacterial endocarditis, severe septicaemia, collagenoses, blood dyscrasias (primary or secondary to drug toxicity), and in patients on high cortisone dosage. In small children the possibility of multiple inflicted trauma must not be overlooked.

Corrosion of the lips and mouth indicate poisoning.

Emaciation suggests advanced malignant disease, or severe deficiency disease, which might, of course, be misleading and merely due to prolonged unconsciousness.

Position of the body

Neck retraction, especially in children, usually indicates meningeal irritation, but it may sometimes occur when there has been a cerebellar tonsillar pressure cone.

Neck retraction and arching of the back (opisthotonos). This is not uncommon in small children with meningeal infections, or advanced degenerative lesions. It may occur in severe meningeal irritation and in tetanus in adults. Extreme degrees of opisthotonos in adults with extension (not flexion) of the hips and knees is rarely organic.

Curling of the body away from the light is seen in meningeal irritation by infection or blood.

The patient who lies with the head drooped to one side, one upper limb pronated and adducted and one lower limb externally rotated, usually has developed an *acute and profound hemiplegia.*

When all limbs are extended, the upper limbs are pronated and the feet plantar-flexed, this represents the *decerebrate attitude* and occurs in lesions of the midbrain between the superior colliculus and pons.

If, however, the upper limbs are flexed and the lower limbs extended, the *decorticate position* is seen in extensive lesions at the level of the basal nuclei, or between this level and the cortex.

Both postures may first be revealed by response to cutaneous stimulation.

INVOLUNTARY MOVEMENTS OF IMPORTANCE IN STATES OF DISTURBED CONSCIOUSNESS

Convulsions

Coma accompanies and follows isolated fits or status epilepticus, of 'idiopathic' or symptomatic origin. The degree of unconsciousness may be far greater than the severity of the preliminary convulsions may lead a layman to expect—so the history again is vital. If convulsions are known to be limited to one part of the body, for all practical purposes this indicates structural disease of the opposite hemisphere. Repeated focal convulsions involving a little more of the limb each time, and particularly if then spreading to the other side, are highly suggestive of a spreading cortical thrombophlebitis or an encephalitis. Minor twitching of the extremities, if unilateral, have localising value, but if bilateral merely indicate diffuse cerebral disorder. Unilateral myoclonic jerks have a similar significance, but see the section on myoclonus (p. 138–9), for their special importance in sub-acute encephalitis.

Attacks of generalised rigidity and decerebrate attacks

These may occur when the brain stem is the site of primary disease, when it is under compression, subjected to trauma, or has had haemorrhage into its substance either primarily or as a result of tentorial herniation. They may also be seen in very advanced diffuse cerebral and basal nuclear disease, especially in children, in whom they may also accompany meningitis.

Rigors and tremors

Intermittent rigors without rise of temperature occur when there is an irritative lesion of the ventricular walls, e.g. by rupture of an abscess or haematoma, and a constant coarse twitching tremor of the hands and arms accompanies this ventriculitis.

FURTHER GENERAL EXAMINATION

Respiration

Stertorous breathing, accompanied by stridor and cyanosis if there is also respiratory obstruction, is common in epileptic fits and cerebro-vascular accidents.

One of the commonest disorders of respiration is the periodic (Cheyne–Stokes) type in which there is alternating hyperpnoea and apnoea. This usually indicates a bilateral cerebral or high brain stem lesion or metabolic dysfunction. The causal lesion is rarely as low as the upper pons. Other brain stem lesions of the midbrain or mid-pons cause central hyperventilation or ataxic irregular breathing patterns. The latter are most commonly seen in lesions of the medulla and lack the rhythmical waxing and waning of the Cheyne–Stokes type.

Shallow, rapid breathing occurs in shock, haemorrhage and hypoglycaemia.

The odour of acetone in the breath in diabetic comas is classical, but not detectable by many people.

Pulse

The pulse is (*a*) rapid and weak in haemorrhage, shock, some stages of syncope and circulatory collapse; (*b*) slow and weak in some stages of syncope and in vaso-vagal attacks; (*c*) very slow and full in complete heart block (when Stokes–Adams attacks occur), and in severely increased intracranial pressure. A weak, irregular pulse is found in low brain stem lesions and a fibrillating pulse raises the possibility of cerebral embolism.

Examination of the head

Injuries may be hidden by hair, but careful palpation may reveal a fracture line, a depression, or a 'soggy' area of a severe contusion. A bony lump may suggest an underlying exostosing tumour. Percussion of the skull in children with hydrocephalus produces a high-pitched, cracked-pot note, and in comatose infants a bulging fontanelle indicates increased intracranial pressure. If burr-holes or a decompression are present they should be palpated, for if tense and bulging this means high intracranial pressure.

Signs of meningeal irritation

Test for neck rigidity and carry out Kernig's test, both at the beginning and the end of the examination, when the stimulation may have roused the patient.

Neck rigidity is the more important sign. It may, however, indicate cerebellar tonsillar herniation at foramen magnum level, rather than frank meningitis. This is important for it would contra-indicate a lumbar puncture, and the history of the onset is vital. In meningitis, Kernig's sign is usually positive as well.

In the earliest stages of subarachnoid haemorrhage, neck rigidity may not have developed, sometimes is delayed even 24 hours, and if coma or collapse is profound, e.g. after massive intracranial bleeding, or in advanced meningitis in childhood, neck stiffness may not develop at all.

The ears

Examine carefully for signs of:

(*a*) Middle ear infection, which may indicate an intracranial abscess.
(*b*) Tenderness and swelling over the mastoid, for the same reason.
(*c*) Bleeding from the inner ear, for this often indicates a basal fracture.

The tongue

A common cause of coma being epilepsy, the tongue should be examined for evidence of having been bitten. The surface and the inside of the cheek, palate, fauces and pharynx should be inspected for the effects of corrosive fluids.

EXAMINATION OF THE NERVOUS SYSTEM

An attempt should first be made to raise the conscious level. This is done by rubbing the sternum vigorously with the knuckles, and by pressure in the supraorbital notch. (The actual *level* or *state* of consciousness has already been recorded.)

The more detailed examination of the nervous system is now designed to differentiate between the two basic causes of altered consciousness (brain stem reticular formation depression *or* bilateral cerebral dysfunction together with brain stem depression) and to seek any evidence for a specific structural lesion. There may be signs of diffuse disease or of a focal lesion in the supratentorial or subtentorial compartment. In addition to evaluation of the level of consciousness itself, and attention to the pattern of respiration, it is the examination of the pupils, ocular movements and motor function that forms the most crucial part of the exercise.

The cranial nerves

The ordinary routine examination is not possible, for all observations have to be objective, and a somewhat different approach must be adopted.

The fundi

These must be most carefully examined in every case, the abnormalities having the same significance as described in Chap. 7. Remember, however, that whereas true papilloedema (in the absence of marked hypertension) indicates increased intracranial pressure, its absence does not in any way exclude a space-occupying lesion.

Visual fields

These cannot be accurately tested, but in stuporose states a menacing movement towards the eye from one side and then the other will normally produce a blink, which may be absent when the gesture is made from the side of a hemianopia.

The pupils

Note the size of each pupil, their comparative size, and their reactions. For full details of pupillary abnormalities, see Chap. 8. In states of disturbed consciousness the following points are of greatest importance:

In *most* cases of toxic or metabolic coma, the *pupillary light reflexes are spared. Their presence or absence is, in fact, the single most important sign in distinguishing metabolic from structural disease.*

Widely dilated pupils (7–9 mm) occur in midbrain lesions that selectively affect the oculomotor complex or third nerves, and do not react to light.

If the sympathetic system, also, is involved, pupils of *medium size* (4–7 mm) which are inactive to light may result from midbrain lesions. These may be primary, or secondary to central pressure herniation as in cases of tumour or haematoma in the supratentorial compartment. Be certain any dilatation is not due to the use of atropine by a previous examiner.

Unilateral pupillary dilatation with deteriorating consciousness should be considered as a sign of unilateral tentorial herniation until proved otherwise. It is commonly, but not invariably, on the side of the expanding lesion and demands prompt surgical action. By the time both pupils are dilated there has usually been a secondary haemorrhage into the brain stem, and even correction of the primary lesion may not save the patient.

Very small pupils (0.5–1 mm) are seen in pontine lesions, and in certain drug intoxications, especially morphia, but also during simple sleep.

Ocular position and ocular movements

Note the position of the eyes, any deviation from the midline, how well sustained this is, any spontaneous ocular movements, and any movements on sudden noise or on command.

Abnormalities of conjugate deviation have an important role in comatose states and are dealt with in Chap. 8. Remember that forced upward deviation of the eyes or oculogyric crises can be caused by toxic doses of the phenothiazine derivatives. Skew deviation of the eyes occurs in pontine or cerebellar lesions.

Because the pathways controlling oculomotor-vestibular reflexes lie adjacent to the reticular formation good use can be made of testing these responses. The reflex eye movements following passive rotation of the head (oculocephalic or 'doll's head' manoeuvre) and caloric stimulation of the ears (oculovestibular) are noted. These observations are of particular value in distinguishing structural lesions of the cerebral hemispheres from those of the brain stem, remembering, of course, that the latter dysfunction is often secondary to central herniation. But in the absence of secondary brain stem compression, cerebral hemisphere lesions do not affect either reflex. Similarly, metabolic suppression of the hemispheres and brain stem spares the oculomotor-vestibular pathways until late, when their abnormality can then be used to identify so-called 'brain stem' death.

In the normal oculocephalic reflex (the 'doll's head' or 'doll's eye' manoeuvre), brisk rotation of the head from side to side or flexion/extension, the eyes show conjugate deviation away from the direction in which the head was moved, before then returning to the primary position. It will be recalled from Chap. 11 that irrigation of the external auditory canal with cold (or warm) water excites nystagmus. (In the unconscious patient, ice-cold water is routinely used to cause maximum effect.) This forms the basis of the oculovestibular (caloric) reflex. In lesions of the diencephalon causing coma, the fast component of that nystagmus is depressed, so that there is, instead, just tonic conjugate deviation of the eyes towards the irrigated ear. Midbrain or upper pontine lesions can cause various abnormalities; deviation may be confined to the ipsilateral eye indicating a contralateral internuclear ophthalmoplegia or be seen only in the contralateral eye suggesting a sixth nerve lesion on the stimulated side. Lower pontine lesions abolish all responses and there will also be absent corneal reflexes. Occasionally such absence of any ocular response is the result of bilateral end-organ poisoning by gentamycin or other related antibiotics.

The face

Facial muscles. Voluntary movements cannot be tested. First study the lines and contours of the face. Flattening and smoothing of the wrinkles on one side, with uncovering of the sclera, are seen in paralysis of lower motor neurone type and sometimes in the acute stages of severe upper motor neurone paralysis. The paralysed side will be blown out and sucked in during expiration and inspiration.

Firm pressure on the supraorbital notch may produce a grimace. Normally, this is most marked on the side stimulated, but when there is facial paralysis it is reduced on the affected side, *no matter which side is stimulated.* Touching the corner of the mouth may produce a sucking reflex and deviation of the corner of the mouth. This is seen in the adult in bilateral cerebral lesions of severe diffuse character.

Facial sensation. The corneal reflex must be tested in each case. It is often bilaterally absent in deep coma or depressed if the cornea has been exposed for a long time.

Painful stimulation of the skin should be carried out by pinprick or pinching, and the relative grimacing on each side compared. Great care in interpretation of corneal reflex and facial sensory tests is required in the presence of facial paralysis (see Chap. 10).

Purely unilateral loss of sensation in comatose patients is usually part of a complete hemianalgesia and indicates a deep-seated hemisphere or upper brain stem lesion. Sensory loss on one side of the face but on the opposite side of the body indicates a lower brain stem lesion, and is especially common in the lateral medullary syndrome, traditionally due to a posterior inferior cerebellar artery thrombosis, but in fact usually a sign of vertebral artery disease.

The motor system

A great deal will have been learnt during the preliminary period of inspection. This applies particularly to the position of the limbs and the degree of movement carried out by each limb. The tone of the limbs can be tested in the normal way, but remember that in the acute stage of a severe intracranial lesion, the tone may be lost, rather than increased, on the side opposite to the lesion.

Raise both arms together and let them fall back. Normally, the fall is checked and slowed, but in unilateral paralysis the arm will fall unchecked. Next raise the legs into the flexed position, so that the soles of the feet rest on the bed, and then allow them to fall back. Unparalysed limbs will remain in that position or slowly extend. A paralysed limb will rapidly fall back to its original position.

Remember, midbrain lesions produce decerebrate posturing, and that this may at first only follow noxious stimulation, and may be unilateral if the other side is paralysed.

The reflexes

Testing the reflexes, being an objective procedure, can be carried out in the normal way and the usual deductions can be drawn, but in states of deep coma the interpretation of the results may be different.

Tendon reflexes may be absent on the paralysed side, or in deep coma, throughout. Superficial reflexes may be unobtainable and have little localising value. The plantar responses may be absent, or bilaterally extensor, and so also have little localising value, except that if there is a unilateral extensor plantar this indicates the side of a pyramidal system lesion.

The sensory system

Sensation can be assessed by observing the patient's response to painful pinching or pricking of the face, arms, trunk and legs, on each side, and it may be necessary to stimulate vigorously. Dilatation of the pupils, grimacing, or movements of the limb will occur if sensation is present. Failure to withdraw a limb may indicate paralysis, loss of sensation, or both. In the former there is usually movement of the *normal* limb even when the *abnormal* side is stimulated. In deep coma these tests are of little value, other than as an indication of the depth of the coma.

Co-ordination

This cannot be tested in the ordinary way, but in stuporose states the patient will often attempt to fight off interference and to brush off the painful stimuli. During these movements, the presence of a marked ataxia can be observed, and assessment can be made of the patient's ability to localise a stimulus and to place his hand correctly on the painful point.

ESSENTIAL INVESTIGATIONS

Obviously, the history and clinical assessment of the case will influence one greatly in the type of investigation to be undertaken, but in every case there must be examination of:

(*a*) The urine (preferably a catheter specimen), for sugar, albumen, ketones and chlorides.

(*b*) The blood, for estimation of blood sugar, blood urea, blood sodium and potassium, and erythrocyte sedimentation rate.

Once these have been done, a major screening process will have been completed and such conditions as hypoglycaemia, diabetic coma, uraemia, and severe electrolyte disturbances should have been detected. In suspected alcoholism, the blood alcohol level may also help.

Drug toxicity is bound to arise, and it is becoming increasingly possible to detect different drugs in common usage in blood and urine and to know whether these levels are compatible with normal or excessive intake. Close liaison with the biochemical laboratory on this point is vital.

If there is evidence of cardiac disease and the ESR is raised, the coma may be due to infected emboli from bacterial endocarditis and a blood culture and careful examination of the urine for red cells will be required. If there is reason to suspect a collagen disease, the plasma proteins should also be estimated and an electrophoretic analysis obtained.

It must be emphasised that in cases of suspected trauma or tumour, time should not be wasted awaiting the results of these investigations. They can be going on while important radiological procedures are being carried out.

The cerebro-spinal fluid

Great care is required in the selection of comatose cases for lumbar puncture. No patient with papilloedema should have a lumbar puncture carried out unless neurosurgical facilities are readily available and preferably in the same hospital. This applies also where, papilloedema or no papilloedema, it is strongly suspected that the lesion is a space-occupying one, and particularly if it is highly likely to be in the posterior fossa, or to be a subdural haematoma, or a cerebral abscess.

If, however, the patient has signs of meningeal irritation, but nothing to suggest a dangerous intracranial space-occupying lesion, such as papilloedema, a slow pulse, gross cerebellar signs, active middle ear or mastoid infection, then the cerebro-spinal fluid should be examined for cells, sugar, protein, and chlorides, in that order of importance. The details of the cerebro-spinal fluid examination are in Chap. 34. In suspected drug poisoning, drug levels should be estimated. In suspected liver coma, the cerebro-spinal fluid glutamine may be raised.

X-ray examination

X-rays of the skull should be carried out in all cases of coma, for, even if the cause is fairly obvious, such as in cases of diabetic or alcoholic coma, the patient may have received complicating trauma to the skull. There should be several aims in the examination (for details see Chap. 36):

(*a*) To demonstrate the site, nature and severity of any fracture. These influence the approach that a neurosurgeon may have to contemplate.

(*b*) To show the position of the pineal, if calcified. Displacement is a contraindication to lumbar puncture and an indication for further contrast radiographic studies.

(*c*) To detect abnormal calcification in a slowly growing tumour.

(*d*) To show the condition of the sella. Erosion should be assumed to mean raised intracranial pressure and contra-indicates lumbar puncture. Ballooning indicates a pituitary tumour and infarction of this may cause collapse and coma with marked meningeal cellular reaction.

(*e*) To show infection in sinuses, mastoids, or petrous bones, which might cause intracranial infection.

X-rays of the chest

Radiological appearances in the chest of comatose patients can give indirect hints as to the possible cerebral lesion. (For details see Chap. 36, p. 281.)

Radio-isotope scanning (gamma-encephalography) (see p. 307).

The isotope brain scan is a rapid simple method of detecting tumours, clots, abscesses in comatose patients, and multiple lesions in metastatic disease may be picked up more accurately than by arteriography. It is of great value in herpetic encephalitis, of less value in recent infarcts.

Computerised axial tomography (CT) (see p. 310)

In centres fortunate enough to possess this facility it is the investigation of first choice for not only has it the virtue of rapidity, and from the patient's point of view, simplicity, but it has the ability to detect virtually all types of cerebral lesion that might require urgent intervention, as well as demonstrating multiple lesions, and ischaemic lesions at a stage often missed by the isotope scan. Subdural haematomata can be more difficult to detect however, and sometimes the isotope scan may be preferable.

Electroencephalography and echoencephalography

The advent of scanning procedures has reduced the value of these in comatose patients but if such facilities are not readily available, the EEG may serve to lateralise a lesion where clinical examination has failed, and may localise it to one part of one hemisphere—this is particularly valuable in cerebral abscesses. In herpetic encephalitis bitemporal focal slow wave abnormality superimposed on the widespread abnormally slow tracing of any encephalopathy may enable an alert EEG technician to suggest the diagnosis. The examination cannot produce diagnostic labels however, though an entirely normal record in an unconscious patient would make a supratentorial lesion highly improbable. The echogram, by showing shift of midline structures, can indicate the side to which further investigations should be directed.

In units where arteriographic facilities are available but CT scanning is not, this form of contrast radiography will normally be utilised to confirm suspected space-occupying lesions, because the nature as well as the site of the lesion can be determined in a high proportion of cases. This applies to subdural haematomata, to many glioblastomata, and to meningiomata, while multiple lesions may be shown in metastatic disease. X-ray findings of this type profoundly influence the next step in investigation or treatment. An arteriogram which shows merely a space-occupying lesion will probably be followed by direct surgical inspection of this area. If the arteriogram shows no more than that the ventricles are dilated, then the chances of a IIIrd ventricle or posterior fossa lesion become much greater, and ventriculography may be required.

Deteriorating consciousness is always a grave sign, but before embarking on extensive investigation, each case must be assessed as an individual problem, always asking oneself whether 'doing something' is, in fact, going to benefit the patient. Remember also that deteriorating consciousness is not the same as failure to regain consciousness. In head injuries, for example, the former is very much more of an indication for further investigation than the latter.

Chapter 28
Disorders of Speech

This part of the neurological examination frightens many physicians, probably because the volume and complexity of the literature on the subject is so great that it is assumed that the examination must be similarly prolonged and complex. Certainly a minute analysis of a speech defect can be both, but for practical purposes the procedure can be both shortened and simplified. Assessment starts while taking the history, continues throughout the physical examination and then is analysed in more detail by the use of specific tests.

Speech defects fall into four main types: dysphasia (or if complete, aphasia); dysarthria (anarthria); dysphonia (aphonia); and mutism. Before any detailed analysis is attempted the disturbance must be placed in one of these groups.

Methods of differentiation

(*a*) If the patient is conscious, but making *no attempt* to speak or make sound, this is *mutism*. It is usually part of a psychological disorder, but may be seen in lesions affecting the anterior part of the walls of the IIIrd ventricle and the posterior medial surface of the frontal lobe bilaterally. Total mutism is sometimes due to profound motor aphasia (Broca's aphasia), but the patient then gives the impression both of paying attention and of trying to communicate even if unable to do so verbally.

(*b*) If the patient, though speaking, fails to produce any volume of sound, or merely whispers, this is *aphonia*. It is due to disorders of the larynx and vocal cords. If, despite this, he is able to cough normally, it is probably of hysterical origin.

(*c*) If the volume of sound and the content of the speech is normal, but the articulation and enunciation of the individual words and phrases is distorted, this is *dysarthria*. It is a disorder of control of muscles producing speech, the lesion lying in upper or lower motor neurones, cerebellar system or the muscles themselves—i.e. at many different levels.

(*d*) If the patient is failing to put into properly constructed words or phrases the thoughts he wishes to express, even if articulation is adequate, this then is *dysphasia*. The lesion is one of the highest mechanisms of speech and must be in the dominant cerebral hemisphere. Dysphasic states also include disturbances of writing (dysgraphia), and failure to comprehend the spoken word (receptive dysphasia), or the written word (dyslexia).

If either dysarthria or dysphasia is present, the defect needs closer analysis, but should not be attempted in any detail at the first interview. If the analysis is difficult it should not all be attempted at one time, for fatigue easily affects both patient and examiner and militates against accurate results.

THE ANALYSIS OF DYSARTHRIA

Correct articulation requires correct bilateral co-ordination of the tongue, lips, palate, larynx and the muscles of respiration. These may suffer from lesions of the upper and lower motor neurones, the co-ordinating influence of the extrapyramidal and cerebellar systems, and the actual muscles themselves.

Examination

(*a*) Listen to the clarity of the patient's enunciation during history taking.
(*b*) Ask the patient to repeat certain phrases. These can be chosen for him from a newspaper. Many tongue twisters are used, but it is wiser to start with easier words, for the normal person may find great difficulty with some of the traditional test phrases. These include 'British Constitution,' 'Methodist Episcopal,' 'The Royal Devonshire Constabulary,' 'Peter Piper picked a peck of pickled pepper,' 'The Leith Police dismisseth us,' etc.
(*c*) Ask the patient to read a paragraph from a simple book.
(*d*) Ask him to count successively to 30 or above to test for muscle fatigue.

Listen to the words, whether they slur into one another; whether the rhythm is jerky, explosive, or monotonous; whether speech is too loud or too soft; whether particular letters present particular difficulty, and which they are; whether there is a nasal tone to the speech; whether the disturbance is constant throughout, variable, or increasing towards the end of each sentence or on prolonged counting.

Varieties of dysarthria

(*a*) SPASTIC DYSARTHRIA

This is caused by bilateral upper motor neurone disease. The tongue is small and spastic; the speech is slurred; excursions of the mouth are limited; the letters 'b,' 'p,' 'd' and 't' suffer particularly. The impression is gained that the patient is trying to talk from the back of the throat. The jaw jerk and palatopharyngeal reflexes are exaggerated.

Common causes: Pseudobulbar palsy, motor neurone disease, upper brain stem tumours.

(*b*) RIGID DYSARTHRIA

This is a result of extrapyramidal lesions producing rigidity of face or tongue muscles, without wasting, and without exaggeration of the reflexes. Speech is monotonous, all inflections and accents disappear, words run into one another and sentences start and stop abruptly. Excursions of the tongue and lips are greatly reduced. The later words in long sentences may come out in a rush. In severe cases, the phenomenon of palilalia, i.e. the constant repetition of a particular syllable, may be heard.

Common cause: Parkinsonism.

(*c*) ATAXIC DYSARTHRIA

Here there is inco-ordination of the muscles of speech, including the respiratory muscles. Speech is irregular, slurred and drunken, sometimes too loud, or too soft, the words run into each other or are spaced too far, the rhythm is jerky, sometimes explosive, staccato, or scanning. There may be accompanying grimaces and gesticulations. It may be quite impossible for the patient to articulate the test phrases. Think of an intoxicated person's speech!

Common causes: Multiple sclerosis, cerebellar disease or tumours, hereditary ataxia, choreas, anti-convulsant and other drug toxicity.

(*d*) DYSARTHRIA DUE TO LESIONS OF THE LOWER MOTOR NEURONES AND MUSCLES

Speech as a whole may be well preserved, but individual words and sounds cause difficulty, the distribution and extent of the muscular weakness governing the particular variety of defect produced.

Facial paralysis causes difficulty with the labials such as 'b,' 'p,' 'm,' 'w'.

Tongue paralysis affects a large number of sounds, particularly those involving the letters 'l,' 'd,' 'n,' 's,' 't,' 'x,' 'z,' and speech is profoundly distorted.

Palatal paralysis produces nasal speech. 'b' and 'd' become 'm,' 'n' and 'g' becomes 'rh,' and 'k' sounds like 'ng'. The position of the head alters the degree of the defect, the patient's speech being worse *when the head is bent forwards*.

Demonstration of which muscle is paralysed also aids in differentiation, but in diseases such as polyneuritis or myasthenia gravis many different muscles are involved and the defects become more complex.

(*e*) MYASTHENIC DYSARTHRIA

In all muscular weakness there is a tendency for the disability to increase as the patient struggles to speak, but in true myasthenia the voice may be normal at the beginning of each sentence, but abnormalities develop as the sentence progresses. These may be of any of the types mentioned above, but particularly palatal weakness and including hoarseness. A few moments of rest will return the voice to normal. This is usually demonstrated by asking the patient to count up to 30. The abnormality is temporarily cured by injections of edrophonium chloride (Tensilon) or neostigmine.

(*f*) DYSARTHRIA IN DYSPHASIC STATES
A degree of dysarthria may accompany expressive dysphasia, non-fluent dysphasia (see below), and may occasionally be found in lesions producing severe apraxia of the muscles of articulation. A combination of dysphasia and dyarthria may accompany internal carotid artery thrombosis, if the other vessels in the neck are diseased as well. It must always be remembered that in mixed speech defects dysphasia is the most important localising element, for it must mean a dominant hemisphere lesion, whereas dysarthria follows lesions at many sites.

THE ANALYSIS OF DYSPHASIA

The development of thought about dysphasia is beyond the scope of this book but it is a subject of great interest and importance, and summaries written by the late Lord Brain are available and eminently readable in his *Speech Disorders*. An attempt will be made here to produce a relatively simple scheme of examination by which the main types of dysphasia can be detected.

Unfortunately, the lesions that usually produce dysphasia are not such as to justify attempts at pin-point localisation, and for similar reasons, though classification of dysphasia aids in its comprehension, in clinical practice a mixture of the different types is the rule rather than the exception.

Preliminary information
One must first know the patient's nationality, native language, and educational level; his previous ability to read, write, spell and calculate; his handedness; whether, if right-handed, this is genuine or was enforced at an early age; and whether there is left-handedness in the family. One must, of course, determine if there is any mental deterioration, hemianopia or hemiparesis which might confuse the tests. Anything up to 99 per cent of right-handed individuals have left hemisphere dominance for language, but bilaterality may be present in some. The majority even (perhaps 60 per cent) of left-handed people may have left hemisphere dominance, but bilateral dominance is probably quite common. The matter is still unclear.

Spontaneous speech
Always be on the alert for dysphasia. Many dysphasic patients find their way to psychiatric departments because a doctor has not realised what it is he is hearing when listening to a patient's apparently incoherent spontaneous speech. The patients are merely described as 'confused'.

Most information is gained from just listening to the patient. Let him try to tell his own story without his relatives interrupting. Is his speech 'fluent' or 'non-fluent'? Listen carefully to the construction of each word and sentence. Are these correct? Is he making sense? Is he using the right and appropriate words? Is he using wrong words or words which are nearly, but not exactly, right (paraphasia)? Is he using word forms which do not exist (neologisms)? Is he involuntarily repeating the same words after having once used them (perseveration)? Is he using long sentences to overcome the failure to find a particular word (circumlocution)?

At the same time, note if he understands the question asked him and the instructions later given during the course of the ordinary examination. Perseveration may be evident both in verbal reply and in response to commands, e.g., a patient who has just shown his teeth may do so again when told to place his finger on his nose.

Comprehension

Note whether his reaction and answers to ordinary conversation are normal and appropriate. With the exception of some patients with 'conduction' aphasia, even the most severely affected patients should be able to answer questions designed to require only an answer 'Yes' or 'No'. For example, one could ask 'is it true that it is raining outside'. Then the patient can be asked to point, on command, to named objects around the room. Lastly, three objects (your pin, cotton-wool and reflex hammer, for example) should be placed before the patient. He is then asked to place the objects around himself in positions designated by the examiner.

These tests should accurately assess comprehension even in patients with gross motor speech deficits and dyspraxias.

Naming objects

Explain to the patient that he is about to be asked the names of a number of common objects. Start by showing such things as a watch, comb, key, pen or pencil. Then go on to component parts of the object, such as the strap, buckle, winder and second-hand of the watch. Note if he gives the right name promptly or hesitantly; if he uses paraphrasia, or neologisms, or if he perseverates. Use about twenty objects before deciding that no abnormality exists. If he fails to give a name, can he choose the right one from a list of alternatives, or if shown several objects, can he pick out the object named? Make a note at the time of any errors.

Repetition

Testing the ability to repeat words or phrases is important and often overlooked (see below). Ask the patient to repeat a complex phrase and if he fails, simpler phrases or even single words.

Reading

Having assessed the patient's normal capacity in this respect in relation to age, education, nationality and visual acuity, give individual words to be read out first, then sentences, then longer passages, and finally instructions to perform certain actions. This will link the sensory and motor side.

Writing

For all practical purposes, writing is always abnormal in a truly dysphasic person. Dysphasia is a disorder of language, not just speech. He may be able to write his name and address, but not construct linguistically correct sentences. Ask him to compose a piece about the weather, or his job, and test the ability to write to dictation. If he has a right hemiplegia, he must try to write with his left hand.

Calculation

Ask the patient to perform simple sums. These have usually been concerned with money, but the change to decimal coinage in Britain means that one's questions must be adjusted to the age of the patient. Start simply by easy addition—2 plus 4, 3 plus 8, and make this progressively harder. How many new pence are there in a pound? How many ten pence pieces in one pound 50? How much would ten first-class postage stamps cost?

Ask him to subtract 7 from 100, then 7 from the answer, and so on progressively down the scale. Most people of average education can do this in 40 seconds or less. One mistake should be overlooked. Listen carefully to their method of doing this, and avoid confusing inability to concentrate with inability to calculate.

Varieties of dysphasia

The first and most noticeable feature of dysphasia concerns the disruption of spontaneous, conversational speech. By and large, patients are either 'fluent' or 'non-fluent' in their speech output. Basically, patients with 'fluent' speech will have a lesion posterior to the sylvian fissure, those with 'non-fluent' dysphasia a lesion anterior to the fissure. There are some exceptions to this rule, however, in that some patients cannot be so simply classified and that also some patients' dysphasia is initially 'non-fluent' only later becoming 'fluent'.

A typical 'non-fluent' dysphasic will utter few words, will struggle visibly, will not be able to use long phrases and there is often associated dysarthria (see p. 223). In contrast, the 'fluent' patient may even be excessively loquacious, but his speech is full of mistakes: paraphasias, neologisms and circumlocution will be present, with very few nouns.

When the immediate peri-sylvian region, both anterior and posterior to the fissure, is involved in a lesion then one of the significant disturbances concerns *repetition*. The presence or absence of normal ability to repeat spoken language is now regarded as an important distinction. Thus, patients with abnormal repetition form an identifiable category of dysphasics which include those with lesions in Broca's area, Wernicke's area and between the two, in the arcuate fasciculus. Conversely, dysphasia with normal repetition indicates pathology sparing the peri-sylvian region, further away from the fissure. Dysphasias with preserved repetition are, similarly, of three types, all forms of so-called 'transcortical' disturbances. Lesions anterior to the fissure, but superior to Broca's area, cause 'transcortical-motor' dysphasia with non-fluent speech and normal comprehension. Lesions posterior and inferior to Wernicke's area cause 'transcortical-sensory' dysphasia, in which repetition is again preserved, but in the presence of fluency and poor comprehension. If there has been a watershed zone infarction (often following sudden haemodynamic disturbances of perfusion) then the whole area surrounding the peri-sylvian regions may be infarcted, and the latter becomes 'isolated' from other cortical structures. The dysphasia that follows is non-fluent, comprehension is also poor, but repetition is still possible leading to persistent echolalia.

Finally, it will have been noticeable to readers that the above remarks do not include the words 'expressive' nor 'receptive'. This is because firstly, as already emphasised in previous editions, most dysphasias exhibit difficulties both of expression and comprehension of language, but also because the more recent classifications of speech disorders stress the importance to the clinician, concerned as he is with anatomical localisation, of considering patients speech as being 'fluent' or 'non-fluent', with or without preserved repetition. On this basis, the main types of dysphasia can be defined:

BROCA'S DYSPHASIA

Speech is non-fluent, even to the point of mutism in extreme examples, with preserved comprehension and poor repetition. Naming ability is also poor, and the lesion, naturally, is in Broca's area. He may have several words, which are used repeatedly and incorrectly to convey an astonishing variety of meanings.*

WERNICKE'S DYSPHASIA

Lesions in Wernicke's area result in a fluent dysphasia, but with profoundly

*A patient encountered by one of us was only able to say 'South Africa vica me' and yet by the use of this phrase was able to ask for a bedpan, complain about the food, and indeed carry on a useful degree of conversation. A skill of this type indicates that the defect has been present for a very long time.

affected comprehension and impaired repetition. 'Naming' is poor. The patient, failing to produce correct words or syntax, so fails to comprehend his own errors, that he produces a jumbled string of meaningless words and neologisms, in fact—jargon. Hence the older term 'jargon dysphasia'.

CONDUCTION DYSPHASIA

As mentioned above, a lesion that disrupts the arcuate fasciculus connecting Broca's and Wernicke's areas, causes a third variety of dysphasia characterised by poor repetition. Speech is fluent and paraphasic because Broca's area is disconnected, and comprehension is also relatively spared thus distinguishing this dysphasia from Wernicke's type.

TRANSCORTICAL DYSPHASIA

Characterised by retained repetition, and subdivided according to fluency and comprehension into 'transcortical-motor' and 'transcortical-sensory' types, as above.

STUTTERING AND STAMMERING

This is too familiar to need description. When affecting children, predominantly boys, it is often (though not always) associated with ambidexterity or with the enforced use of the right hand in a left-handed child. How much it has a psychogenic basis, and how much associated psychogenic features are secondary to the stutter, is still uncertain, but there is no doubt it can occur as a manifestation of a mild dysphasia, not infrequently in the recovery phase of a definite dysphasia.

There are other forms of speech disturbance considered formerly to have localisational significance. Recent experience puts this in considerable doubt, but the terms have become familiar, and for the sake of completeness are included below, with the locations originally thought responsible.

ECHOLALIA

The involuntary repetition of words and phrases, spoken by someone else without the intention of doing so, and without understanding their meaning. The lesion lies in the temporo-parietal region.

PURE WORD DUMBNESS

Ranging from total inability to articulate to mere slurring of speech, this uncommon defect is accompanied by normal reading, writing, copying and ability to tap out syllables. The muscles unable to articulate are able to perform their other functions. This is an apraxic speech defect and the lesion may be widespread in the left hemisphere.

PURE WORD DEAFNESS

Spontaneous speech, reading and writing are normal, but the patient cannot recognise the spoken word, even as words or as a familiar language. This is a rare defect and is due to a lesion in the middle of the first temporal gyrus.

DEVELOPMENTAL AUDITORY IMPERCEPTION

Frequently a hereditary disturbance predominantly affecting males with normal hearing, this is suspected if they appear to pay no attention to spoken words, and therefore fail to learn to imitate, and therefore to speak. A speech of their own may develop which is very difficult to understand and forms one type of 'idioglossia'—a similar defect occurring in patients deaf from earliest years.

Alexia

This, the inability to understand written speech, is further divided into *alexia without agraphia*, or pure word blindness, and *alexia with agraphia*.

Pure word blindness is rather rare. The patient is able to speak, understand and write, both spontaneously and to dictation, but cannot understand or copy the written word. It is an example of a 'disconnection syndrome', similar to conduction dysphasia already described. In this instance, a lesion of the left occipital cortex and splenium of the corpus callosum 'disconnects' the language area of the left hemisphere (in right-handed people) from both the visual cortices. There is an associated right homonymous hemianopia, and the usual cause is infarction in the territory of the posterior cerebral artery.

Alexia with agraphia, also known as visual asymbolia, is very much more common. The patient cannot read, or write spontaneously with either hand, but may be able to copy to some extent. The lesion lies in the left angular gyrus, and is usually accompanied by nominal aphasia, acalculia, hemianopia, and possibly visual agnosia.

Developmental dyslexia is usually seen in children as a slowness in learning to read. Their vision being normal they may be thought to be mentally retarded, though intelligence can be quite normal and all other speech functions normal, though mirror writing may be present. The child may indeed try to read words from right to left. The defect may be familial, and may possibly be due to an incomplete left hemisphere dominance.

Agraphia

As one of the symptoms of other aphasic states, writing defects are common. A pure agraphia, without the other features of speech disturbance, may occur in lesions which lie between the angular gyrus and the motor area, but may sometimes be anterior or posterior to this.

An apraxia of the hand, due not to a disturbance of language so much as to an inability to make the correct movements for writing, produces a form of dysgraphia, the lesion lying in the region of the left angular gyrus, or if limited to the left hand, in the corpus callosum.

Acalculia

The recent development of an inability to manipulate figures may be part of any of the major aphasias. If acalculia is not associated with other speech defects, it indicates a lesion of the left angular gyrus (see Gerstmann's syndrome).

It will be seen that there is considerable overlap between these different states and the sites of the lesions responsible. Where tumours are concerned, the lesion is usually much larger than the type of speech defect might suggest. At other times, the position of the main bulk of a lesion appears rather far from the area known to produce particular defects, It must be remembered that tumours, for instance, have remote effects due to displacement, vascular compression, or oedema, as well as the effects of direct local invasion. For these reasons attempts at pinpoint localisation from dysphasic defects often become frustrating to the perfectionist because the pathological process involves, directly or indirectly, so wide an area. Computerised axial tomography sounded the final death-knell of the would-be pinpoint localiser—but the academic intellectual exercise in the attempt still has its merits in the logic of neurological appraisal. Stroke syndromes, on the other hand, are more precise and do allow very accurate localisation.

No apology is made for repeating the necessity of detecting *dysphasia* in any speech disturbance—for the lesion responsible for this lies in the dominant cerebral hemisphere, no matter what other lesions the patient may have as well.

Chapter 29
Apraxia

Apraxia is a failure of the ability to carry out well-organised voluntary movement correctly despite the fact that motor, sensory and co-ordinative functions are not significantly impaired. It is *not* the word, as is the modern tendency, to delineate any improper motor response resulting from paresis or incoordination.

Methods of testing

First make sure that if there is any weakness, sensory defect, or ataxia, it would not interfere seriously with voluntary movements, and that the patient understands instructions.

Ask him to hold out his arms, put out his tongue, show his teeth, etc. If he fails, note whether, despite this, these movements are normal when they are automatic, e.g. licking the lips, smiling or responding to an obvious offer to shake hands.

Next ask him to make a fist at someone, to scratch his arm, and, more difficult, to use a pair of scissors, a pen, a comb, making sure first that he recognises these things. Ask him to open a box of matches and to take out a match; to go through the motion of lighting a cigarette; to show how he would hammer a nail, play a violin, put in a corkscrew and take a cork out of a bottle. Any test requiring three or four different movements can be used, both with and without objects.

Give him a series of matches and ask him to form a triangle, a square, or more complex patterns. If this appears difficult, do it for him and ask him to copy it. Ask him to write his name and address. Note how he manipulates buttons or studs; how he takes off his coat and jacket and puts them on again.

Forms of apraxia

Four types of apraxia are usually recognised, the first two of which cause most difficulty because their names are similar and the difference between them is a fine one.

IDEOMOTOR APRAXIA

The patient performs automatic acts normally, such as blowing his nose, shaking hands, pushing back hair, etc., and is able to formulate the idea of an act and to describe how it should be done, but when it comes to carrying out the movement on command, he is unable to do it correctly. This is probably the commonest form of apraxia, and usually just referred to as 'apraxia'. The basic disturbance is an inability to imitate or mime an act involving the use of objects. There is a common tendency to substitute a body part for the object, for example using the index finger *as* a toothbrush rather than pretending to *hold* one.

IDEATIONAL APRAXIA

The formulation of the method of carrying out the whole of a complex act is defective, though the execution of different parts of the complete act may be normal. The popular description is of the patient who, when told to do each of these actions separately, will take a match box, hold it correctly, open it correctly, take out a match correctly, and do the same with a cigarette box, but when told to go through the motion of lighting a cigarette, will be unable to do so or will try some manoeuvre such as striking the cigarette on the match box. So this form of apraxia is recognised by the patient's inability to use objects properly and not tested for by imitation or miming. In clinical practice, ideomotor and ideational apraxia frequently co-exist.

CONSTRUCTIONAL APRAXIA

The patient is defeated by attempts to make designs with, for instance, matches, either spontaneously or by copying. Often in writing he cramps everything into one small corner of the paper.

Koh's blocks. This is a series of blocks with colours occupying the whole or half of one side, which can be so arranged as to make simple or complex patterns. The patient with constructional apraxia is unable to make or copy the simplest design. The side of the figure opposite the lesion may be omitted altogether.

DRESSING APRAXIA

The patient becomes hopelessly muddled in trying to dress and undress, puts his clothes on the wrong way round, or may be quite unable to start the necessary motions. This defect, which is also possibly present if ideational apraxia is present, may be found entirely by itself.

Lesions producing ideomotor apraxia interrupt connections running between the dominant parietal cortex and the motor area, and also with the opposite motor area through the corpus collosum. Therefore a lesion situated:
(*a*) In the dominant supramarginal gyrus should produce bilateral apraxia.
(*b*) Between this gyrus and the left motor cortex should produce right-sided apraxia (in right-handed people).
(*c*) In the corpus callosum could produce left-sided apraxia.

In practice, however, the lesions are often more diffuse, though the dominant parietal lobe is most heavily involved. Constructional apraxia occurs in angular gyrus lesions of either hemisphere, but when isolated is usually from non-dominant parietal lesions. Dressing apraxia may also occur in a non-dominant posterior parietal lobe lesion. Vascular and degenerative diseases are more often responsible than neoplasms.

Chapter 30
Agnosia and Disorders of the Body Image

Agnosia, though a remarkable phenomenon, is not an unfathomable mystery, and it is, in short, a failure to recognise some object or sound when the sense by which it is normally recognised remains intact. This defect may be present in the field of any of the normal sensations, but agnosia for smell and taste are doubtful entities.

Examining for agnosia

Visual recognition

First show the patient a number of common small objects. Ask him to (*a*) name them, (*b*) describe their use, (*c*) pick out others named for him.

If he is unable to do so allow him to feel the object in a hand in which the sensation is normal and ask the same questions.

Next show the patient several different colours and ask him (*a*) their names, (*b*) to pick out duplicates from a separate set, (*c*) to arrange them in shades of increasing lightness.

Now show him some familiar objects, holding them in one or other homonymous visual field.

If the patient is well enough, ask him to walk towards a particular point, having placed some chairs in the way, and observe whether he is able to find his way to the correct place and around the obstructions.

VISUAL AGNOSIA

(*a*) The patient is unable to name or describe the use of the objects shown, but is able to identify them when he touches them, or by their characteristic noise or smell. (A patient with nominal aphasia will be unable to find the exact name, whichever sense is used.) This defect is called *visual object agnosia*. It may vary according to the size of the objects, the patient's environment, and even from examination to examination.

The site of the lesion lies in the second and third occipital gyri and the adjacent subcortical white matter in the dominant hemisphere.

(*b*) He may be unable to identify, match or arrange colours. This is often associated with object agnosia and is termed *visual agnosia for colours*. The lesion is in a similar situation.

(*c*) He may be unable to find his way around an obstruction or to find his way to a given point. This is *visual agnosia for space* and results in visual disorientation. It is most marked in bilateral postero-inferior parietal lesions, but unilateral lesions can cause an agnosia for one-half of space, so that the patient will turn always to the opposite side and is liable eventually to return to the point of starting. This is most clearly demonstrated when the non-dominant hemisphere is affected.

Tactile recognition

First ensure that sensation is normal in both hands. Ask the patient to close his eyes and then place a number of common objects in turn in one or other hand. Ask him to name them, to describe their shape, size and texture and to indicate their use.

If he fails to do this, allow him to look at them or to hear or smell them, and see if he is then able to recognise them.

TACTILE AGNOSIA

The patient may be unable to recognise any detail of the object at all. In such a case it is probable that discriminative or postural sense is defective, and the defect becomes one of astereognosis. If he is able to describe its size, shape and texture, but is not able to give its name or its use, and particularly if on seeing it he is then able to name it, this is true *tactile agnosia*. It is a defect which commonly co-exists with visual object agnosia.

The site of the lesion is in the contralateral supramarginal gyrus. It is possible that left-sided agnosia in a right-handed person may also be caused by a lesion of the corpus callosum.

Auditory recognition

First determine that the hearing in both ears is normal. Ask the patient to close his eyes and to identify sounds made by striking a match, ringing a bell, shaking money, tearing cloth, etc.

AUDITORY AGNOSIA

The patient who is unable to recognise these sounds, but can recognise the objects on sight or touch has *auditory agnosia*. As there is often word deafness as well, it may be necessary to write out the instructions. If there is an associated aphasia which might confuse his answers, he should be told to illustrate the sound himself, if he recognises it.

The site of the lesion is in the posterior part of the temporal convolutions of the dominant hemisphere.

THE PARIETAL LOBE AND DISORDERS OF THE BODY SCHEME

A normal individual is able, without looking or having to give much thought to the matter, to tell at any moment where each part of the body is, and where it lies in relation to objects around it. If there is a defect of postural sensibility some other sense, such as vision, may be necessary to determine where the defective limb lies. There are situations, however, when, despite the use of other senses, the normal appreciation of the shape, size and position of one or other part of the body is disturbed, sometimes to such an extent that if that part is diseased the patient may be quite unaware of it, and may even deny that it is part of his own body.

Examination

First determine if the patient knows which is his right and left hand and leg. Then ask him to point to different major parts of his own body, using each hand in turn if possible. Next ask him to point to the ring finger of his left hand, the forefinger of his right hand, to point to the little toe, etc. Make this more difficult by asking him to place his fingers behind his back and pick out individual digits. Ask him then to pick out individual digits on the examiner's hand, and finally, the examiner should interlock his fingers with the patient's and ask him to pick out the various digits.

During the course of the general examination, observe whether the patient does or does not appear to be aware of any disability, such as a hemiplegia, which may be present. If he seems unaware of this, draw his attention specifically to the paralysed limb and ask him to explain his inability to move it.

Disturbances of body scheme

Difficulty in remembering which is right and left is a common problem especially if the question is suddenly asked, but when once reminded most people continue to answer correctly afterwards. Persistent right-left disorientation is seen in parietal lobe disorders.

Patients may be unable to identify any part of their body. This is termed *autotopagnosia*. A lesser degree of this is found in the inability to pick out individual digits and is termed *finger agnosia*.

Gerstmann's syndrome, which consists of finger agnosia both for the patient's own fingers and the examiner's, acalculia, right–left disorientation, and agraphia without alexia, is found in lesions of the dominant hemisphere, in the region of the angular gyrus.

In lesions of the parietal lobe of the non-dominant hemisphere, which present an easier situation for examination as there is less intellectual defect and no aphasia, there may be complete lack of awareness of the opposite half of the body. If that side is paralysed the patient may be unaware of, and even deny the existence of, the hemiplegia. He may say the limbs do not belong to him and may even complain that the arm in his bed belongs to someone else. This is known as *anosognosia*, and may exist in relation to hemiplegia, blindness, deafness, or any other disability.

At the other end of the scale there is the phenomenon of the *phantom limb*, so common in amputees as to be considered normal, which is a retention of the whole body image after the removal of one member, a retention sufficiently vivid for pain and parasthesiae to be felt in the fingers or toes. Over the years the phantom tends to shrink in size.

Sensory inattention

Neglect of one side may be present, but not in the gross degree described above. It is then necessary to present to the patient simultaneous bilateral stimulation of one of the common senses in order to detect the defect which has been called by Macdonald Critchley 'Inattention'.

VISUAL INATTENTION

First determine by confrontation that the visual fields are individually intact. Then face the patient, both patient and examiner having both eyes open. Place the forefingers of both hands so that they can be seen in the patient's temporal fields equidistant from the midline. Ask the patient to point to the finger he sees moving. Move first one finger, then the other (not alternately), and finally, move both together, when the patient with visual inattention on one side will point to one finger as if that one alone had moved.

Next use movements of the whole hand. If the attention defect still persists, tell him positively that at times both hands will be moved together. This will make no difference in the fully developed case.

Now move both hands for a few moments and then stop moving the hand on the normal side. The patient may, after a short delay, appreciate the movement on the abnormal side which he had previously failed to do.

Ask the patient to draw some symmetrical object, such as the head of a flower, a house, a clock face, or a bicycle. If necessary give him a model to copy. If defeated by complexities of this type, simple geometrical designs could be copied. The patient with an attention defect will leave out, or incorrectly space out, the petals on one side of a flower, the figures on one side of a clock face, one wheel of a bicycle, the window on one side of a house, or he may fail to join up the angles to one side of a rectangle. If there is an associated constructional apraxia (see p. 231), this test may, of course, be completely impossible.

AUDITORY INATTENTION

First determine that hearing in each ear is approximately equal. Then ask the patient to close his eyes and to point to the side from which he hears a noise. Shake a bunch of keys, irregularly, first on one side and then the other and every now and then on both sides simultaneously. If auditory inattention is present only the sound from one side will be appreciated. At times unequal sounds can be used, quite a slight sound being heard on the normal side, while a loud sound is simultaneously produced, but not appreciated on the abnormal side.

TACTILE INATTENTION

First determine that the patient's superficial sensation is normal, and that he is able to recognise right from left. Then ask him to close his eyes and, with a pin, prick one or other arm at irregular intervals. He should say, or move the arm that is being stimulated. Assuming he locates the side of these pricks correctly, then prick on both sides simultaneously. A patient with tactile inattention will indicate one side only. The stimuli can then be changed to stroking, pinching, and quite painful tapping of a limb, and still only one side is appreciated.

Ask the patient to hold both hands out, keeping the eyes closed, and to say into which hand an object is placed. Put similar objects, e.g. oranges, into each hand simultaneously. The patient with tactile inattention will only appreciate one. Take this one away and after a short time he will draw attention to the other.

Note how he puts on his coat and jacket. He may be entirely satisfied with a situation in which one arm is left out. If dressing apraxia is present, this is only of value if it is consistently on the same side.

This phenomenon of inattention is described by Bender and many other authors as 'extinction'. It is most commonly seen after vascular accidents, in cerebral atrophic lesions, sometimes in parietal lobe tumours, including meningiomata, when it may recover after removal, and rarely in other conditions. Isolated cases have been described in which a similar phenomenon is present in lesions of a large variety of other parts of the nervous system, but usually it can be taken to mean a lesion of the parietal lobe of the contralateral hemisphere.

Chapter 31
The Autonomic Nervous System

Only a limited amount of the mass of information available regarding the autonomic nervous system (ANS) is applied with any frequency during the practice of clinical neurology. However, recent years have seen the evolution of several simple and non-invasive tests of both sympathetic and parasympathetic function. These can be applied with reliability using only straightforward equipment and requiring little time. Detailed testing of autonomic function remains highly complex and is really the preserve of specialised units. New advances have revealed a system abounding with neurotransmitters within a very complicated neural organisation such that full investigation involves expertise in physiological, pharmacological and biochemical laboratory techniques.

Whereas the ANS is concerned with virtually every organ in the body, from skin to brain, it has been in the study of *cardiovascular reflexes* that tests of a 'bedside' nature have been recently devised. That is not to forget, naturally, the many autonomic reflexes that are examined within the *cranial nerves* (see pupils, lacrimal response, salivation, etc.). *Bladder* and *bowel* dysfunction is prominent amongst the manifestations of autonomic failure, and there are also the changes in *respiration, skin,* and *sweating* to record.

General inspection

Note the colour of the skin, especially of the extremities, both when first seen and after exposure. Look for local or general flushing or cyanosis, and feel the temperature of the skin in different parts of the body. Recent sympathetic lesions produce warmth and redness in the affected areas. Note whether sweating is unexpectedly profuse or abnormally slight, and if there is a localised abnormality, what its distribution is in relation to sensory dermatomes.

Complete sympathetic lesions result in the absence of sweating, but partial lesions may produce excessive sweating. Notice any changes in colour, texture and quantity of hair or nails. Look especially for signs of any well-recognised local autonomic lesions, such as Horner's syndrome (p. 51).

CARDIOVASCULAR REFLEXES

The simpler physiological tests here are based upon the responses of the

heart rate and blood pressure to various stimuli. Sympathetic and parasympathetic function is involved.
(*a*) *Postural hypotension:* a fall of more than 20–30 mmHg systolic blood pressure on standing is abnormal. Causes can be central or peripheral; if the latter, severe sympathetic dysfunction is present.
(*b*) *Blood pressure response to pressor stimuli:* mental arithmetic, sustained handgrip or exposure to cold cause a rise in blood pressure. The use of a handgrip dynamometer allows a quantifiable test. Less than 10 mmHg rise in diastolic pressure is abnormal. Both central and peripheral (sympathetic) lesions affect these tests.
(*c*) *Heart rate responses:* (i) in the normal person, a change of posture from lying to standing is followed by an immediate increase in heart rate and then a relative bradycardia. This can be quantified by using continuous ECG recording. A parasympathetic lesion will slow down or abolish the response, a situation found in diabetic or other autonomic neuropathies. (ii) With an intact parasympathetic nerve supply, the heart rate varies *with respiration* (sinus arrhythmia). This is reduced or abolished in the presence of an autonomic neuropathy. (iii) Massage of the carotid sinus stimulates the baroreceptors and vagal parasympathetic activity should then slow the heart rate. Afferent or efferent lesions abolish the response. Care should be taken in this test; severe bradycardia and hypotension can result in hypersensitive persons.
(*d*) *The Valsalva manoeuvre:* here there is a response in both blood pressure and heart rate. In the first exhalation (against a closed glottis), the blood pressure drops and the heart rate increases. On releasing (by opening the glottis) the blood pressure 'overshoots' the resting value and the heart slows.

The test can be performed by the patient exhaling into a mouthpiece connected to a manometer or sphygmomanometer to hold the pressure at 40 mmHg for 15 seconds. An ECG records the heart rate response.

Afferent or efferent parasympathetic lesions impair the response. (Patients with lesions at the foramen magnum such as cerebellar ectopia develop a characteristic headache.)

These clinical tests of cardiovascular function can be augmented by biochemical or pharmacological methods. Intravenous infusions of noradrenaline and atropine test for sympathetic and parasympathetic function respectively. Plasma noradrenaline and renin can be measured directly.

SKIN RESPONSES

Erythema. Scratching the skin will produce a line surrounded by a spreading flare and followed by a wheal with central pallor. This is often exaggerated below the level of a transverse cord lesion, and, according to the lesion, may be unilateral or bilateral, often becoming apparent after testing cutaneous sensation to pin prick. At the level of the lesion, even the normal response may be absent. Exaggerated responses unfortunately can occur in normal or psychoneurotic individuals—this 'dermatographia' is, however, not simply limited to the skin below a segmental level.

Temperature. The measurement of skin temperature by means of accurate skin thermometers can show:
(*a*) Increased temperature below a recently denervated level.
(*b*) Decreased temperature following chronic neurological lesions which have caused prolonged immobility.
(*c*) Increased response to warming of the part or of distant parts over the denervated area in sympathetic lesions, but
(*d*) Decreased response to warming in areas where the deficit is circulatory rather than neurogenic.

Pilomotor responses. These are similar in significance to the erythematous responses. They are produced by sharp scratching, or by touching the warmed body with cold metal.

Scrotal response. Touching the scrotum with a cold object normally results in a vermicular contraction of the dartos, without elevation of the testicles, thus differing from the cremasteric reflex. This is absent in sympathetic paralysis.

A sweating test

The areas to be tested are first thoroughly dried, and then liberally dusted with Quinizarin powder. The patient is placed under a heat cradle, and given a hot drink combined with 0.5 g acetylsalycilic acid. Areas of sweat production are clearly outlined as the powder turns black when exposed to moisture.

In sympathetic lesions there will be a segmental loss of sweating corresponding to the distribution of the affected sympathetic fibres. Below a transverse cord lesion, sweating may be absent in the early stages, but may later become abnormally profuse. At the segmental level of a recent transverse lesion the response is often exaggerated.

This is a good test for the results of sympathectomy, of section or injury to peripheral nerves, and for demonstrating and photographing denervated areas. It can show, objectively, areas of sympathetic denervation in syringomyelia. It is a capricious test, however, and requires a lot of experience before it can compare in value with the assessment of cutaneous sensation for the purpose of determining the level of a cord lesion.

Thermography

Infra-red photography of part or whole body surfaces will give detailed areas of temperature difference undetectable clinically, and again objectively is useful for localisation and comparison. Again, great experience in interpretation is required and artefacts may abound.

EXAMINATION OF BLADDER FUNCTION

Normal urinary continence and voiding requires a balance between the so-called 'forces of expulsion' and the 'forces of retention'. Detrusor and abdominal muscle contraction, on the one hand, needs to be balanced against the activity of the bladder neck (internal) and urethral (external) sphincters on the other. This balance does not depend exclusively on nervous control—there are physical factors involved also, such as the inherent distensibility of a given detrusor muscle. So not all disorders of micturition are the result of faulty nervous control; but they are certainly common in neurological disease.

Lesions of the superior frontal and anterior cingulate gyri, whether the result of stroke, tumour or hydrocephalus, reduce awareness of bladder function and cause incontinence. More posterior lesions of the frontal lobes may cause spasticity of the striated muscle (external) sphincters and therefore produce retention. Incomplete lesions of the upper motor neurone pathways above the sacral spinal cord interfere with the storage and voiding of urine. Frequency and urgency of micturition are the rule, with incomplete bladder emptying. A complete transection of the spinal cord in the first place causes retention with 'overflow incontinence' and then later a 'reflex bladder' may develop with automatic emptying induced by abdominal pressure. Lesions of the sacral cord itself or the outflow in the cauda equina lead to a flaccid neurogenic bladder which enlarges and again can cause 'overflow incontinence'. With impaired parasympathetic function in the sacral segmental supply, sensation is lost in the S2–4 dermatones. In tabes dorsalis, damage to the sympathetic and parasympathetic sensory side of the reflex arc results in painless bladder enlargement.

In investigating bladder function the exact history is absolutely vital. All but the more complex problems can be reasonably assessed with a good history and appropriate neurological examination. Some questions would include: Is there normal sensation of bladder filling and voiding? Can voiding be interrupted voluntarily by sphincter action? What is the force of the stream like? When does incontinence occur?

The examination, naturally, should always include testing the sacral segments (see p. 156, Fig. 67). Bladder swelling may be palpable. The superficial anal reflex should be tested (p. 191). The condition of the motor and sensory pathway to the lower limbs will testify to any spinal cord, conus medullaris, or cauda equina lesion.

A useful assessment of detrusor function can be made by asking a patient while passing urine to breathe deeply, thus interrupting abdominal muscle straining. If the detrusor is not functioning the flow will cease.

Residual urine can be assessed by a post-micturition X-ray of the bladder as part of an intravenous pyelogram, without catheterisation.

Urodynamic studies

In the narrower sense of the word, 'urodynamics' refers to the investigation and assessment of the bladder and lower urinary tract. In its broader concept, we now have a whole new discipline embracing the total management of bladder disorders. Rather like good neurophysiological investigation of, say, a case of suspected muscle disease, the ideal urodynamic assessment is tailored to the clinical situation.

But the essential requirement is to measure intravesical pressure during bladder filling (the 'filling cystometrogram'), and the relationship between intravesical pressure and urinary flow rate during voiding (the 'micturition cystometrogram'). Sophisticated urological departments will now use a four-channel recording of abdominal pressure (via rectal catheter), total bladder pressure (via bladder catheter), subtracted true intravesical (detrusor) pressure and flow rate. The filling volume and voiding volume will be recorded. A note is made of the patient's awareness of bladder *sensation*, the *capacity* before a strong desire to void is appreciated, the *compliance* of the bladder (the volume change for a given pressure), and the *contractility* of the detrusor (e.g., spontaneous contractions before complete filling). If the bladder is filled with contrast medium, then video-radiological screening is possible, detecting abnormalities of structure and visualising the bladder contraction and sphincter mechanisms. These can then be interpreted alongside the pressure-flow measurements. In this way, the assessment of neuropathic bladder dysfunction has become much more detailed and accurate. Surgical intervention or other treatments can be advised on a more rational basis.

The pressure in the normal almost empty bladder is about 1 cm of water, and if quantities of about 50 ml are introduced at a time the pressure steadily rises, with rhythmical variations as the bladder wall accommodates. Vesical sensation is felt at about 100–150 ml when a pressure of about 6 cm should be registered. The bladder can usually be distended to 400–600 ml. The rhythmical contractions which are accompanied by a slight sense of urgency will build up until reflex micturition occurs accompanied by a sharp rise in pressure. This may, however, not occur in patients who are tense and nervous. If the bladder is atonic and known to be insensitive great care must be taken not to over-distend it and risk rupture.

RESULTS

These are expressed in terms of the observed bladder sensation, capacity, contractility and compliance together with the pressure and flow measurements during filling and voiding. A 'functional profile' is thus obtained.

In a *complete* lower motor neurone lesion one finds a senseless, high capacity (flaccid), acontractile and hypercompliant bladder with low pressure. Voiding requires straining.

In a *complete* upper motor neurone lesion, one finds a senseless, low capacity (spastic), hypercontractile (hyper-reflexic), hypocompliant bladder with high pressure. There will be a hyperactive sphincter, and reflex voiding.

In practice, lesions are often not complete; they can be 'mixed' and the urodynamic findings can become modified by local changes in the bladder wall, chronicity of disease and the degree and duration of any bladder distension. However, some generalisations can be made:

In *bilateral lesions* of the pyramidal system of some standing, i.e. cord or brain stem lesions, the bladder is small in capacity, contracts rapidly on stimulation, so that discomfort is felt early, but the sensation is poorly localised. In *recent lesions of the spinal cord,* there is often a period of paralysis of bladder musculature with atonia and easy distension before these features develop.

In lesions of the *cauda equina, conus medullaris,* or *peripheral nerves,* there is loss of bladder sensation, the pressure is high, the capacity not greatly increased, and contractions may occur infrequently. These may be large enough to cause evacuation, which, however, is incomplete.

In severe lesions of the *sensory roots* or *posterior columns,* there is total loss of bladder sensation, the muscle is atonic, distends easily so that the pressure is low, contractions are absent, evacuation is absent and the residual urine high. In such cases, great care must be exercised.

In *cerebral lesions,* the results are variable. There may be retention or incontinence at the outset, but as the cerebral lesion recovers, urinary symptoms also recover. Bladder sensation is normal, but the capacity is reduced and micturition is precipitate. Retention with overflow is a rare finding in high spinal or cerebral lesions.

Lesions of the *dominant hemisphere, demyelinative lesions,* and some *diffuse cerebral lesions* result in the so-called uninhibited bladder, in which the contractions, capacity and sensation are normal, but micturition occurs precipitately as soon as contractions reach a size large enough to produce evacuation.

As a group, patients with multiple sclerosis often develop a 'mixed' picture of disturbance. The typical pyramidal tract type disorder of bladder function may be combined with external sphincter occlusion (spasticity or dyssynergia). There will follow a combination of frequency and urgency of micturition with a tendency to retention. Alternatively, the detrusor itself may be weak, with low intravesical pressure. Symptoms will then vary in accordance with the state of the sphincters. Some patients will tend towards incontinence, others towards retention. It will be seen that in any one given patient, a variety of mechanisms may underlie an apparently simple complaint. Full urodynamic evaluation is then essential.

THE RECTUM

Acute lesions of the spinal cord, especially of the sacral segments, cause laxity of sphincters and incontinence. If the sacral segments or the pelvic nerves are involved the gripping of a gloved finger by the internal anal sphincter will be absent even in the chronic state. Stroking the skin near the external sphincter will not produce reflex contraction. Higher spinal lesions or pontine lesions of chronic type usually allow tonic contraction of the sphincters and result in constipation.

SEXUAL FUNCTION

Either diffuse autonomic failure, local spinal, or root lesions may interfere with sexual function. The history alone may be of considerable diagnostic value. There are occasions when potency is disturbed before bladder function in a male with a developing spinal cord disorder. Relevant questions include enquiring whether erection is absent or occurs normally, or whether just reflexly (noctural tumescence)? If ejaculation is present, is it of normal force or not? Is orgasmic sensation normal?

Proper, psychically induced erection is a function of the parasympathetic hypogastric nerves. Reflex erection is mediated by the pelvic nerves from sacral roots. Spinal lesions may cause initial priapism (reflex painful erection). Subsequently, spinal disorders above T12 may cause impotence with retained reflex erection but without ejaculation. A complaint of impotence with retained reflex erection and ejaculation is characteristic of a psychological disorder. (Never forget the many drugs which may cause impotence.) Cauda equina lesions will usually result in failure of both erection and ejaculation with impaired sensation.

THE USE OF DRUGS

The amount of additional information gained by the use of sympathomimetic or parasympathomimetic drugs is not very great in routine investigation, but there are a few specific responses which are of occasional value.

In suspected sympathetic lesions an injection of adrenaline causes excessive vasoconstriction in the affected zone.

Intracutaneous injection of 0.1 ml of 1/1000 histamine will not produce the normal wheal and flare in a totally denervated zone, but will in an area of hysterical anaesthesia.

The ganglion blocking agents can distinguish between vasoconstriction due to autonomic overaction and structural disease of the vessels. In the latter, administration of the drug makes no difference to the blood flow and temperature of the extremities.

Peperoxane, or phentolamine, given intravenously will produce a fall in blood pressure in cases of hypertension due to phaeochromocytoma, but not in hypertension of other causes, and can be used as a diagnostic test.

Ergotamine tartrate given early in an attack of true migraine may abort the pain, and given prior to an expected attack of true periodic migrainous neuralgia (which usually occurs at the same time each day), will stop the attack from developing, and is of value as a diagnostic test.

Amyl nitrite, given during the vasoconstrictive phase of migraine, may stop the symptoms experienced during the aura, but increases the headache.

Neostigmine and Tensilon are used in the diagnosis of myasthenia gravis and have autonomic side effects which are undesirable. In the case of neostigmine the concurrent injection of atropine will reduce these effects considerably.

SYMPATHETIC BLOCK

Though sympathectomy has little value in cerebral thrombosis or arteriosclerosis, the injection of local anaesthetic into the stellate ganglion can be useful in certain limited circumstances. If a patient with a hemiparesis has an occlusion of the internal carotid artery, arteriography may show the intracranial portion of the carotid artery filling with blood by anastomosis from the external carotid, through the orbital plexus, and in a retrograde manner along the ophthalmic artery. A sympathetic block may temporarily improve this anastomosis and cause a measurable improvement in speech and in the power of the arm. Sympathectomy might then benefit that patient.

Similar blocking of the middle or inferior ganglia can be used to assess the possible results of sympathectomy in Raynaud's disease, and in the curious condition called Sudeck's atrophy, where there are painful wrist and finger joints, trophic changes in the hand, weakness, limitation of movement, increased reflexes, X-ray changes showing osteoporosis and apparent coalescence of the carpal bones, and, oddly enough, increased peripheral blood flow to the superficial tissues.

FOR DETAILED READING

Bannister R. (1983) *Autonomic Failure: A Textbook of Clinical Disorders of the Autonomic System.* Oxford University Press, Oxford.

Johnson R.H. & Spalding J.M.K. (1974) *Disorders of the Autonomic Nervous System.* Blackwell Scientific Publications, Oxford.

Plum F. (1962) Bladder dysfunction. In: *Modern Trends in Neurology No. 3,* pp. 151–172. Butterworths, London.

White J.C., Swithwick R.H. & Simeone F.A. (1952) *The Autonomic Nervous System.* Macmillan, New York.

Part VII
The Investigation of Neurological Problems

Chapter 32
Towards A Balanced Attitude
(some introductory observations)

Over the last 20 years there have been gradual changes in the attitudes of clinicians towards neurological investigations, which on the whole have been all to the good. However, a dark cloud is looming on the horizon warning of a potential further change which could be a serious reversal to the thoughtful physician, and to neurology as a whole. Forty years ago the neurologist had few measures at his command outside his clinical acumen, a number of X-ray procedures, the ability to do certain relevant blood tests, and to examine the cerebrospinal fluid. So big a part did this latter element play that in the first edition of this book I implied that the indications for lumbar puncture would be any neurological condition in which the clear-cut *contra-indications* did not apply. This is no longer an acceptable dogma either in respect of lumbar puncture or of any other investigation. As more diagnostic measures become available one needs to ask oneself even more closely 'why, in this particular patient, am I suggesting this particular investigation? Is it truly likely to give relevant information, and is the information so obtained going to be of value in the management of the case? Indeed, is it so important to know that information, that if the investigation carries with it some risk to the patient, is that risk justified?' It often is (maybe in experienced hands usually is), but sometimes it is not, and if it is not justified, then it should not be carried out.

This line of thought has brought new terms into medical language. One that one hears on all sides is the classification of procedures into 'invasive' and 'non-invasive'. While all of us know more or less what we mean when we use these terms, they seem sometimes to have rather artificial definitions. For instance, to put a needle into an artery is invasive; to put it into a vein apparently is non-invasive (or sometimes the thoughtful person says 'relatively' non-invasive). Presumably a skin electrode for electromyography is non-invasive, an intramuscular electrode invasive. Shining a light in the eyes is non-invasive, but is it non-invasive to flash a stroboscope during electroencephalography to stimulate cortical responses, and maybe on a rare occasion to precipitate a major epileptic fit?

Some sense of proportion needs to be brought to the use of these terms, for it is the implications of the very terms themselves that could be a foretaste of the further change of attitude referred to earlier. This is the development of what is becoming widely known as 'defensive medicine'—i.e.

doing everything one can think of in the way of investigation for fear of not doing something that might just conceivably have been important, the fear being these days, unhappily (and somebody has got to say this), not so much of missing information that might be of value to the management of the patient, but that of being exposed at some later date to litigation for not having done it. This is a major problem in some countries whose legal system encourages actions for so-called negligence against doctors, with the potential for enormous damages if found proven; and, like a malignant growth, it is spreading.

In those parts of the world where this fear has as yet not become so prominent, there is gradually developing a desire to find and limit methods of investigation to those which are of the least discomfort to the patient, and which expose him to minimal danger of complications. The trouble here is that these methods may or may not be as good at demonstrating what is required as those that are older and well-established. So one has to be convinced that one has used not only a relevant method, but one that has been enough.

Nowhere more than in the field of neuroradiology does this apply, and each five-year period has seen the most dramatic advances in this field. There are those of us who, when first introduced to intracranial contrast arteriography, assisted in the exposure by a surgeon of the carotid artery in the neck, probably in an operating theatre; the transporting then of the patient to the X-ray department, where injection of the contrast medium was carried out under direct vision while the X-rays were being taken; the return of the patient for wound closure, with the almost certain guarantee that a repeat of the procedure on that side would be impossible. To us the development of percutaneous techniques seemed almost to be the ultimate (even if one did in earlier years have excellent, if unwanted, views of the vertebro-basilar system unilaterally due to the wrong vessel being entered). Barbarous though the cut-down techniques may have seemed, whether they had the same occasional complications is dubious—at least one knew which vessel one was injecting, and that one was in the lumen of the artery and not producing dissection of the wall. When direct puncture of the vertebral artery was required, it was not only difficult, but potentially dangerous—what if, for instance, unknown to the examiner, the other vertebral artery was vestigeal or occluded. Into this field came the evolution of the femoral or brachial artery catheterisation techniques under X-ray monitoring, which avoided direct puncture of a vital cerebral artery, enabled the origin of the vessels to be seen, and was of course invaluable in four-vessel arteriography where both carotid and vertebro-basilar systems were visualised. But it still involved the puncture of an artery and was therefore an 'invasive' investigation. To avoid this, attempts were made to develop techniques of intravenous injection of the media, but haemodilution was a great problem, so that large quantities had to be used; and there was filling of so many vessels, arteries and veins, rather faintly, that a useful degree of definition was rarely obtained. This method of introducing the medium has now been reborn under the technique of Digital Subtraction Angiography which is described on p. 294. A relatively risk-free procedure, this method gives good, if black-on-white, pictures and shows atheromatous lesions clearly. It is not yet really good enough to satisfy the surgeon for undertaking such measures as aneurysm surgery, and so-called 'conventional' arteriography may have to be done as well. So if aneurysm is under suspicion as a diagnosis, why not do it in the first place? Clearly in other conditions, such as carotid stenosis, this is a safe and viable technique and it is being improved all the time.

But other methods are being adopted where no 'assault' upon the vascular tree is necessary. By the use of sonic techniques and computerising the results the major vessels can be visualised in an almost three-dimensional manner, and stenoses, atheromatous plaques, and occlusions can be clearly demonstrated to those who know how to read the pictures. Are they good enough for an arterial surgeon to decide which way he will handle the problem? Some think they are; others demand confirmation by 'conventional' arteriography. One realises in writing this that by the time this book is published these new techniques may be the 'conventional' ones, and others may have advanced still further.

When one comes to intracranial lesions such as tumours, haematomata, infarcts, oedema, abscesses, and atrophy, computerised axial tomography (CAT or CT scanning) is now accepted, if not necessarily available, world-wide. Nuclear magnetic resonance (NMR) or magnetic resonance imaging (MRI) has been restricted purely by problems of finance and space, for its value is unequalled in showing intrinsic lesions of the brain, brain stem and spinal cord, and the ability to reconstruct views in different planes is impressive to a degree. To be able to demonstrate lesions of multiple sclerosis in areas unsuspected clinically is of inestimable value diagnostically when there appears clinically to be only one single lesion. (See pp. 310–315 for these procedures.) Positron emission tomography (PET scanning) produces pictures easy to interpret only to the initiated, but enables a dynamic view of cerebral metabolism, normal and abnormal, to be obtained, and must have widespread application in the future (p. 314).

We have therefore a wealth of techniques, but few of these are widely available. Some are extremely exciting, but will they stand the test of time and cost-effectiveness? Maybe, but until this is certain we have to maintain an acquaintance with all those techniques that have been of proven value over many years, and try and see where the newer methods may give better information, possibly be safer, and may lead to even further advances in the years to come. Holography, for instance, has not yet played the major role one might expect—perhaps it yet will.

To the wealthily endowed, highly sophisticated, modern clinical research unit, a lot of what follows in subsequent chapters will be 'old hat' but the great majority of neurological or suspected neurological patients in this world are not admitted to such units and these pages are directed at those who have to make their decisions unaided by technological magic.

Chapter 33
Blood, Urine and Faeces

The good neurologist will use laboratory investigations as part merely of the collection of evidence to differentiate between the 'short list' of possible conditions into which his history and examination has grouped the patient's condition.

Certain of the more simple examinations may justifiably be carried out in each case. In the blood these include estimation of haemoglobin, a blood smear, a total white cell and differential count, an erythrocyte sedimentation rate and serological tests for syphilis. The urine should be tested for albumen, sugar and acetone, microscoped for cells and casts, and the specific gravity measured.

In the course of such investigations, however, there may be certain findings which give rise to a train of diagnostic thought which may or may not move one from one's original impression and may focus attention on possible further lines of investigation which may be required.

This chapter should be read as a notebook relating laboratory investigations with particular problems. A great deal must of necessity be omitted, as are most tests outside the scope of the average general laboratory.

THE BLOOD

The red cells

An abnormal haemoglobin or blood film may call for absolute red cell measurements. Microcytic anaemia is too common to be of great significance, but may, if severe, be a cause of syncope, or may indicate blood loss from a cryptogenic primary neoplasm. Macrocytic anaemia is important, and must be further investigated by sternal marrow examination, serum Vitamin B_{12} and folate levels, and gastric secretory studies.

Vitamin B_{12} deficiency can cause not only subacute combined degeneration of the spinal cord, but also dementia or even optic atrophy. Intestinal absorptive defects associated with steatorrhoea and macrocytic anaemia cause polyneuropathy and spinal cord degeneration. Folic acid deficiency can cause neurological lesions, especially dementia. Disturbances of blood folate with red cell macrocytosis may follow heavy anticonvulsant dosage, and so may not be too uncommon in neurological practice.

Polycythaemia is accompanied by a darkening of the fundus and vascular congestion not unlike early papilloedema, and intracranial vascular occlusions are common, even in relative youth.

Sickle-cell anaemia may be associated with multiple micro-infarcts in the nervous system.

The white cells

High polymorphonuclear leucocytosis can accompany pyogenic lesions of the nervous system (meningitis, intracranial or spinal abscess), polyarteritis nodosa and the collagenoses. The latter diseases cause multiple lesions in the nervous system, particularly multiple peripheral nerve lesions.

Leukaemia can cause bizarre exudative and haemorrhagic fundus appearances. Lymphatic leukaemia may be associated with a similar type of multifocal leucoencephalopathy to that seen in the later stages of Hodgkin's disease, with profound neurological deficit, hemiplegia and aphasia.

Infectious mononucleosis can be complicated by a Guillain–Barré syndrome usually during the phase of recovery, but local cranial or peripheral nerve lesions due to direct glandular pressure may occur during the acute stage of the illness; occasionally there may be an encephalitis.

Eosinophilia is found in parasitic infestation (cysticercosis, hydatid disease, trichiniasis) and so may be important in epilepsy, recurrent encephalitis, or space-occupying lesions in individuals who may have been exposed to these possibilities.

Lupus erythematosus cells should be looked for in the blood in cases of diffuse cerebral disease with pyrexia, fits and mental change, for these may be presenting features in systemic lupus erythematosus. Screening for anti-nuclear factor is the standard investigation in these cases, with the finding of anti-DNA antibody the most specific, positive result.

The platelets

Diffuse central nervous system lesions, with haemorrhages, fits, dementia and coma, result from thrombocytopaenic purpura or the platelet thrombosis syndrome, both conditions showing low platelet counts.

In the syndrome of diffuse intravascular coagulation which may accompany septicaemias, and result in multiple cerebral infarcts, the platelet count will progressively decrease.

Erythrocyte sedimentation rate

The particular value of the ESR corrected for anaemia is the tendency for it to be high when a cerebral or spinal tumour is metastatic and not primarily originating in the nervous system. Unfortunately, it is not a constant enough finding to be diagnostic. In tumours thought to be benign (e.g. meningiomata or pituitary tumours) a high ESR should raise the suspicion of malignant change. Very high figures are obtained in collagen disease (diffuse central and peripheral neurological lesions), in temporal arteritis (severe headache and visual loss in the elderly), in sarcoid (multiple cranial nerve palsies, diabetes insipidus, polyneuropathy), and in myelomatosis (bony collapse, spinal compression, or predominantly motor polyneuropathy). The ESR is also raised in infective lesions, in active meningovascular syphilis, in bacterial endocarditis with cerebral emboli, in absorbing haematomata and in pregnancy, known or unsuspected.

In some laboratories the *plasma viscosity* is preferred to the ESR as being open to less error but it may be some time before this is widely adopted.

Serum proteins

There are three main conditions capable of affecting the nervous system in which serum protein estimation is of value by virtue of a reversal of the albumen/globulin ratio. These are the collagen diseases, sarcoidosis and myelomatosis. The ratio is also altered in liver failure, which may be a cause of recurrent coma and organic dementia.

Serum protein analysis should include electrophoresis, and if possible, immuno-electrophoresis. The significance of information obtained in neurological disease is still in the realm of exploration, but the demonstration, identification and quantitative assessment of the globulins has yielded some important information. Macroglobulins should be looked for in cases of obscure retinopathies or unexplained papilloedema, especially if accompanied by spinal cord lesions. Myeloma protein appears as a band near the gamma band. More and more neurological conditions are thought to represent antigen/antibody reactions, and in obscure diffuse lesions of the brain, cord or peripheral nerves increases in the gamma-globulin may be found. There is a suggestion this may be so in multiple sclerosis—but see under CSF electrophoresis, p. 270.

Blood urea

Stupor, coma, or exudative fundus appearances may be due to renal failure. Polyneuropathy can occur in uraemia and peripheral nerve abnormalities are not uncommon after renal dialysis.

Blood sugar

In any case of coma this should be estimated *at once*. Severe hypoglycaemia, if allowed to continue, will, within a few hours, cause irreparable cerebral damage. Neurological lesions rarely occur unless the blood sugar falls below 45 mg/100 ml (less than 2.5 mmol/litre). Very high figures occur in ketotic coma, but can also be present in other types of coma if the patient happens also to be a diabetic.

If recurrent attacks of loss of consciousness are accompanied by ataxia, sweating and tingling around the mouth, the possibility of hypoglycaemia arises. Blood sugar estimations should then be taken after an *absolute* fast of 24 hours, which if the diagnosis is strongly suspected, may have to be prolonged to 72 hours before a significant lowering of blood sugar occurs. A period of prolonged fasting should also be followed by a glucose tolerance test extended for at least 5 hours in an attempt to show a reactionary hypoglycaemia. If facilities are available an electroencephalogram should be taken before the fast, and when low sugar levels are reached. If an abnormal tracing is produced sugar should be given while the tracing is in progress to see if it reverts rapidly to normal. If low levels are produced or symptoms develop, plasma insulin levels should be taken at the same time.

The high blood sugar levels of diabetes may have important relevance in peripheral neuropathies and amyotrophies, and may explain the multiple small, button-like 'haemorrhages' in the fundus due to microaneurysm formation. These may also be of relevance when vascular occlusions have occurred at an age generally considered too young for arteriosclerosis.

Serum electrolytes

These should be estimated in any case of unexplained coma, circulatory collapse, or weakness of the muscles. This applies particularly to patients with renal disease, diarrhoea, pituitary tumours, to those who have been treated by hypophysectomy, and to all patients on steroid therapy. The potassium is of particular importance.

Serum potassium

Variations in the level of the serum potassium can be associated with recurrent episodes of flaccid weakness of muscles. The level is low in periodic paralysis, in potassium-losing nephritis, in aldosteronism and in some cases of steatorrhoea and during cortisone treatment. It is high in a rare condition, in other respects clinically similar to familial periodic paralysis, which has been called *adynamia episodica hereditaria.*

Serum calcium and phosphorus

Tetany, either of organic origin or due to hyperventilation, may be mistaken for epilepsy. Low serum calcium is found following parathyroidectomy and also in the condition of idiopathic hypoparathyroidism which is often associated with calcification of the basal ganglia.

High calcium figures occur in hyperparathyroidism which may produce a syndrome not unlike motor neurone disease; in myelomatosis and in sarcoidosis. In most cases the phosphorus varies inversely to the calcium.

Serum cholesterol

Hypercholesterolaemia is sometimes associated with sudden cerebrovascular accidents in young people who have no apparent cardiovascular disease. It is helpful in identifying myxoedema, which may easily be forgotten when considering the causes of mental torpor, hoarseness and sometimes ataxia.

Serum T3 and T4

Measurements of tri-iodothyronine (T3) and thyroxine (T4), the use of commercial kits such as Thyopac-3 to measure T3 resin uptake, the estimation of thyroid-stimulating hormone (TSH) and the effect upon this level of intravenous thyrotrophin-releasing hormone (TRH) are all *in vitro* tests which can indicate overactivity of the thyroid or hypothyroidism. These are important investigations in muscle wasting (for possible thyrotoxic myopathy) and in exophthalmos even when only unilateral. Myxoedema can mimic the mental slowing of pre-senile dementia, and may be associated with ataxia. The *in vivo* radioactive uptake examinations can be used to distinguish hypopituitarism from primary hypothyroidism for an injection of TSH will cause a rise in uptake in the former but not in the latter. Many other tests of even greater complexity are available, but they are costly and should not be utilised without careful previous thought.

Serum acid and alkaline phosphatase

In male patients with spinal compression or peripheral nerve lesions in the lower limbs, a high serum acid phosphatase will suggest metastases from a carcinoma of the prostate.

High alkaline phosphatase may be found in Paget's disease, multiple bony metastases, advanced liver disease and collagenosis, all of which may be associated with obscure puzzling and often diffuse neurological problems.

Serum transaminase

The two enzymes estimated, glutamic oxaloacetic transaminase (GOT), and glutamic pyruvic transaminase (GPT), are widely distributed throughout the body, the former being greater in heart and liver, and the latter in liver. The serum levels are abbreviated to SGOT and SGPT. They are raised in massive cerebral haemorrhage and thrombosis. A rise occurs in both enzymes in liver disease, so that in suspected metastatic disease, collagenosis, or hepatolenticular degeneration, high figures hint at hepatic involvement otherwise not apparent. They are raised in muscular dystrophies, but are of less value than the creatine kinase. A rise in SGOT alone is most common following coronary thrombosis and may suggest the source of a cerebral embolism.

Serum creatine phospho-kinase (CPK)

The serum level of this enzyme is very high in pseudo-hypertrophic muscular dystrophy and in those siblings of known cases who are likely later to develop the disease. It may be slightly raised in female carriers. It rises in polymyositis and after injury to muscle. The enzyme occurs in muscle and brain, but they differ, and whereas raised figures may be found in the blood after severe cerebral trauma, infarction, and sometimes neoplasia, these figures are influenced by so many factors that the main value of the investigation at the moment remains in helping to distinguish primary muscle disease (e.g. dystrophies) from neurogenic disturbances (e.g. polyneuropathy).

Serum B_{12}

A low serum B_{12} (below 100 μg) should be sought in any case in which there is a combination of peripheral nerve and spinal cord disease, and also in organic dementias, for Vitamin B_{12} deficiency presents one of the few remediable causes of dementia.

Serum folate

Folic acid deficiency can cause dementia and possibly a polyneuropathy. A low folate may be found in patients on heavy and prolonged anticonvulsant medication, and very occasionally in carcinomatous neuropathy.

Serum pyruvic acid

A pyruvic acid tolerance test may show a rise to abnormally high figures in Vitamin B_{12} deficiency, and should be carried out when investigating a polyneuropathy, or when cerebral symptoms may be the result of thiamine deficiency complicating chronic alcoholism.

Serum copper, copper oxidase and caeruloplasmin

These are all very low in hepato-lenticular degeneration. The examination is complex and should not be requested lightly, but is justified in obscure cases of involuntary movement, especially if familial.

Agglutinations

There are many agglutination tests available against bacterial and viral agents which should be applied in obscure cases of meningitis and in encephalitis, and a rising titre during the course of the disorder is particularly significant. In meningitis the tests for brucellosis and leptospirosis (including *Leptospira canicola*) must not be overlooked, for they are often not carried out routinely. In acute encephalitis the titres of herpes simplex are vital, and in any chronic encephalopathy the titre against measles, for this is raised in most cases of subacute sclerosing panencephalopathy (inclusion body encephalitis).

THE URINE

Routine examination

The urine must be examined in every case for albumen, sugar, acetone, cells and casts.

Red cells in the urine may suggest polyarteritis nodosa, or a primary renal tumour, as well as acute or chronic nephritis.

Chronic renal disease may explain exudates in the fundus, or account for a hypertensive vascular accident in a young person.

Diabetic glycosuria can explain peripheral nerve lesions, polyuria, muscle wasting and states of disturbed consciousness. Note, however, that glycosuria may follow subarachnoid haemorrhage and could cause confusion in comatose patients. Under these circumstances there is no ketosis unless vomiting has been excessive and it then does not compare with the degree of ketosis in diabetic coma.

Bence-Jones protein

Bence-Jones protein is excreted in myelomatosis, but in this disease greater diagnostic value comes from serum electrophoresis, for the urinary abnormality is an irregular finding.

Porphyrins

The urine should be tested for the presence of porphobilinogen in any obscure polyneuropathy, especially if relapsing and associated with abdominal pain, or dementia, and even if the urine remains of normal colour.

Creatine and creatinine

The output of these two substances is raised in active muscle degeneration, in the myopathies, but not in motor neurone disease. Muscle enzyme studies have largely supplanted this investigation.

Amino-acids

Chromatographic studies should be carried out in suspected cases of *Wilson's disease*, when amino-acid output is high, and in mental retardation in infants, as amino-aciduria accompanies *galactosaemia*. The output is raised also in *Hartnup disease*, an error of metabolism characterised by ataxia, dementia and light-sensitive skin eruption and sometimes by fits. Indicanuria is also present.

Copper

High daily excretion of copper is characteristic of Wilson's disease.

Lead

Lead intoxication (with high daily output) is a possible, but now rare, cause of polyneuropathy (especially wrist-drop), encephalopathy, or a syndrome not unlike motor neurone disease. This should be looked for especially in obscure encephalopathies in childhood.

Phenylpyruvic acid

Tests for the phenylketones should be carried out in the urine of all children showing mental retardation. Phenylpyruvic oligophrenia is usually clinically evident at the age of 7–12 months after apparently normal early development.

Sulphatides

Metachromatic material is present in the urine in the 'metachromatic leucodystrophy' and should be sought in any syndrome suggestive of a diffuse encephalopathy in childhood, particularly if there is a familial history.

Phytanic acid

Refsum's disease—progressive ataxia, peripheral neuropathy, and retinitis pigmentosa—is associated with abnormal excretion of phytanic acid in the urine.

Hormone studies

When this book was first written there were relatively few hormone estimations available. This has now become so complex and wide a subject that it is beyond the scope of these pages and full details must be sought from endocrinological publications.

THE FAECES

There are four main ways in which faecal examination helps in neurological diagnosis:

(*a*) For virus studies in cases of meningitis or encephalitis.

(*b*) For estimation of daily fat excretion in possible cases of steatorrhoea with peripheral nerve or spinal cord lesions.

(*c*) In demonstrating occult blood when searching for a primary neoplasm.

(*d*) In demonstrating parasitic ova in suspected infestation of the nervous system.

Laboratories have limited time and resources, so select those estimations which may be truly relevant to the problem under investigation.

Chapter 34
The Cerebro-Spinal Fluid

It is not so very long ago that analysis of the cerebro-spinal fluid (CSF) was the main ancillary investigation available to the neurologist. In modern practice the value of information gained from this examination needs to be critically assessed, for the advances of neuroradiology and neurophysiology, together with the increasing relative ease and safety of surgical exploration, have combined to make lumbar puncture a far less important manoeuvre than formerly. It can be dangerous, indeed lethal, under certain circumstances. The information gained is often of dubious value—a protein level of 80 mg per 100 ml imports one piece of information only, namely that the patient has a raised protein in the CSF; it tells nothing of the cause of the rise, the site, nature or extent of the lesion, if such exists. Negative findings exclude very few diseases, and casually carried out lumbar punctures sometimes make more important subsequent investigations very much more difficult. This chapter is an attempt to show when this investigation is of value, when it may be misleading, and when it is positively contra-indicated.

LUMBAR PUNCTURE

Indications for lumbar puncture

In brief, a lumbar puncture should be carried out if some specific piece of information is likely to come from the CSF examination which would *substantially* contribute towards diagnosis, treatment, or assessment of the progress of the disease, *and where the clear-cut contra-indications are not present.* In each case, the question must be asked, 'What exactly is the information I hope or expect to obtain from this procedure?' If one has no clear idea of the answer, then there is no justification for lumbar puncture.

Contra-indications for lumbar puncture

The contra-indications to the procedure are quite clear, are of the greatest importance and yet are ignored with frightening regularity.

(*a*) *Local sepsis.* Infected material from a lesion such as a bedsore near the lumbar puncture site can be transferred to the meninges, with disastrous results.

(*b*) *High intracranial pressure* as shown by bilateral papilloedema. Persistent disregard of this rule sooner or later causes avoidable fatalities from cerebellar tonsillar herniation through the foramen magnum or uncal herniation through the tentorial hiatus. A special neurological or neurosurgical hospital resident becomes distressingly familiar with urgent requests from other hospitals for the admission of a previously alert patient with papilloedema 'who has a CSF pressure of over 300' and has suddenly become very drowsy. It must be said that in some rare cases of meningitis papilloedema may develop, yet the CSF needs to be examined to confirm the diagnosis and isolate the responsible organism. If this is to be done neurosurgical facilities should be immediately available if conscious level deteriorates.

(*c*) Symptoms and signs suggesting a *tumour in the posterior fossa* causing incipient brain stem compression whether there is papilloedema or not. This would be judged by drowsiness, vomiting, slowing of the pulse, or episodes of faintness on change of posture in addition to cerebellar or other localising signs. The danger of tonsillar herniation and severe brain stem compression is acute.

(*d*) Patients already showing signs of *tentorial* or *tonsillar herniation*. This should be suspected when a patient with symptoms suggestive of an intracranial space-occupying lesion suddenly becomes drowsy, develops neck stiffness and the pupils dilate. There is danger here also to the patient with the Arnold Chiari malformation where the tonsils may already be well below the foramen magnum. CT scanning should be a preliminary step.

(*e*) Patients whose attitude towards investigative manoeuvres is such that the lumbar puncture is likely to be blamed for all future ills. This is not uncommon and unless truly vital information is likely to be obtained, house physicians should remember that their contact with the patients is unlikely to last more than twelve months, while their chief may have to suffer for a lifetime.

(*f*) In practice it is also wise to refrain from lumbar puncture if either myelography or air encephalography is expected to be the next step, because the CSF can be examined at the same time, the patient is saved two punctures, and a recent puncture often causes technical difficulties in satisfactorily introducing contrast media into the theca. If the CSF is going to be examined at the time of air encephalography, the specimen for cell count must be the very first drops removed, for a pleocytosis develops during the procedure.

TECHNIQUE OF LUMBAR PUNCTURE

For the normal diagnostic procedure the patient should lie on his side, the back at the extreme edge of a firm bed. One iliac crest must be maintained vertically above the other. The body is curled up to separate the spinous processes, and two lines are drawn, one joining the tops of the iliac crests, and the other running down the spinous processes. These intersect at the L3–4 space, and the puncture can be carried out at this space, or the next above or below. The higher spaces are usually easier to enter.

Mark the space, cleanse the skin thoroughly (asepsis is as important as in any surgical operation) towel off the selected space, scrubbing the hands thoroughly before and after the skin preparation, and drying the hands on a sterile towel.

After warning the patient that he will feel a stinging sensation, with a fine needle raise a bleb of local anaesthetic in the skin. Wait a few moments, and then inject a little more under the skin, into the ligament between the spinous processes and a little to either side of it. Withdraw the needle, massage the area, and then allow at least two minutes to elapse for the anaesthetic to have its effect. The majority of painful lumbar punctures are due to failure to follow this last rule.

Now warn the patient he will feel pressure, and may at one point have a sharp stab of pain—on piercing the dura. Insert the needle exactly in the midline midway between two spines, and pointing very slightly towards the patient's head, remembering that in this lateral position the midline is not necessarily halfway between the upper and lower sides of the body. Push the needle slowly but firmly forwards. A distinct jerk will be felt as it passes the inter-spinous ligament, and a smaller one as it enters the dura. After this second point withdraw the stiletto and allow a few drops of fluid to escape. If none appears push the needle a few millimetres further in and turn it slightly. When fluid is obtained the manometer is quickly attached to the needle either directly or by using a three-way tap, and an assistant can hold the upper end.

Interpretation of lumbar puncture findings

The CSF pressure

Normally the fluid rises in the manometer to about 110–115, moves up and down on respiration, jerks upwards on coughing, and moves freely upwards on abdominal compression. Test each of these features.

A very low pressure is most commonly due to faulty placing of the needle, in which case abdominal compression will cause no rise. A slight alteration of its position by advancing, withdrawing or rotating the shaft will be necessary. The pressure is also low below a complete spinal block and when there is a block at the foramen magnum. A state of idiopathic CSF hypotension is recognised in some countries, but has never achieved popularity in England.

A high pressure is most commonly due to tension, or to abdominal compression in a plump patient. Straighten the back and legs slightly and assure the patient that all discomfort is now over.

If the reading still remains high this may be due to a genuinely high intracranial pressure.

Two common fallacies

(*a*) Pressure cannot be assessed by observing the speed with which the CSF drips out of the needle. A manometer must always be used.

(*b*) No significance can be attached to a high reading if the puncture is done under a general anaesthetic.

The Queckenstedt test

The assistant places his hands on either side of the patient's neck, and presses over the jugular veins, first with one hand, then with the other and then both together. Raising the intracranial venous pressure also raises the intracranial CSF pressure, and this rise is reflected in the manometer providing that the pathways between the skull and the lumbar puncture needle are patent. The fluid will rise quickly by about 100 mm and fall rather less quickly, but still quickly, on release.

If there is a complete spinal (or foramen magnum) block, no rise will take place on jugular compression, though the pressure may have risen on abdominal pressure. If there is a partial block, the fluid may rise slowly and remain at the new level, or may rise and fall very slowly. If, clinically, the block might lie in the cervical region, the test should be repeated both with the head flexed and extended. A partial block may be temporarily converted into an obvious block.

If no rise occurs on either the Queckenstedt test or abdominal compression, this is most likely to be due to faulty needle position.

A common fallacy

A difference between the effects of compression on the two sides is important only if one suspects thrombosis of a lateral sinus or jugular vein, or neoplastic infiltration at this site. It is not uncommon in normal patients, due to anomalies of the course of one lateral sinus, so that compression of the corresponding jugular vein does not cause enough intracranial venous congestion to raise the CSF pressure.

Collection of the fluid

Disconnect the manometer and allow the fluid to drip slowly into a container, removing 5–8 ml. If the sugar content is likely to be important and there is a delay before the analysis is carried out, the fluid should be collected in a fluoride-coated tube.

If the pressure should be unexpectedly high (over 200), and the precautions mentioned above have failed to lower it, then only the fluid in the manometer should be removed.

If the pressure is extremely low, enough fluid to examine the cells and protein only should be removed. One cannot too strongly deplore the practice of withdrawing fluid by means of a syringe in such cases. This can make a previously incomplete spinal compression complete, or can convert incipient cerebellar tonsillar herniation into an irremediable impacted pressure cone.

The obese patient

In a fat patient it may be impossible to identify the landmarks. It is then justifiable to carry out the puncture with the patient seated astride a chair, with pillows in front to cause the back to curve backwards. The exact midline can be better established and it is very rare for the spinous processes to be impalpable. Pressure readings are, however, of little value and the danger of a pressure cone forming in high-pressure states is even greater.

CISTERNAL PUNCTURE

This procedure, which should never be undertaken lightly, or by anyone not already very skilled in lumbar puncture, is only very rarely required for CSF examination, and is these days more used by radiologists than in the wards.

Indications for cisternal puncture

(*a*) When CSF examination is absolutely vital (e.g. in meningitis), but lumbar puncture has failed due to technical difficulties, or has not been carried out due to local sepsis.
(*b*) In order to inject opaque material for myelography above a block, for good examination of the cervical region, or for modern methods of cisternography, and sometimes simply because myelography has failed by the lumbar route.

Contra-indications to cisternal puncture

These are the same as those for lumbar puncture, but in addition it should be avoided if the clinical picture suggests that there may be a lesion in the cisterna magna itself or a developmental anomaly at the foramen magnum level (e.g. the Arnold–Chiari deformity).

Technique of cisternal puncture

Cisternal puncture can also be carried out with the patient either lying or sitting. Stringent precautions for sterility are required and these must include shaving the occipital region. Little of routine value is to be gained from pressure reading or manometric studies.

The head is well flexed. The first palpable spinous process (which is the spine of the second vertebra) is identified and the local anaesthetic introduced into the skin and subcutaneous tissues 0.5 cm above this. The needle is then introduced exactly in the midline, 0.5 cm above the second spinous process in the plane of a line running from this point, through the external auditory meatus to the nasion. The cisterna magna lies 4–6 cm from the surface. As the needle is introduced it will be felt to pass through the atlanto-occipital membrane at about 3 cm. The stilette should be withdrawn. If no fluid escapes, it is replaced and the needle advanced another 0.5 cm. This is repeated at 0.5 cm distances until the fluid appears. *It is not wise to persist beyond a depth of 6 cm*. If the needle encounters the base of the skull, as it often will on first introduction, withdraw it appreciably, depress it slightly and introduce it again.

VENTRICULAR PUNCTURE

This is a surgical procedure, requiring surgical equipment, environment and skill, whatever the age of the patient.

Indications for ventricular puncture

(*a*) To obtain CSF for examination in cases of raised intracranial pressure.
(*b*) To insert contrast media for ventriculography.
(*c*) To insert antibiotics if lumbar injection is contra-indicated.
(*d*) For temporary reduction of intracranial pressure in emergency.

Because it is possible, in an infant, to perform ventricular puncture through the fontanelle before it is closed, this has in the past been carried out in some hospitals, in the authors' opinion, too readily. The amount of information likely to be gained from this procedure should be most carefully and critically considered. One is still passing an instrument through brain tissue, and the amount of damage that one has seen done to an infant's brain by its liberal use in relatively inexperienced hands is enormous. The authors consider that ventricular puncture requires the same skill and experience in all age groups.

EXAMINATION OF THE CEREBRO-SPINAL FLUID

Hold the container first up to the light and then against a white surface.

A cloudy fluid

(*a*) Most commonly, if regrettably, due to inadequately cleaned apparatus.
(*b*) An increase in the cell count above about 400 per mm^3.
(*c*) If also smoky in appearance this may be due to the presence of large numbers of red cells.

A blood-stained fluid

The first few drops must be watched most carefully. A blood-stained CSF is due most commonly to trauma to local vessels during the puncture. If the first few drops are clear and the fluid then becomes blood stained this is due to damage to the vertebral venous plexus. If the first few drops are blood stained and the fluid then runs clear it is due to damage to the superficial vessels.

If the fluid remains evenly blood-stained, it may

(*a*) Still be due to a traumatic tap or

(*b*) Represent genuine spontaneous subarachnoid haemorrhage.

In order to distinguish the fluid must be centrifuged *immediately*. If the supernatant fluid is colourless this is unlikely to be anything but traumatic. If it is xanthochromic, blood is likely to have been in the fluid already. This is a good working general rule, but not invariably correct.

If a perfectly conscious and alert patient has no signs of meningeal irritation, be very wary of attributing a very heavily blood-stained fluid to subarachnoid haemorrhage—it is nearly always traumatic.

A xanthochromic fluid

This is due to the entry of blood pigments into the CSF. It may occur in several ways:

(*a*) Following haemorrhage into the CSF. It usually does not develop for 6 hours, but may persist up to 20 days.

(*b*) In a highly proteinous fluid, e.g. below a complete spinal block; in the vicinity of a neurofibroma; in some cases of the Guillain–Barré syndrome.

(*c*) In some cases of subdural haematoma.

A fluid which clots

(*a*) The blood from a traumatic puncture usually clots.

(*b*) A highly proteinous fluid may clot if it becomes contaminated by a drop of blood.

(*c*) A cobweb clot may form in tuberculous meningitis. This is a rich source of tubercle bacilli, but not commonly seen.

The cells

If there are more than five cells per mm^3, or if any of them are polymorphonuclear, the fluid is abnormal.

A wholly or predominantly polymorphonuclear pleocytosis indicates acute meningeal irritation, but gives no indication as to the cause.

A wholly mononuclear pleocytosis occurs most commonly in sub-acute irritative or degenerative processes affecting the parenchyma of the nervous system, with or without meningeal involvement.

Polymorphonuclear pleocytosis

Very high counts (many thousands) can be found in most pyogenic bacterial meningitides, and these are associated with a low sugar content.

High counts (thousands), in addition to the above, occur in leptospiral meningitis, in acute haemorrhagic necrotising leuco-encephalopathy, in allergic meningeal reactions to parasitic infestation, and occasionally when cerebral haemorrhages or softenings have occurred in close relationship to the ventricles or surface of the brain, and in infarction of a pituitary tumour. In these cases, the sugar content is normal, but in other respects they may resemble a bacterial meningitis.

Moderately high counts (hundreds) are seen in the earliest stages of several conditions which are usually characterised by a mononuclear pleocytosis, such as acute lymphocytic choriomeningitis, or tuberculous meningitis, and also in some very acute disseminated demyelinative lesions.

Raised polymorphonuclear counts (below 100) usually form part of a rise in both types of cell, and this can be found in a wide variety of sub-acute infective lesions (e.g. cerebral abscess or tuberculous meningitis), granulomatous lesions (e.g. syphilis or sarcoid), metastatic neoplastic lesions, and following the introduction of irritant substances such as blood or air into the subarachnoid space.

Needless to say, these divisions and those that follow are artificial. They are intended merely to indicate the train of thought that may be started when figures of a particular order are obtained.

Mononuclear pleocytosis

Mononuclear counts in the thousands are very rarely seen.

Hundreds of mononuclear cells per mm^3 are found in viral meningitis and encephalitis, in tuberculous meningitis, in some very acute demyelinative conditions, especially in young children, in parasitic infestation and in the presence of a cerebral abscess. A rise in the polymorphonuclear cells frequently accompanies the infective lesions in the earliest stages.

A mononuclear count of less than 100 per mm^3 is very common in a variety of sub-acute degenerative and granulomatous lesions, the commonest of which are multiple sclerosis, neurosyphilis, and in metastatic cerebral or spinal disease.

High cell counts may occur if a necrotic tumour lies in close contact with the ventricular system.

N.B. A mononuclear pleocytosis with a sugar content below 40 mg per 100 ml (2 mmol/litre) occurs to all practical purposes only in *tuberculous meningitis, torulosis, carcinomatosis of the meninges,* and *multiple spinal seedlings from a medullo-blastoma.*

A raised mononuclear count may be seen if another lumbar puncture has been performed recently (as may be the case prior to transfer from a general hospital to a special unit). In these circumstances it is most important to find out if the original CSF was normal.

An important precaution

The cells must be counted as soon as the fluid is removed. If CSF is allowed to stand in a glass tube for some hours, many of the cells present adhere to the glass and a misleadingly low count may be obtained. (See also under Sugar content.)

Distinguishing cell types

The normal method of counting cells only differentiates rather vaguely between multinuclear and mononuclear cells. The millipore technique used in many laboratories is invaluable in differentiating cells types, and staining the centrifuged deposit from a cellular CSF is another simple additional test. Appropriately stained deposits may show the cells to be malignant cells (in metastatic disease and some gliomas), plasma cells (in myelomatosis), of the plasmacyte series (in acute necrotic encephalitis), or eosinophils (in parasitic disease), to mention only a few conditions in which information of diagnostic value may be obtained.

The protein content

Normally this lies between 0.15 and 0.4 g/l. It is lower in the cisterna magna and lower still in the ventricular fluid. If, as is not infrequent, figures of 0.1 g are consistently recorded in the lumbar fluid, there is something wrong in the laboratory and the methods and standards need reconsideration. This applies equally if figures are persistently above 0.6 g.

A low protein

In practice this has only negative value. It is, for instance, very uncommon, but by no means unknown, for a neurofibroma to be in contact with the CSF pathways and yet for the protein to remain normal or low.

A raised protein

This occurs in so many diseases of the central nervous system, the meninges, or the blood vessels, that there is no purpose to be gained simply by listing them. Figures over 1.0 g/l are usually only seen below a complete spinal block, in 'infective' polyneuritis (the Guillain–Barré syndrome), and sometimes in carcinomatosis of the meninges. Figures over 0.1 g/l are seen in the three conditions just mentioned, but are also found without a complete block in spinal neurofibromata, and with acoustic neuromata, spinal or cerebellar haemangioblastomata, and occasionally with meningiomata and subdural haematomata, in neurosyphilis and the collagenoses.

A rise in protein merely indicates abnormality and cannot be considered diagnostic of any one particular disease process. Even in multiple sclerosis, figures of 1.5–2 g/l may be seen in the more acute stages, but such diagnoses as progressive muscular atrophy, subacute combined degeneration of the spinal cord, or heredofamilial ataxia should be earnestly reconsidered if the protein is appreciably raised.

If the CSF is blood-stained, an allowance of 0.01 g/l of protein should be made for each 750 red cells per mm^3.

Globulins

The Pandy test (addition of carbolic acid) and the Nonne–Appelt test (addition of saturated ammonium sulphate) detect excess of globulin without qualitative differentiation. These tests have been supplanted by electrophoresis of the CSF proteins. Globulins are raised in inflammatory diseases such as tabes dorsalis and meningovascular syphilis; in demyelinative disease; and in any condition producing very high total protein.

Electrophoresis of the cerebro-spinal fluid

This allows quantitative measurements of the protein fractions after concentration of the CSF, to be carried out, especially of the globulins, and this has become diagnostically helpful in certain situations. If a patient is clinically suspected of having multiple sclerosis a gamma-globulin of over 12 per cent of the total protein is considerably in favour of this diagnosis, and if over 25 per cent is very strongly in favour if there is no reason to suspect neurosyphilis or collagenosis. The importance is that it may be shown when the disease is clinically quiescent, when the total protein is normal, and a Lange curve, if carried out, normal. The gamma-globulin may contain two characteristic bands. Further analysis by immunoelectrophoresis will show it is the IgG fraction that is raised. These IgG bands are called oligoclonal, because when antibody is synthesised within the CNS the response is limited to a small number of B-cell clones. Oligoclonal bands are present to some degree in all CNS infections and are an especially prominent feature in chronic infection such as sub-acute sclerosing panencephalitis. (In this case nearly all the IgG is measles specific.) There is bound to be elevated IgG in the presence of many CSF lymphocytes. In MS it is the finding of IgG bands *in the appropriate clinical setting* that is important, together with a lack of any abnormal IgG in the serum. In established cases, up to 95 per cent will show this response, and even after just one suspected episode, the figure is 50–60 per cent.

Electrophoresis is not the only means to demonstrate IgG bands, and in recent years more experience of *isoelectric focusing* has accumulated. This test is particularly sensitive for the detection of oligoclonal IgG, commercial 'kits' are available but the technique is more expensive than electrophoresis.

The sugar content

Normally this lies between 0.5 and 0.75 g/l. The estimation must be carried out quickly, especially if there is a pleocytosis. If a highly cellular fluid stands overnight the sugar content may be greatly reduced, unless a fluoride tube is used.

A high sugar

The sugar is said to be slightly raised in some encephalitides, but usually such a reading merely reflects a high blood sugar, e.g. in diabetes, and this diagnosis has been made in this way on more than one occasion!

A low sugar

The sugar is lower in some, but not all, cases of meningeal infection. In active pyogenic meningitis the level is usually below 0.4 g/l. In virus meningitis it does not fall.

Unless one of the other conditions mentioned on p. 268 is obvious, a lymphocytic meningitis with a CSF sugar below 0.4 g/l should be treated as tuberculous meningitis without waiting for confirmatory investigations, for these cause delay and delay may spell disaster in a now curable disease. Only someone who was in neurological practice before the advent of streptomycin can appreciate the incredible drama contained in those last four words.

The chloride content

Many laboratories no longer estimate CSF chlorides. This is probably unwise. Tuberculous meningitis still occurs in many disguises, and, if suspected, the chloride content should be specifically requested. Normally this is 7.0–7.5 g/l. Increases are not of neurological importance and reflect conditions causing a rise in blood chlorides.

Chlorides are decreased slightly in systemic infections and in meningeal infections as well as in conditions characterised by low blood chlorides, e.g. after prolonged vomiting.

Very rarely does any condition other than tuberculous meningitis reduce the chlorides below 6.25 g/l. In the early stages, however, they may still be normal, but the sugar is usually diagnostically low, and the treatment must not await their fall.

Other estimations

Many other substances may be measured in the CSF, but the value of these estimations, except as part of a specific research project, is very limited. Barbiturate and other drug estimations are important in cases of unexplained coma. The glutamine level is often raised in hepatic coma. It may well be that certain enzyme systems will come to be studied routinely, but, as yet, the high hopes of this line of investigation have not been realised.

Chromatographic studies and electronmicroscopy are likely in the future to add to our knowledge.

The Lange curve

Many young physicians have never heard of the Lange curve, or think it is a style of golf swing, electrophoresis of CSF proteins having virtually replaced it in all well-equipped laboratories. In some cases however it still may need to be carried out. Of the various colloidal precipitation reactions, it was the simplest and the best, depending upon the colour changes resulting from the precipitation of colloidal gold solutions by varying dilutions of CSF.

It almost certainly does depend upon the presence of abnormal globulins and the degree of precipitation is recorded as ranging from 5 if complete to 0 if no colour change occurs. Ten dilutions are tested and normally no figure above 1 should appear.

The main changes are:

(*a*) The so-called *first zone* or *paretic curve*, where precipitation is greatest in the lowest dilutions and is recorded as, for instance, 5544321000. This is seen in general paralysis of the insane and taboparesis (when the WR will also be positive), in disseminated sclerosis, certain infective conditions such as encephalitis and infective polyneuritis; in inclusion body encephalitis and in parasitic diseases such as cysticerosis. It may occur in the presence of a very high protein level, such as occurs when there is a spinal block.

(*b*) The *mid-zone* or *luetic curve*, represented as 0112332100, characteristically occurs in tabes dorsalis and meningovascular syphilis, but in minor degree may be found in a number of different conditions.

(*c*) The *end-zone curve,* or the *meningitic curve*, is of little practical value, and it would be a poor physician who relied on this to make his diagnosis of meningitis.

If the techniques of electrophoresis and immunoelectrophoresis are not available, the Lange curve remains a useful investigation, even if the level of the CSF protein is quite normal. It has always been difficult to persuade laboratories to accept this, but neurologists know it to be true.

Serological tests for syphilis

One used to say that the Wassermann reaction was invariably positive in untreated general paralysis of the insane, but the widespread use of penicillin in treatment of minor disorders nowadays can reverse the WR in many cases of neurosyphilis without stopping progression of the disease.

A positive WR remains of great value but one often needs to use the more elaborate tests when it is negative, before excluding syphilis. Like the WR, the VDRL slide test has the drawback of all other flocculation tests, namely false-negative results are not infrequent. The first truly specific test was the treponemal immobilisation (TPI) test, but it is time consuming, costly, and can still be negative even in late syphilis. A simpler alternative is the fluorescent treponemal antibody-absorption (FTA-ABS) test. It is more specific and sensitive, very reliable although very occasionally false-positive results do occur.

The flocculation tests, WR and VDRL, should be positive in late syphilis, but may be negative in tabes dorsalis or in patients who have received penicillin (as above). Conversely, in only a very small number of patients with neurosyphilis does the FTA-ABS test become 'converted' by treatment. If the FTA-ABS test is positive in the blood, it needs to be performed on CSF, and in active neurosyphilis is then *almost always* reactive. It follows that to perform the test on CSF in patients with negative blood FTA-ABS tests is totally unproductive!

If, in addition, the CSF contains more than five polymorphonuclear leucocytes/mm, then the diagnosis of neurosyphilis is secure in the correct clinical context. Most patients with old yaws have a positive FTA-ABS test, and monospecific tests (IgG and IgM) may then be required to diagnose new syphilitic infection.

Bacteriology and virology

If an infective condition is suspected, advice should be sought from the laboratory before the puncture is carried out, for immediate inoculation of culture media with the fluid often gives a better chance of identifying an organism. All cases of pyogenic meningitis must have the organism identified by every possible means and its sensitivity to various antibiotics determined. In tuberculous meningitis, the use of both culture and guinea pig inoculation is often essential to prove the diagnosis beyond doubt.

In viral disease it is disappointingly rare to recover the virus from the CSF, but it may be possible in lymphocytic choriomeningitis and herpes simplex encephalitis. More value comes from examination of the blood, urine and faeces, though agglutination tests may sometimes give positive results.

The roles of ECHO and Coxsackie viruses in meningoencephalitic disease is becoming increasingly appreciated.

In cases of suspected torulosis, the organism must be grown on Sabouraud's medium and it is wise to attempt this in any lymphocytic meningitis having a low CSF sugar content.

Iatrogenic changes

(*a*) Blood introduced in the CSE by a traumatic lumbar puncture causes a white cell pleocytosis within 12 hours which may persist in decreasing degree up to 20 days, and long after the blood itself has disappeared. Xanthochromia appears here as well.

(*b*) Air may be introduced through a lumbar puncture needle either purposely, at pneumoencephalography, or accidentally due to faulty apparatus, or due to movements and straining by the patient causing air to be sucked through the needle. Either will cause a pleocytosis similar to that produced by blood.

(*c*) The mononuclear count rises during the course of pneumoencephalography, so that only the first drops of fluid are of value for cytology if this procedure is being carried out.

Chapter 35
Biopsy

Very few parts of the body are now exempt from investigation by biopsy and the nervous system presents no exception. However, neurological diagnosis is more often aided by biopsy taken from some other system, than by direct examination of nervous tissue itself. A biopsy is a surgical operation, it should be treated as such, and should only be carried out if genuinely valuable information may thus be obtained.

Before a biopsy is performed the examiner should be clear in his mind as to what he hopes to learn from the procedure, and whether, when he has learnt it, it is, in fact, going to influence his management of that particular patient's problem, or aid the diagnosis and treatment of other cases. If not, it is doubtful whether it is an examination which is truly justified.

The purpose of the biopsy

(*a*) In *nervous tissue*. To establish a diagnosis when radiology and direct inspection have been uncertain.

(*b*) In *other organs*. To discover a pathological process known also to affect the nervous system.

(*c*) To supplement routine histology by electronmicroscopy, biochemical, histochemical, and virological analysis of the specimen.

The adequacy of the specimen

As histological, biochemical and histochemical studies develop, the use of minute fragments of tissue becomes less valuable, particularly in the brain and muscles, where abnormalities absent from the fragment taken may be florid in neighbouring areas. Another source of error, applying particularly to the brain, is that if needle biopsy is used, the normal tissue may enter the needle more easily than the abnormal, and tumours can easily be missed if this technique is commonly employed. The pathologist and biochemist should be asked about the minimum size of specimen they require in each case.

Indications for biopsy

(*a*) BRAIN

Biopsy of tumours is a common procedure in the course of surgical exploration, and needs no further elaboration. The popularity of biopsy of the brain itself has waxed and waned. At first thought an unnecessarily dangerous procedure, there then developed a tendency 20 or so years ago for it to be requested too casually, often without adequate thought of the true value of information to be obtained, and without remembering that an adequate and therefore sizeable specimen was required. This produced a lesion, and that lesion could potentially be epileptogenic, and apart from this the areas from which biopsy is feasible often do not show the diagnostic histology for which one is searching.

The pendulum then swung the opposite way as it became appreciated that certain, previously thought to be degenerative, diseases (such as Jakob–Creuzfeld disease) were due to an agent transmissible to primates and therefore potentially to the human, and therefore potentially to neurosurgeons and pathologists. Suspicions were also aroused about other diseases such as Alzheimer's disease, with less acceptable evidence, but the result has been a gradually increasing reluctance to perform brain biopsies on puzzling non-space-occupying conditions and progressive dementias, particularly as the procedure rarely leads to useful therapy.

Each case needs to be most seriously assessed and most neurosurgeons will wish to have such cases well investigated neuroradiologically before embarking on the procedure. If it is done it should be either by turning down a flap, which also allows direct inspection of the brain, or by making a large burr-hole. Needle biopsy, through an ordinary burr-hole, though undeniably popular, more often than not gives unsatisfactory information by missing, or displacing, the relevant histology.

In children showing a combination of progressive dementia, fits, tremors and visual impairment, possible causes include sub-acute inclusion-body encephalitis, lipoidosis or leucodystrophy. Biopsy may be the only certain way of diagnosis during life, and prognosis depends on this. A large trephine or a small flap is required so that a piece of brain of adequate size can be taken for both histological and biochemical examination.

In an acute encephalitis where the herpes simplex infection is suspected inspection of the temporal lobe allows the typical naked eye appearances to be seen, which are quite different from an abscess, and a biopsy can, by use of fluorescent staining techniques, give confirmation of the diagnosis within hours so that treatment may be instituted before permanent destruction has occurred.

Even here the increasing ability of CT scanning to differentiate these conditions is reducing substantially the need for this procedure.

It is in the progressive dementias of later life where the desire is to differentiate from an infiltrating glioma, that the greatest reluctance to use this method has grown. Fortunately serial scanning has become equal in value, if delayed sometimes in definitive results.

(*b*) PERIPHERAL NERVE

Merely demonstrating a fall-out of nerve fibres is not fundamentally helpful. However, in obscure chronic polyneuropathy, sural nerve biopsy is indicated in some patients. Amyloid infiltration, sarcoidosis, and primary hyperoxaluria, for example, cause specific recognisable abnormalities. Biopsy can distinguish between the demyelinating and axonal forms of hereditary neuropathies, but so do the clinical and electrophysiological features. Sural nerve biopsy is also of value in showing the characteristic deposits in metachromatic leucodystrophy, and methods of teasing out individual nerve fibres have shown the importance of segmental demyelination in certain polyneuropathies, such as in diabetes and some toxic states.

(*c*) MUSCLE

Muscle biopsy offers an opportunity of examining (i) muscle fibres, (ii) nerve fibres, and (iii) blood vessels. Here again, an adequate sample is essential, including a portion of skin if dermatomyositis is suspected. If one of the collagen diseases is suspected, perivascular infiltration, hyaline change or necrosis in vessel walls, and areas of myositis may be shown, alternating with entirely normal muscle.

In muscular dystrophy the variation of muscle fibres from greatly enlarged to markedly wasted will distinguish this condition from simple neural atrophy.

Other dystrophic changes include areas of necrosis, abnormalities of sarcolemmal nuclei and evidence for some fibre regeneration. In neurogenic atrophy, for example in the spinal muscular atrophies, the characteristic picture is of groups of uniformly atrophic fibres in the midst of other fibre groups displaying quite normal or even hypertrophied features. This is so-called 'type-grouping'. As is so often the case, however, myopathic-looking changes do occur in essentially neurogenic conditions and mistakes can be made.

In myasthenia gravis some parts of the specimen may show atrophy, others basophilic change in the muscle fibres, and others the collections of round cells which have been called lymphorrhages.

In trichiniasis and other parasitic diseases the organism may be shown in the muscle when the cerebral symptoms are merely those of an encephalitis.

Coërs and Woolf elaborated a technique which widens the scope of this procedure by making it possible to demonstrate the terminal nerve endings and nerve end-plates following injection of methylene blue into the nerve fibres at the time of biopsy. Concurrently with this specimens are taken for conventional histological staining, for histochemical studies both of the cholinesterase in the subneural apparatus, and of the enzymatic changes in the different types of muscle fibre.

The technique has not given the differential diagnostic proof that was at first hoped. It is largely of research value, but it has shown the degree and mechanism of re-innervation following disease or injury to the lower motor neurone, and has allowed the terminal nerve endings to be located sufficiently accurately for them to be included in the minute specimens required for electron microscopy. Interesting neural changes have been shown in diseases previously thought to be purely muscular, e.g., myasthenia gravis, myotonic dystrophy. Such 'motor point' biopsy (the correct site has to be determined by EMG) may show the abnormal motor end-plates in the former. There is abnormal terminal branching, and destruction of the ACh receptors can be seen on electron microscopy.

Histochemical study now plays a vital part in muscle biopsy investigation. It is by this means that 'type-grouping' is identified, for example. A whole new field of muscle disease has been recognised in the form of the 'mitochondrial myopathies', and the list of specific disturbances in muscle biochemistry is growing year by year.

Various types of phosphorylase deficiency exist (McArdle's disease amongst them) alongside such other entities as acid maltase and carnitine deficiencies. Nemaline (and myotubular) myopathy, central core disease and others have been recognised since the burgeoning of histochemistry and electron microscopy.

(*d*) BIOPSY OF OTHER ORGANS

The liver

In suspected hepatic coma biopsy may show advanced cirrhosis, and in hepato-lenticular degeneration may, by showing more cirrhosis than suggested by the liver function tests, greatly influence the prognosis. Typical changes can be shown in sarcoidosis or lymphoma.

The kidney

In children with a familial diffuse encephalopathy, metachromatic leucodystrophy is a possibility and metachromatic deposits can be demonstrated in the glomeruli and tubules.

The lungs

This is justifiable in cases where clinical features suggest cerebral or spinal neoplastic disease, and in which there is a peripherally situated lung shadow which is not characteristic of a bronchial neoplasm. Biopsy may show the condition to be granulomatous or neoplastic, and the former finding would greatly influence treatment.

The glands

If there is evidence of multiple lesions in the central nervous system, accompanied by glandular enlargement, biopsy of one of these may show malignant invasion, a granuloma such as sarcoid, or a reticulosis.

In suspected sarcoidosis, biopsy of the scalene muscles may include affected glands not palpable on clinical examination.

The blood vessels

These are normally examined by means of muscle biopsy (q.v.). In cranial arteritis, however, excision of a small section of the superficial temporal artery or external occipital artery will not only confirm the diagnosis, but is also likely to relieve the pain in that area.

The skin

It is important to examine the skin in cases of possible myositis, for most commonly this is only part of the whole syndrome of dermatomyositis, though naked eye skin changes may be minimal. The skin can be examined at the time of muscle biopsy.

The stomach

Biopsy of stomach mucosa through the gastroscope is sometimes a justifiable procedure in cases of suspected sub-acute combined degeneration of the spinal cord in which the blood picture is dubious or confused by previous therapy.

The jejunum

In obscure polyneuropathies in which steatorrhoea is discovered in the course of routine investigations, jejunal biopsy may show characteristic appearances of adult coeliac disease.

The rectum

In metachromatic leucodystrophy the characteristic deposits may be demonstrated in the nervous tissue in the rectal wall, and recognisable changes may occur in lipoid storage disorders.

The bones

Apart from examination of the bone marrow in suspected Vitamin B_{12} deficiency, biopsy is usually limited to proving the nature of a radiologically demonstrated abnormality which might have relevance to nervous system disease. This will apply to rarefactions in the skull which might be due to metastases, xanthomatosis, myelomatosis, or to an eosinophil granuloma. Solitary myelomatous lesions can also occur in various bones and be associated with polyneuropathy which can be purely motor. Bony tumours may compress peripheral nerves.

Chapter 36
The Practical Use of the Neuroradiographic Services

Each time a new edition of this book has been planned the sections on neuroradiology have required the major revision, because so rapid have been the advances and improvements in this field that even the journals, let alone a textbook, barely succeed in keeping up with them.

The first edition carried no mention of CT scanning. The fourth edition prophesied that nuclear magnetic resonance might soon become a household word. The enormous value of these two advances would make much of this section irrelevant were it not (a) that the expense of obtaining, housing, and operating these two facilities is so great that in most countries they are concentrated in a very few specialised areas, if one looks at hospitals worldwide; and (b) that wonderful though they are, they must not be allowed to suppress analysis of a problem so that the correct investigations for that problem are undertaken. Blunderbuss investigation is not worthy of a hitherto noble profession.

However, it will be a decade before all neurological units will have immediate access to these two scanning procedures and in any case the basic principles dealt with in the following pages remain highly relevant, though it will be indicated which paragraphs may be rendered obsolescent by this new technique.

Despite the transformation in the ease and accuracy of diagnosis that all new developments in neuroradiological technique have offered to the profession, the cost and practical value of this service is often not properly appreciated, many patients being exposed to unnecessary, uneconomical, uninformative and at times potentially dangerous amounts of radiation.

The site of the lesion in the nervous system must be determined as accurately as possible before X-rays are requested. The examiner must then ask himself if he is satisfied he is requesting an X-ray (*a*) of structures truly relevant to this site and (*b*) with some specific purpose in mind. For instance, pointless X-rays of the *whole* spine are too often requested. Again, patients with difficulty in walking often have the lumbosacral spine X-rayed though all leg reflexes have been found to be exaggerated and both plantar reflexes extensor, and a moment's thought would have shown that the lesion must be above the termination of the cord and hence above the vertebral level T12/L1.

The reason and purpose for each X-ray must be clearly thought out and equally clearly stated in the request. If a radiologist's only contact with the clinical details of the patient is a hurriedly written request form saying 'Skull.? CT' it is very tempting for him to issue a curt and totally nonsensical report such as 'No CT seen'.

If the post-graduate feels offended by these elementary remarks, let him spend half a day in a neurological X-ray department and then read them again; and though originally written a quarter of a century ago, regrettably the need to write them still remains.

All clinicians should have a working knowledge of which variations from normal require neurological investigations and for this reason, space is first devoted to films routinely taken in every general X-ray department. This is followed by the main indications for requesting more elaborate techniques and an outline of the help that they can be expected to give.

PLAIN RADIOGRAPHS

The chest

Every case of suspected intracranial or spinal cord disease should have a postero-anterior film of the chest taken. This procedure is quick, easy, carries only a small radiation dose, and may sometimes give an immediate diagnosis, eliminating the necessity for special investigations.

The following list briefly relates neurological abnormalities to certain findings in the chest X-ray:

(*a*) Carcinoma (primary or secondary)—cerebral or spinal tumours.
(*b*) Pancoast tumour—brachial plexus compression.
(*c*) Bronchiectasis, abscess, empyema—intracranial abscess.
(*d*) Tuberculosis—meningitis.
(*e*) Sarcoid—multiple cranial nerve palsies, polyneuritis.
(*f*) Polyarteritis nodosa—multiple focal neurological lesions.
(*g*) Mitral stenosis—cerebral embolism.
(*h*) Severe emphysema—papilloedema.
(*i*) Thymoma—myasthenia gravis.

The skull

Films should be taken in standard projections which are designed to display different anatomical structures. Careful radiographic technique and high photographic quality are essential to avoid false interpretation. *A 'straight X-ray' should be an X-ray that is straight.* The standard projections are a lateral, postero-anterior with 20° tilt downwards, and the Towne's projection. To these are added a basal projection and an antero-posterior as required.

INDICATIONS

(*a*) Trauma—to detect fracture lines, pineal displacement from intracranial haematoma, and the presence of air.

(*b*) When intracranial disease appears, after careful thought, to be a real possibility, i.e. not just every headache.

(*c*) When systemic disease is suspected which is known to produce skull changes, e.g. the abnormal calcification in hypoparathyroidism.

There is a body of opinion which believes that X-raying the skull in cases of relatively minor trauma without loss of consciousness so rarely shows abnormalities which influence the management of the patient that, if only for reasons of economy alone, they should not be carried out simply as a matter of routine. The arguments for and against this view would fill pages, but it should be remembered that in a number of cases both of extradural and subdural haematomata the evacuation has to be carried out in the absence of modern scanning procedures, and it will be at the site of a fracture, if demonstrated, that the operator will wish to make his first burr-hole.

Skull appearances and their possible significance

When each film is examined attention is directed to the calvarium, the sella turcica and clinoid processes, the sphenoidal wings, the petrous bones, the basi-occiput, and any normal or abnormal intracranial calcification.

THE CALVARIUM

Normal rounded translucencies caused by arachnoid granulations lie very near the sagittal suture. Symmetrical bilateral rounded translucencies, more laterally placed, can be caused by persistent parietal foramina and they may mimic burr-holes.

Localised thinning of the vault occurs normally at the frontoparietal junction, in the low occipital region and in the grooves of the sinuses. Smooth generalised thinning is rarely significant. Diploic venous lakes in the parietal region are often dramatic, but rarely important.

Abnormal rounded translucencies, irregularly distributed, are produced by metastases, especially myelomata, and by xanthomatosis. Single rounded translucencies of varying size can be caused by diploic dermoids; by haemangiomata of the skull itself (giving an appearance similar to a spider's web); by simple developmental defects, and sometimes following long after a localised injury.

In long-standing raised intracranial pressure, the skull may be thin and a 'beaten silver' appearance produced. This is however, quite common in children normally and may persist into early adult life, so that 'beaten silver' without other signs of raised intracranial pressure is rarely important.

Normal thickening is seen in the frontal region and at the torcula; generalised thickening is rarely significant.

Abnormal thickening is seen locally in relation to exostosing tumours, fibrous dysplasia of bone (especially above the orbits), and in Paget's disease. Here there are usually areas of rarefaction as well, and the thickening has a 'fluffy' appearance. The undulating thickening in the frontal region of hyperostosis frontalis interna is very striking, but is not itself responsible for intracranial disease.

Separation of the sutures occurs in children with high intracranial pressure and in young people following head injury.

Abnormally early closure of the sutures is the fundamental lesion in craniosynostosis.

N.B. Meningiomata can produce bone destruction, hyperostosis, excessive vascularisation, and enlargement of meningeal artery grooves and foramina, or any combination. It has been assessed that 85 per cent of frontal meningiomata produce these changes and as this is a benign, operable tumour, it is most important that they should not be overlooked.

THE SPHENOIDAL WINGS

These are best seen through the orbits in the postero-anterior film with 20° tilt. Asymmetry can be quite normal. If the bone is appreciably thickened on one side this can be caused by a meningioma-en-plaque, or by fibrous dysplasia of bone. Enlargement or erosion of the superior orbital fissure may be caused by meningiomata, optic nerve gliomata, pituitary tumours or aneurysms. If there is any suspicion of abnormality in this site, views of the *optic foramina* should be taken which can confirm the bony erosion or thickening.

THE PETROUS BONES AND BASE OF SKULL

The petrous bones are best examined in the Towne's view and basal projections, but when the internal auditory meati may be of importance, a complete examination should include Stenver's views, and an antero-posterior film, when the internal auditory meati can be seen through the orbits. Erosion occurs in malignant tumours arising in the naso-pharynx, petrous epidermoids, acoustic neuromata, tumours of the glomus jugulare and neuromata of the trigeminal nerve (when an enlarged foramen ovale may be seen in the basal view). The foramen spinosum may be enlarged by a middle meningeal artery feeding a meningioma.

THE BASI-OCCIPUT

Neurological interest in this area is greatest in cases of basilar invagination which may be a primary developmental disorder, may be associated with syringomyelia, or may occur secondary to Paget's disease. Platybasia, where the posterior fossa is flat and the basal angle increased, may be a normal variation. In basilar invagination, however, when compression of medulla, cerebellar tonsils, and upper cervical cord can occur, the atlas is closely applied to the base of the skull, and the odontoid process projects more than 6 mm above McGregor's line. This line joins the tip of the hard palate to the lowest part of the occipital bone and utilises landmarks easier to define in lateral films than many of the other measurements recommended.

THE SELLA TURCICA

The lateral view of the skull must indeed be truly lateral. Slight obliquity gives the sella a disorganised appearance, and it is wiser to reject than to try to interpret such a view.

Look at the anterior and posterior clinoids, the cavity of the sella itself, the definition of its floor, and its relationship to the sphenoidal sinus.

Erosion of the anterior part of the dorsum sellae occurs in increased intracranial pressure. Supra-sella and para-sellar lesions (e.g. cavernous aneurysms) can produce local destruction. In generalised osteoporosis and sometimes in arterial hypertension erosion may appear to be present, but the cortex of the dorsum sellae remains intact, though faint. Asymmetrical thickening occurs in meningiomata of the anterior fossa and medial sphenoidal wing.

Enlargement ('ballooning') of the cavity of the sella is seen in pituitary tumours. In advanced intracranial hypertension and in the presence of large suprasellar masses decalcification of the clinoids may give a similar appearance. Gross destruction can occur in long-standing raised intracranial pressure, pituitary neoplasms, carcinoma of the sphenoid, and chordoma.

Bridging of the sella, a small sella, and linear calcification behind the dorsum sellae are rarely of clinical significance.

Normal intracranial calcification

Displacement of normally calcified structures is capable of giving indirect evidence of a change in the size of one part of the brain.

THE PINEAL GLAND

This structure, normally lying in midline and best seen in the Towne's view, is calcified in about 55 per cent of people over the age of 25, but may be calcified at 6 or uncalcified at 90. Its position must be measured, for a displacement of more than 2.5 mm from the midline is pathological. It may, however, calcify more on one side than the other, which can be confusing and give a false impression of displacement.

Displacement laterally occurs in any space-occupying lesion including unilateral cerebral oedema, when it is away from the lesion, and in unilateral cerebral atrophy, when it is towards the lesion.

Displacement downwards occurs in parietal tumours and large subdural haematomata.

N.B. A central pineal gland does not exclude a space-occupying lesion, and bilateral cerebral swelling, bilateral subdural haematomata, or bilateral metastases may 'cancel out' any potential displacement.

THE CHOROID PLEXUSES

It is not uncommon for these to be calcified, when they appear as two mottled, grape-like bodies, symmetrically placed, seen best in Towne's view. Their relative positions vary too much for apparent displacement to be of much value.

THE FALX

Again, the falx is not uncommonly calcified. This appears in the lateral view as a rather indefinite, patchy mottling over the upper part of the skull, but in the antero-posterior views it can be seen as a densely calcified, sometimes linear, sometimes pear-shaped, body in the midline with a tendency to form a V-like structure as it approaches the sagittal sinus. The calcification itself is of no significance, but may, by displacement, occasionally indicate a space-occupying lesion. It may cause confusion in the lateral view and be mistaken for some pathological structure, but its shape and position in the antero-posterior plane is very characteristic.

Abnormal intracranial calcification

The presence of calcium in a lesion can be taken as an indication of chronicity and therefore is most likely to be seen in relatively benign lesions or lesions which started relatively benign even if recent anaplastic change has taken place.

NEOPLASMS

It is most common for calcification to be seen in meningiomata and in oligodendrogliomata. In the latter there is often a curious serpiginous appearance resembling the outlines of gyri or blood vessels. Ten per cent of gliomata calcify. Calcification almost resembling a 'cast' or the trigone of the lateral ventricle is seen in the posterior parieto-temporal region in a particular childhood tumour of mixed pathology.

Dense calcification above the sella is common in craniopharyngiomata, and small calcified areas located near the ventricles may be seen in subependymal gliomata and hamartomata.

VASCULAR LESIONS AND ANOMALIES

Serpiginous speckled calcification is sometimes seen in arterio-venous angiomas, but not very frequently. If the gyri are clearly outlined by tramline calcification the anomaly is more likely to be of the type seen in the Sturge–Weber syndrome. A ring of calcification (Albl's ring) related to the sella turcica may occur in aneurysms, this often being much larger than the present cavity of the sac. Old intracerebral haematomata frequently show mottled calcification and have in the past been mistaken for tuberculomata, which are rare lesions in this country.

Curvilinear or parallel streaks overlying the sella turcica are frequently seen in the elderly with atheroma of the carotid artery, but may be an indication of more widespread cerebral atheroma.

BASAL GANGLIA CALCIFICATION

Calcification outlining the basal ganglia and usually including the dentate nuclei is seen in toxoplasmosis, hypoparathyroidism and pseudo-hypoparathyroidism and in a rare familial condition of unknown aetiology. Rounded balls of calcification ('brain-stones') occasionally occur in tuberous sclerosis but more often are found incidentally, no known explanation being forthcoming.

Intracranial air

Air inside the cranial cavity is seen following air encephalography, ventriculography and occasionally lumbar puncture, but also following fractures which have involved the sinuses, and occasionally in osteomata of the frontal sinus. A 'brow-up' film is important in all cases of CSF rhinorrhoea for this may show a frontal collection of air.

TOMOGRAPHY

Simple tomography (i.e. not computerised), once the province mainly of chest radiography, is now well established in neuroradiography. Suspected erosion of the sella, of the petrous bones, of the sphenoidal wings, enlargement of the optic or internal auditory foramina, and anomalies at the foramen magnum, all offer themselves particularly for this investigation on plain X-rays. Combining this with air-encephalography outlines suprasellar extension of pituitary tumours, acoustic neuromata, and the position of the cerebellar tonsils in relation to the foramen (and also cerebellar atrophy) probably better than any other method though the more advanced CT scanners, especially using contrast enhancement, produce excellent pictures, and nuclear magnetic resonance is, so far, unequalled in demonstration of the anatomy and abnormalities in the posterior fossa.

CONTRAST RADIOGRAPHY

The use of X-rays alone has, in the past, been only capable of detecting major differences in tissue density such as calcified structures (e.g. bone) as opposed to muscles, skin, brain tissue or cerebro-spinal fluid. In order therefore to show the intracranial blood vessels and ventricles it has been necessary to introduce a contrast medium denser than bone into the arteries, or a less dense medium than brain (e.g. air) into the ventricles and subarachnoid space. The introduction of CT scanning has overcome part of this problem because it is now possible to show the ventricles clearly without contrast media, the subarachnoid spaces if enlarged, and the presence of abnormal structures of densities different from brain, such as tumours, haemorrhages, infarcts, abscesses or simply oedema of brain tissue. The need for the introduction of air by means of air-encephalography or air-ventriculography has therefore, in areas equipped with CT scanning, been reduced to such a degree that the younger radiologists and neurosurgeons have little experience of these procedures. Arteries, unless calcified, or containing contrast media, are not clearly shown by CT scanning however, so that arteriography remains a reduced but nevertheless important investigation. Even here attempts are continuously being made to reduce the need actually to puncture the artery, but at the time of writing these measures have not produced the clarity of pictures required if active intervention involving the cerebral vasculature is contemplated. The following sections therefore deal with contrast radiography as if CT scanning were not available, as indeed in many parts of the world it is not. Indications are given as to where the methods described have been, or are being, supplanted by these newer techniques.

When investigations are requested which are time-consuming for the X-ray department, possibly painful for the patient and not without risk, the scope and indications of each method must be understood and an even more careful assessment made of their justification.

CAROTID ANGIOGRAPHY

Once percutaneous techniques had been developed by which radio-opaque contrast media could be injected directly into the carotid artery, or even the vertebral artery, in the neck, without the need for open operation, angiography became a procedure which, in experienced hands, was relatively simple, immensely valuable, and relatively safe.

However, there still was the danger of damaging still further a vessel whose walls were already the site of disease, such as atheroma. Other techniques soon were developed, which were rather more time-consuming, but safer, and capable of giving information about the origin of the vessels, and of more proximal vessels as well. These apply particularly to the introduction of a catheter via the femoral (or sometimes the brachial) artery, and guiding it under X-ray control to precisely the point desired for injecting the media. Once in the common carotid, if the bifurcation is free of disease, the catheter can be advanced to give selective internal, or sometimes external, carotid artery pictures. In cases of internal carotid stenosis or thrombosis, anastomoses can be shown by purely injecting the media into the common carotid artery.

The external carotid is sometimes cannulated to show lesions such as tumours of the glomus jugulare and other chemodectomata lying high in the neck (which are supplied by this vessel and not by the vertebral artery as is sometimes thought), and to demonstrate certain arterio-venous communications usually at the vertex or in the occipital region. It can be particularly valuable in showing the external carotid supply to a meningioma when differentiating between this and a superficial glioma.

The internal carotid is selectively cannulated when better detail is required to show aneurysms, ventricular size and the circulation in tumours.

By means of apparatus for rapidly changing the films, the early arterial, later arterial, capillary, early venous and late venous phases can all be shown from one injection. The procedure is first carried out in the antero-posterior plane and then repeated in the lateral plane, and to experienced eyes the results give information far beyond the mere demonstration of a space-occupying lesion or vascular anomaly.

In cerebral tumours, the size, position and the pathological type may be diagnosed with a high degree of accuracy in many cases. This made the process of ventriculography as a preliminary to craniotomy rarely necessary unless intraventricular extension of the tumour was suspected or the findings were equivocal as regards site. The advent of CT scanning has of course reduced this need very much further still. In cases of aneurysm, additional oblique projections show its shape and origin, and the presence or absence of a neck—invaluable to the surgeon.

The main indications are listed below, the type of problem being mentioned first, the purpose of the examination following.

Clinical indications for carotid angiography

(*a*) *Spontaneous intracranial haemorrhage.* The patients should be those in whom demonstrating the cause would lead to a therapeutic procedure. They should not be too old, nor too ill, and their cardio-vascular systems must not be in a state of advanced disease.

The aim is to demonstrate cerebral aneurysms, arterio-venous anomalies, or intracerebral haematoma which might be treated.

CT scanning has virtually replaced the procedure for showing haematomata, and gives a very high index of suspicion as to the presence of an angioma, but more detailed arterial and venous pictures are required if surgery is contemplated.

(*b*) *Epilepsy starting over the age of 30* used to be an important reason if there had been focal features to the attacks, focal EEG changes, focal paresis following the attack, or any new abnormal physical signs between the attacks. Indeed, focal epilepsy at any age, unless known to follow perinatal cerebral damage.

The aim was to demonstrate a cerebral tumour or vascular anomaly.

(*c*) *Increased intracranial pressure.* To demonstrate a supratentorial tumour, if present; to determine its site; to deduce, from the vascular pattern shown, the likely pathological type. Sometimes the demonstration of dilated but normally placed ventricles by the arteriographic appearances can suggest that the tumour or cerebro-spinal fluid obstruction lies in the IIIrd ventricle, aqueduct or posterior fossa.

(*d*) *Sudden hemiplegia in young people* with no cardiac disease, to demonstrate, if possible, the mechanism, e.g. intracerebral haemorrhage from a minute anomaly.

(*e*) *Head injuries* who have developed hemiplegia, fits or increasing drowsiness after a normal interval. To detect subdural or extradural haematomata.

(*f*) *Signs of chiasmal compression* even if almost certain to be due to a pituitary adenoma. It is not unknown for a large aneurysm unexpectedly to be shown and it is better that this should be a surprise to the radiologist than to the surgeon during operation.

In (*b*) to (*f*) the use of the CT scan has virtually replaced arteriography, and is capable, in all these situations, of detecting small lesions which arteriography might have missed.

(*g*) *Recurrent unilateral paralysis.* To demonstrate the internal carotid artery in the neck as well as intracranially and detect stenosis, or thrombosis. This type of presentation may also follow (*b*) or (*c*) above.

(*h*) *Unilateral IIIrd or VIth nerve palsies* of sudden or very rapid onset. To detect vascular anomalies.

Contra-indications to carotid angiography

(*a*) Patients showing marked atheroma and hypertension who are in the later age groups, unless some life-saving measure is likely such as the evacuation of a subdural haematoma or removal of a meningioma. Damage to a diseased carotid artery can convert a narrowing into a complete occlusion.

(*b*) If, on mature reflection, there is no real likelihood of any of the conditions mentioned above being demonstrated, e.g. cases of constant headache for 25 years (a common reason for referral). Arteriography should never be done 'just on the off chance.'

(*c*) If no experienced arteriographer and no experienced interpreter of results is available, or if the quality of the films is likely to be so inadequate that the whole process will have to be repeated when the patient is moved to a special unit.

VERTEBRAL ANGIOGRAPHY

At one time this procedure was carried out by direct percutaneous arterial puncture, as in the case of carotid arteriography, but this carried a higher risk, particularly in the arteriosclerotic patient, and did not show the origin of the vessel, which is where the pathology frequently lies. By developing the technique of passing a catheter through femoral, brachial or axillary arteries, and guiding it under X-ray screening control until its tip lies at the entrance of the vertebral artery, the whole vessel can be visualised and the procedure, in good hands, is very much safer. The femoral route is the best, but it has the disadvantage that only the left vertebral artery can easily be outlined, and the brachial has the disadvantage of occasional complicating occlusion of the vessel punctured, so that arch aortography is often preferable (see p. 291).

Indications for vertebral angiography

(*a*) To demonstrate vascular anomalies in the territory of the vertebral and posterior inferior cerebellar arteries, and also in the territory of the basilar or posterior cerebral arteries, when these have not been shown adequately by carotid angiography. In the young, therefore, it is justifiable in cases of subarachnoid haemorrhage where no anomaly has been seen in the carotid circulation. Conversely if several aneurysms have been shown on the carotid circulation vertebral arteriography is frequently indicated, for if further aneurysms are present it is doubtful if operative interference is justified.

(*b*) To investigate occipital tumours, when carotid angiography has not filled the posterior cerebral arteries. Now that more is known about the anatomy of the vessels, particularly the veins, in the vertebro-basilar distribution, posterior fossa tumours can be investigated by vertebral angiography. This requires considerable expertise both to produce high quality films and to interpret them, and if these are not readily available ventriculography remained the most useful procedure in tumours in this site (prior to NMR).

(*c*) In differentiating between extrinsic tumours lying anterior to the stem (e.g. clivus meningiomata), and intrinsic gliomata of the stem. Either appear to push the aqueduct and IVth ventricle back, but the former displaces the basilar artery backwards as well.

(*d*) To demonstrate stenosis or occlusion near the origin of the vertebral artery, if such a demonstration would significantly alter the management of the case, e.g. it is important, when the question of operating on one stenosed carotid artery arises, to know the state of all the other major vessels to the brain.

Everything written earlier about the supplanting of carotid arteriography by CT scanning applies to vertebral studies as well, especially where tumours are concerned. However, when nuclear magnetic resonance becomes more widely available, this will almost certainly be the investigation of choice in posterior fossa lesions.

Contra-indications to vertebral angiography

(*a*) In patients over 65, in hypertensive patients, or in the presence of marked atheroma unless the knowledge obtained would fundamentally influence management of the case.

(*b*) In cases where the history has suggested a definite brain stem softening in the past. There is a real danger of worsening the condition.

(*c*) In any case at all unless the indications have been fully assessed, for this is not a procedure to be embarked upon lightly.

FOUR-VESSEL ARTERIOGRAPHY AND ARCH AORTOGRAPHY

When the question arises of surgical treatment of a stenosed vessel in the neck; as it has become apparent that the abnormalities responsible for transient cerebral ischaemic attacks may be even more proximal than the origin of the carotid and vertebral arteries; and as the influence of a stenosed subclavian artery upon vertebral artery flow has been appreciated, the need for visualisation of all the main vessels at their origin has encouraged the process of catheterising the aortic arch from the femoral artery, and injection of large quantities of dye to fill all vessels simultaneously. This gives valuable information in the situations described, may show anomalies of development of these vessels, as well as thrombosis or stenosis, but unless special techniques are used, does not show the detail of the intracranial circulation. Even this is possible by this method, but it is time consuming, and it should never be used as a form of blunderbuss arteriography. The procedure has a definite morbidity rate either due to damage to large vessel walls and subsequent thrombosis or embolism; to the blockage of small vessels supplying the cord; or sometimes to idiosyncrasy to the large amounts, or to some constituent, of the contrast medium used. Here again, therefore, it is an investigation for which there must be a real necessity in the particular case, and it must be carried out under experienced hands.

What angiography can show

Angiography is not infallible, and the results are easily misinterpreted unless the angiographer and interpreter deal with several cases each week. Given films of high quality, the diagnostic value is outstanding.

(*a*) DISPLACEMENT OF VESSELS

Displacement of arteries and veins from their normal anatomical positions can be brought about by intrinsic or extrinsic tumours, cysts, intracerebral or subdural haematomata, dilated ventricles, or oedematous brain. Occasionally vessel displacement in the immediate vicinity of the mass gives exact localisation. A unilateral lesion readily causes herniation of vessels across the midline anteriorly where the falx is deficient. Posteriorly the brain is splinted, but displacement of the deep cerebral veins may be seen even when the position of the arteries remains unaltered. This is particularly true in deep intrinsic tumours. Marked unilateral atrophy displaces the vessels *towards* the side of the lesion.

(*b*) ABSENCE OF VESSELS

Arteries fail to fill as a result of thrombosis, embolism, anomalous development of the Circle of Willis, or of its haemodynamics, and of course, technical faults. One anterior cerebral artery often fails to fill from its own side, but contralateral angiography usually shows bilateral filling and the finding is then of no significance. Absence of filling of veins or dural sinuses due to thrombosis is a vital angiographic diagnosis, since this condition may mimic cerebral tumour and may be made worse by surgical interference.

(*c*) ALTERATIONS IN ARTERIAL LUMEN

Local narrowing is due usually to atheromatous plaques (e.g. carotid stenosis), but may also be due to constriction from local tumours (e.g. sphenoidal wing meningiomata). Arteritis—either as part of a polyarteritis, or secondary to local infection (e.g. in meningitis) may give localised constriction and beading of arteries and arterioles. Intense constriction may persist for many days following subarachnoid haemorrhage and results in cerebral infarction and hemiplegia. Whip-lash injuries of the neck can produce carotid narrowing due to mural haematomata and should be suspected in delayed post-traumatic hemiplegia of sudden onset.

(*d*) VASCULAR ANOMALIES

Aneurysms, arterio-venous angiomata and other developmental abnormalities are the most easily and dramatically shown causes of intracranial haemorrhages, focal fits (angiomata), and cranial nerve palsies. Techniques have now been developed for demonstrating spinal angiomata. These are referred to on p. 302. They are by no means universally available, and have a much higher potential morbidity in inadequately experienced hands.

(*e*) THE MOYAMOYA APPEARANCE

This is a leash of small vessels resembling a puff of smoke (moyamoya) seen at the site of an absent vessel such as an occluded or maldeveloped middle cerebral artery. Though resembling an angioma, one is looking at an attempt at collateral circulation.

(*f*) TUMOURS

Meningiomata sometimes show great vascularity, and contrast medium dye may remain in the tumour throughout the venous phase, producing the so-called 'blush'. External carotid vessels are often shown to participate in the tumour's blood supply. Local arteries tend to be displaced in a circumferential manner. Drainage veins from vascular meningiomata are usually well formed. Ironically the arteriographic appearances most closely resembling a meningioma are given by a hypernephroma metastasis.

Glioblastomata may also show great vascularity, but mainly in the arterial phase with many arterio-venous shunts and larger draining veins. Metastases may behave similarly. Cystic astrocytomata and oligodendrogliomata are usually shown more by the displacement of normal vessels that they bring about than by any vascular pattern of their own. An avascular area may be a cystic or solid tumour, abscess or haematoma. It may be impossible to tell arteriographically and exploration was at one time the inevitable next step. This has been modified appreciably by the use of brain scanning—see pp. 305–315.

What an angiogram will not show

(*a*) Very small tumours in certain situations may escape detection, so that it cannot *positively* exclude a tumour.

(*b*) Extensive tumours, if infiltrative, may be difficult to localise unless there is a pathological circulation.

(*c*) Thrombosis of, or small haemorrhages from, very minute vessels, such as the lenticulo-striate group.

(*d*) Brainstem lesions, unless they are vascular anomalies or are due to clivus meningiomata.

In (*a*), (*b*), and (*d*), air studies, either from the lumbar route, or by ventriculography, were required as the usual next stage. Now however CT scanning obviates this need, and if used first, in many cases has obviated the need for the arteriogram at all.

Angiography and anaesthesia

Although carotid and vertebral angiography can be carried out under local anaesthesia, a skilful general anaesthetic makes it a procedure the patient has no fears of having repeated (as is often necessary), enables films of particularly good quality to be obtained, and allows hyperventilation techniques to be used which further improves the quality of the angiograms.

Subtraction techniques

A major problem while using contrast media in skull and spinal radiography is that in certain areas (such as the petrous bones) the density of bone shadow may obscure the contrast medium. If a plain film of the area taken under exactly the same circumstances is superimposed on one showing the contrast medium (e.g. an arteriogram), and then the two are printed onto a further X-ray film, the bony shadows cancel each other out and the contrast medium stands out clearly, though as black on white rather than the familiar appearance. This makes it much easier to see small vascular anomalies, or defects in a column of contrast medium, in areas normally very difficult to see. It is purely a photographic manoeuvre, but of immense value, and there are pieces of quite sophisticated apparatus available by which this can be viewed as well as photographed.

The most advanced of these techniques is called 'digital subtraction angiography (DSA). By the use of high speed computers, the subtraction is virtually instant. Data can be manipulated, by computer, so that particular areas can be studied under magnification and very small differences of shading can be shown. The concentration of contrast required is considerably lower, and an intravenous injection only is required to view the extracranial vessels. This means a very much reduced risk to the patient, less expense (contrast media are very costly—top of the 'drug expenses' list in our hospital) and the technique is rapid. Problems do occur, however, with vessels becoming superimposed on each other, and from movement artefacts.

Non-invasive investigation of the carotid arteries

Although with the advent of digital subtraction techniques (DSA), carotid angiography is now far safer and cheaper, much useful information can be gathered by out-patient tests with entirely non-invasive means.

Phonoangiography and oculoplethysmography have now been surpassed by *'Doppler' ultrasound* and so-called *'B-mode' ultrasound.* There are a variety of Doppler ultrasound instruments but the basic principle employs the use of a probe emitting sound waves which are directed, by the examiner, towards the blood vessel under examination. The movement of red blood cells alters the frequency of the reflected ultrasound such that a Doppler 'shift' is recorded and this can be converted into an audible signal.

'B-mode' ultrasound provides an image based on echo ultrasonography. This shows blood vessels, both in longitudinal and transverse section. A two-dimensional image is provided and can be stored on video tape.

Perhaps the best ultrasonic test available is the 'Duplex' scan, a combination of the 'B-mode' and 'Doppler' techniques. Blood flow and the vessel itself are displayed using a single probe. When suitable patients (those with potential for surgical treatment) then undergo DSA, the combined battery of tests will have provided information about the state of many blood vessel walls and their flow, identified plaques of atheroma with or without ulceration, and shown any points of significant stenosis.

Pyelography following angiography

The contrast medium is excreted quickly through the urinary tract, and in cases where a possible metastasis has been shown by intracranial angiography films of the renal area taken at the conclusion of the procedure may indicate a source of a primary lesion, and save the patient from another extensive (and expensive) radiographic procedure.

PNEUMOENCEPHALOGRAPHY (AIR ENCEPHALOGRAPHY)

Investigations involving the introduction of a *negative* contrast medium (i.e. air) into the CSF pathways, either by the lumbar route or through burr-holes, have been those most rendered obsolete by the CT scanner. Not before its time either, for pneumoencephalography, never pleasant, used to be a barbarous procedure, all the CSF being replaced by air, with resultant severe meningeal irritation. The development of techniques by which no more than 30 cc of air need be used, or even less, made the whole process much less unpleasant, and by careful positioning of the head all the ventricles and the subarachnoid space could be visualised with only minor after-effects.

Though written in the past tense this still remains a technique of considerable diagnostic value, and of course has the advantage over ventriculography that it avoids burr-holes, and brain needling, and shows the subarachnoid spaces and basal cisterns.

Air is introduced through a lumbar puncture needle with the patient sitting with the head *accurately positioned* for air to enter the ventricles. Films taken during the filling stage show the IVth ventricle and aqueduct. Lateral and antero-posterior views then follow with varying degrees of tilt, the air flowing at one time into the anterior and temporal horns, then into the occipital horns, and so on. To make the appearances around the sella turcica, the brain stem, the posterior fossa and foramen magnum region even more clearly defined, tomographic procedures in the lateral plane are now of great practical value. In fact a very simple method, named autotomography, is readily available in which the patient's head is simply rocked laterally while the air is injected and films taken. Midline structures remain in focus (such as the IIIrd and IVth ventricles and the aqueduct) while the surrounding masking bone shadows are blurred.

Indications for pneumoencephalography

The most practical help coming from this procedure if CT scanning is not available is in cases coming under the following categories:

(*a*) Suspected cerebral maldevelopment.

(*b*) Suspected cerebral atrophy.

(*c*) Suspected low pressure hydrocephalus.
(*d*) Epilepsy of onset after the age of 30, in whom there is no family history and no sign of tumour.
(*e*) Some cases of post-traumatic epilepsy, to identify local scarring.
(*f*) Pituitary, supra- or para-sella neoplasms, not causing a rise in intracranial pressure. This assists the surgeon by showing the degree of suprasellar extension, and so influencing his approach.
(*g*) In some cases of suspected acoustic neuroma, without rise in intracranial pressure, using special tomographic techniques to visualise the air over the internal auditory meati, and with a neurosurgeon fully cognisant of the case.
(*h*) In suspected syringomyelia, where the descent of the cerebellar tonsils through the foramen magnum may be clearly demonstrated.
(*i*) When an arteriogram has shown a suspicion of a tumour, but the findings are very dubious, and there is no evidence of raised intracranial pressure.

Contra-indications to pneumoencephalography

(*a*) The presence of signs of increased intracranial pressure. Opinions differ about this and some radiologists introduce air without removing any cerebro-spinal fluid, so reducing the danger of cerebellar pressure coning. As a working rule, however, such activities are best left to those having both special experience and *immediate* neurosurgical facilities available.
(*b*) A suspicion of a posterior fossa tumour or abscess. There is here a very real danger of pressure coning.
(*c*) Cases of stabilised congenital hydrocephalus. Disturbing the hydrodynamic balance often seriously upsets the patient and gives no truly useful information.

VENTRICULOGRAPHY

This is a surgical procedure requiring burr-holes, ventricular puncture, full surgical conditions and an experienced surgeon, whether the patient is a small infant or an adult. To show the size, shape, and position of the ventricles, the media introduced may be translucent (air), or opaque. The latter is of particular value in demonstrating the IIIrd and IVth ventricles and the aqueduct.

The particular advantage of ventriculography is that it does not carry the hazard of tentorial or cerebellar pressure coning. The disadvantage is that it requires a surgical team and facilities, shaving the head and making burr-holes. The brain has to be needled and sequelae, particularly in the young delicate brain, are not unknown. CT scanning has so reduced the need for ventriculography that it is now quite a rare procedure but this type of scanning does not, as yet, give the lateral views of the IIIrd and IVth ventricles, and aqueduct, which are of such value. Here NMR scanning is proving to be, so far, unrivalled.

Indications for ventriculography (CT scanning being unavailable)
(*a*) Any case in which there is raised intracranial pressure, or strong evidence of a cerebral space-occupying lesion, and arteriography has failed to demonstrate or adequately locate the cause.
(*b*) A case in which there is a posterior fossa or cerebello-pontine angle tumour; to locate its position, gain an idea of its size and guide the surgeon in his choice of approach.
(*c*) A case of suspected obstruction to the IIIrd or IVth ventricles or aqueduct, especially by an intra-ventricular body.

Contra-indications to ventriculography
(*a*) Any case in which it will be possible to obtain the same and *adequate* information safely by some other means.
(*b*) The presence of scalp or skull sepsis.
(*c*) The presence of marked arterial hypertension, when there is an increased danger of intracranial bleeding.
(*d*) In cases of cerebral abscess, if localisation is possible by other means, to avoid infection of the ventricular system.

Information gained from air encephalography and ventriculography

(*a*) DISPLACEMENT OF THE VENTRICLES
A neoplasm or other space-occupying lesion will deform and displace the ventricles away from the lesion. An atrophic or scarred area will draw and deform the ventricles towards the lesion.

(*b*) FILLING DEFECTS
Tumours lying in, or adjacent to, ventricles will alter their normal shape and allow the size of the lesion to be estimated and its position to be located.

(*c*) OBSTRUCTION OF THE CEREBRO-SPINAL FLUID PATHWAYS
Air may be held up by obstruction at the foramen of Munro, in the aqueduct, IVth ventricle, or at the foramina of Luschke and Majendie, and the exact site of the obstruction may then be clearly defined by the introduction of opaque contrast media.

(*d*) CEREBRAL ATROPHY
Characteristically this is shown by the presence of large pools of air over the

cortex, which, if very localised, may be associated with drawing of the ventricles towards this site. There may, however, be simple generalised enlargement of the ventricles, or both features may occur together. Cerebellar atrophy is best shown by the use of tomographic radiography in the lateral plane, demonstrating enlargement of the IVth ventricle and cisterna magna, and shrinkage of the cerebellar folia.

(*e*) LOW PRESSURE HYDROCEPHALUS

The ventricles will be large, the subarachnoid space not filled, and no evidence of obstruction at aqueduct level. Such patients will go on to a RISA scan (see p. 309).

(*f*) CEREBRAL MALDEVELOPMENT

Agenesis, porencephaly, atresia of the aqueduct are only a few of the abnormalities easily shown.

THE SPINE

The routine examination includes lateral and antero-posterior views, for all regions, and oblique projections in the cervical region if there is evidence of nerve root disease and it is desired to show the root foramina.

Indications for X-ray of the spine

In any case in which a careful clinical assessment has suggested that the lesion lies in the spinal cord, the spinal nerve roots, or the cauda equina. The highest level of neurological abnormality must first be determined. The X-rays requested can then be limited to those parts of the spine above that level, remembering that spinal segmental levels and vertebral levels do not correspond and the difference increases as lower levels are reached (see p. 160).

Abnormalities of possible neurological significance

This is not the place to attempt to give a detailed description of the many abnormalities of bone which may be seen in X-rays of the spine and only those features commonly of relevance to neurological disease will be noted.

VERTEBRAL BODIES

Collapse due to fracture, osteoporosis, advanced tuberculosis, or metastases may cause root and cord compression. Osteolytic destruction is most commonly due to metastases, but may occur in myeloma.

Altered bone pattern or density. Increased density occurs in Paget's disease, osteoblastic metastases, reticulosis, the sclerosing form of myeloma, and in Charcot's disease. An angioma causes characteristic vertical trabeculation.

Hollowing of the posterior surfaces is seen in long-standing lesions such as intraspinal dermoids, syringomyelia, benign tumours or cysts.

Hemivertebrae causes gross scoliosis on flexion. In the lumbar region they may be associated with disc disease. At higher levels the scoliosis if severe can cause deformity of the cord sufficient to produce paraparesis.

Kypho-scoliosis can be a cause of cord distortion and paraparesis.

Fusion of cervical vertebrae (Klippel-Feil syndrome) is often associated with congenital abnormalities at the base of the skull such as platybasia, or basilar invagination causing cord lesions at foramen magnum level.

THE INTERVERTEBRAL DISCS

Narrowing of the disc spaces is more often due to degenerative changes than to disc prolapse and is so common that it need not necessarily be significant. Once having decided a definite level of the lesion, however, narrowing of a disc space and associated osteophytic outgrowths at that level may mean compression of roots, cord, or spinal vessels. When a disc space is narrowed and adjacent bodies show destructive changes, the lesion is usually inflammatory. In metastatic disease the disc is preserved.

THE PEDICLES

These are thinned and eroded over one or more segments in the presence of an expanding lesion. The importance of perfect radiography is very great in assessing minor differences. Metastasis is a very common cause of pedicle destruction.

THE VERTEBRAL CANAL

(*a*) *Narrowing*. This may be a feature of spinal deformity, spondylosis, Paget's disease, achondroplasia, basilar impression, all with resultant cord compression.

(*b*) *Widening*. Expansion occurs from lesions of long standing such as dermoids and astrocytomata.

The antero-posterior diameter of the mid-cervical spinal canal averages 17 mm on a film taken at 6 feet (almost 2 metres) with remarkable regularity. In syringomyelia this diameter is usually enlarged, and if it substantially exceeds 22 mm it is almost diagnostic of the disease.

THE INTERVERTEBRAL FORAMINA

Enlargement is almost always associated with neurofibromata, either single foraminal enlargement due to a tumour at that site, or multiple enlargement from widening of the root sheaths seen in von Recklinghausen's disease.

In cases of cervical root compression, encroachment by osteophytes may be shown in oblique views.

MYELOGRAPHY

In this country myelography by the introduction of air or oxygen under positive pressure into the subarachnoid space has not gained much popularity, as it is time consuming, tomography is necessary and the radiation dose is high. However, in cases of syringomyelia, the Arnold-Chiari malformation, and in some foramen magnum tumours, air-myelography used in conjunction with tomography can show the position of the tonsils, the size of the cord and its dynamic collapse or expansion, with great clarity.

Positive contrast media are more commonly used. A lumbar puncture with careful Queckenstedt tests is carried out. If there is a complete block, only a small volume of the medium is introduced and the patient is tilted under fluoroscopic control until the site of the obstruction is demonstrated. If no block has been demonstrated, 5–6 cc (and sometimes more) can be introduced and the patient remains sitting upright until fluoroscopy is carried out.

Cisternal injection can be used to define the upper limit of a complete obstruction or where lumbar puncture has been technically impossible. This is best carried out on the X-ray table so that screening can follow at once and if there is a serious possibility of a spinal block, preferably immediately before any operative procedure that is contemplated, for introducing contrast media above a block can convert a weakness of the legs into a paraplegia.

If there is any doubt about the position of the needle, no contrast media should be injected. Extradural media are not only useless but the less absorbable compounds obscure for a long time all attempts to visualise the theca at subsequent myelography.

Certain preparations have developed a bad reputation, usually on the flimsiest of evidence, for producing chronic post-myelography symptomatology. As a result new media are constantly being introduced which are easily absorbable. They do not give as good pictures, but appear to satisfy those so critical of the older substances, and certainly are of great value in showing root sheaths, and when combined with spinal CT scanning.

Indications for myelography

If there are any suspicions of spinal cord or root compression and, therefore, in:

(*a*) Cord lesions with complete or partial pyramidal and spinothalamic tract

involvement, or posterior column sensory less, *when a definite level of abnormality has been established.*
(*b*) Cases suspected of cervical spondylosis with cord compression.
(*c*) Cases of severe kypho-scoliosis with pyramidal tract involvement.
(*d*) Cases suggestive of an intrinsic cord lesion, in which the diagnosis between syringomyelia, cord tumour or angioma is important.
(*e*) Lesions at foramen magnum level when cerebellar ectopia or Arnold-Chiari malformation is suspected. Here it is particularly important to screen the patient supine as well as prone in order to outline the tonsils.
(*f*) In suspected syringomyelia the head should be positioned to try and allow contrast to enter the IVth ventricle. This often will not occur in syringo-myelia, for the exit foramina may be blocked, but in intrinsic tumours filling is normal.
(*g*) Some cases of lumbar disc prolapse when operation is contemplated but the physical signs do not give a single precise level.
(*h*) Cases of spinal block (see contra-indications (*a*).

Contra-indications to myelography
(*a*) In subtotal or total obstruction of the spinal canal, *unless operative exploration is to follow very soon.* Myelography may convert a subtotal into a total obstruction or hesitancy of micturition into total retention.
(*b*) In the presence of lumbar skin sepsis.
(*c*) In patients known to perpetuate complaints, unless there is an essential reason for carrying out the procedure. The root discomfort frequently experienced for a few days afterwards may be magnified into the major symptom of the patient's life, and considered responsible for all and any illnesses that may follow. In fact this has become so much of a medico-legal problem that many radiologists prefer to remove the non-absorbable media at the end of the examination. In the authors' opinion if it is to be removed it is then that it should be done, and the removal months later because of continued complaints of back pain is a procedure that is not likely to relieve that pain, or remove all the media, and it entails at least one more lumbar puncture and maybe others.

Myelographic findings
An experienced radiologist can produce helpful information under several circumstances.
(*a*) The upper and lower limits of a partial spinal block can be defined by careful manoeuvring of the contrast medium column. By combining lumbar and cisternal injections these limits can also be shown in a complete spinal block.
(*b*) If a tumour is suspected it may be possible to tell if it is extradural or intradural.

(*c*) The cord itself may be shown to be expanded due to an intrinsic tumour or a syrinx.
(*d*) Serpiginous defects suggestive of an excess of tortuous vessels can be shown in angiomata of the cord.
(*e*) Indentations of the column of medium will show disc protrusion in the cervical or lumbar regions, lateral views being of greatest value.
(*f*) Rounded defects just below the foramen magnum will suggest cerebellar tonsillar descent in the Arnold-Chiari malformation.
(*g*) Irregular obstruction breaking up the medium suggests an arachnoiditis.
(*h*) The examination may be completely normal, which in certain circumstances is a finding of utmost value to the clinician, if frustrating to the radiologist.

MYELOGRAPHY WITH CT SCANNING

The combination of spinal CT scanning with the introduction of contrast media has now become a major investigative procedure. The original rather small pictures obtained have now advanced to considerable enlargement and much greater ease of interpretation. Clearly only available to departments having the later generation scanners it is of great value in demonstrating tumours, intrinsic and extrinsic, cord enlargement by cavitation, and disc lesions. It can be refined to show meningeal thickening and areas of arachnoidal adhesion, while the early part of the nerve root sheaths can be clearly visualised.

SPINAL ARTERIOGRAPHY

Beautiful techniques have now been developed whereby radio-opaque material can be injected, via aortic catheterisation, into the vessels supplying the spinal cord. Used with subtraction films (see p. 293) spinal angiomata can be vividly demonstrated, and their arteries of supply defined. This is no longer only of academic interest because a number of these malformations can be removed. At first there was an unacceptably high rate of spinal complications from the investigation, but with improvements of technique, the nature, strength and quantities of the media used, it plays a vital role in the diagnosis of suspected spinal vascular anomalies. It is still however a manoeuvre requiring great expertise, and should not be embarked upon purely because a hospital has a capacity to carry out aortography.

X-RAYS IN SPECIAL CIRCUMSTANCES

In neurological disease the answer to the diagnostic problem may come from radiological investigation of other parts of the body. The importance of the chest has already been mentioned.

THE ABDOMEN

Plain films of the abdomen may show evidence of a phaeochromocytoma or enlargement of the renal shadow by a hypernephroma. Barium meals and enemata often need to be used in a search for primary neoplasms. A characteristic 'deficiency pattern' in the small intestine accompanies steatorrhoea, a condition associated with neurological complications.

THE PELVIS

This is a good site for demonstrating Paget's disease if it is only suspected in skull or spine, and is a common site for demonstrating bone metastases.

THE JOINTS

The shoulder and knee are the most common sites for Charcot's joints (occurring in tabes dorsalis, syringomyelia, or any cord or root lesion causing severe sensory denervation). The sacro-iliac joints show changes early in ankylosing spondylitis, a condition which may present in young people as sciatica; or may be accompanied by a cauda equina syndrome—both with high sedimentation rate.

THE MUSCLES

The thighs should be X-rayed in cases of epilepsy in patients who have lived in the Far East, Eastern Europe and Central or South America, for it is here, not in the skull, that the typical calcification of cysticercosis is seen.

THE NASOPHARYNX

Indentations of the air shadow from the posterior wall of the nasopharynx are seen in carcinoma and lymphosarcoma, conditions which extend upwards through the base of the skull causing cranial nerve palsies.

THE POST-TRACHEAL SPACE

Enlargement of this area occurs in infections, carcinomatous and myelomatous lesions of the vertebrae, with possible cord or root compression.

PARAVERTEBRAL SHADOWS

In cases of cord compression a paravertebral shadow would suggest tuberculosis (especially if calcified), osteomyelitis, reticulosis, myeloma, haematoma (following fracture), or the dumb-bell type of neurofibroma.

LYMPHANGIOGRAPHY

Hodgkin's disease and reticuloses can give rise to various puzzling neurological syndromes without superficial glandular enlargement being evident. Lymphangiography may show paravertebral, pelvic or abdominal adenopathy clearly, and this should be considered in unexplained root or peripheral nerve compressive syndromes (especially if the symptoms are strikingly exaggerated by alcohol).

To take a 17×14 in (43×36 cm) X-ray plate is a very costly procedure. If a patient is to be cured of his disability as a result of multiple X-ray examinations, then they are worth every penny, but when their multiplicity merely reflects inadequate preliminary clinical localisation of the lesion, then they represent an appallingly unjustified expenditure.

Chapter 37
Scanning

It is the advances in neuroradiology which have dominated the field of neurological diagnosis over the last 40 years as regards both intracranial and spinal neoplastic, atrophic or vascular disease. But apart from plain X-rays, often completely normal in the presence of gross disease, the procedures have been technically complicated, not always devoid of danger to the patient in certain groups, usually require admission to hospital, the services of a full radiological team, and often an anaesthetic. From many of these studies one had to suspect the presence of a radiolucent cerebral lesion such as an uncalcified tumour more by inference (displacement of other structures, patterns of blood supply, absence of vessels) than by the direct demonstration of the nature of the lesion, while small abnormalities could escape entirely. It is not surprising therefore that the search has continued for simpler and cheaper methods of detecting intracranial lesions, and for pinpointing their location when there are no physical signs to guide one, or when what signs there are do not accurately indicate even the side on which the lesion lies. Indeed a very cheap, totally reliable, screening procedure would be an invaluable asset in out-patient departments where so often one is asked to adjudicate on the possible presence of a tumour purely on some symptom such as a headache or a single epileptic attack. Unfortunately no procedure yet exists giving an unequivocal negative, and screening tests cannot give absolute exclusion of intracranial lesions.

However, over the years the gradual evolution of different scanning procedures has brought us slowly nearer to this goal. At first there was the valuable adjunct whereby one could measure and photograph the uptake of a radio-isotope given previously, and show tumours, including multiple small tumours such as metastases, and infarcts, without subjecting the patient to an 'invasive' procedure. When Sir Geoffrey Hounsfield developed the process of computerised axial tomography scanning, it seemed likely to take over radiodiagnosis, as this enabled tumours, infarcts, haemorrhages and atrophic processes to be differentiated and demonstrated so clearly without subjecting the patient to anything more than a rather claustrophobic experience. Admission to hospital was no longer necessary, symptoms such as headache and epilepsy could be investigated over a much wider range of patients, and, once the initial cost of the apparatus was borne, at less expense. The whole-body scanners then came along enabling the spine (and of course all other organs) to become accessible to this form of investigation as well, and in the brain at any rate it became possible to suspect areas of demyelination. With the advent of nuclear magnetic resonance, intracranial areas poorly demonstrated by CT scanning, projections difficult to obtain by other methods, good spinal cord imaging, and even clearer demonstration of demyelinative lesions, all have become possible.

The next stage has to be the ability to show cerebral metabolic processes, and their abnormalities, and to some extent the positron emission scanner fulfils this role, but the interpretation of the pictures obtained is far from easy, and the need to have close association with a cyclotron limits the installation sites available. At the moment this is largely a research facility, but not so long ago this was said about NMR whose ready availability is now limited purely by money and space.

The application of these and other measures can now be considered in greater detail.

ECHOENCEPHALOGRAPHY

If a sonic pulse is directed laterally through the skull it will be reflected from certain structures, and the reflected pulses can be recorded on an oscilloscope. They arise not only from the skull walls on both sides, but also from the ventricles and from central structures midway between these two. If the midline structures are displaced to one or other side the pulse will be reflected either earlier or later than expected according to whether displacement is towards or away from the side of the stimulus. The oscilloscope trace can be photographed and it is an easy, quick and painless method of detecting the side of a space-occupying lesion providing it is in the anterior portion of the hemispheres. The method has many limitations, produces both false positives and false negatives, and cannot be used in isolation from other more sophisticated methods, which in any event have almost completely replaced it. It never had the same success in neurological cases as it did in obstetrics, but it is a cheap, almost 'first-aid' investigation which can be carried out in accident and emergency departments, where those accustomed to its use have been able to detect subdural and extradural clots, or the presence of other space-occupying lesions when there are no localising signs, and may indicate the side to which further investigations should be directed.

A positive echoencephalogram may be very helpful. A negative one means nothing at all.

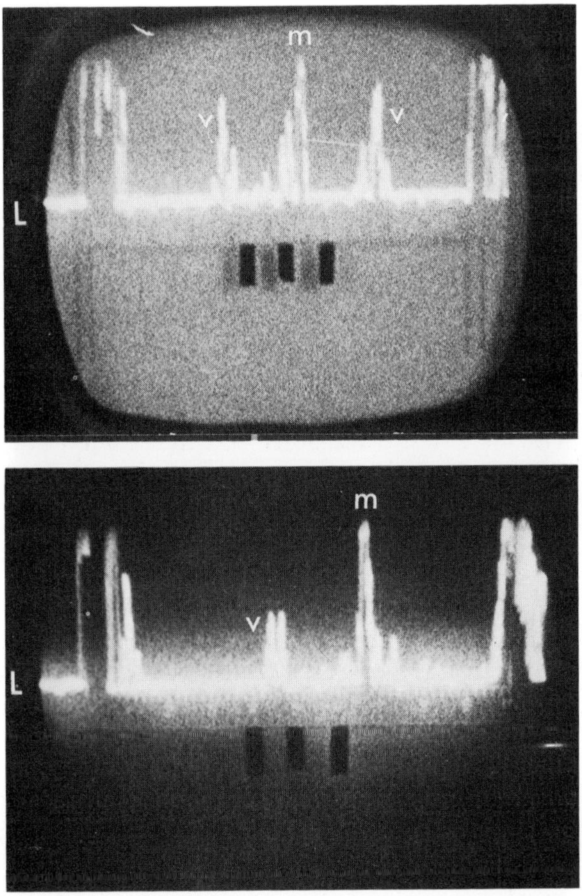

(a)

(b)

Fig. 80. Echoencephalogram. (a) Normal. Sonic pulse transmitted through skull from left side. Vertical deflections represent reflected pulses from (reading from left to right): left skull wall; left lateral ventricle (v): midline structures (m); right lateral ventricle (v); and right skull wall. (b) Left temporal lobe tumour. Note marked displacement of left ventricle and midline echoes from left to right.

ISOTOPE-ENCEPHALOGRAPHY

This technique takes advantage of the fact that certain radio-isotopes, taken orally or injected intravenously, are, after an interval, concentrated in abnormal brain tissue but not in normal brain. They then emit gamma radiation which can be detected by scanning apparatus and the intensity of the uptake recorded as marks on a chart or photographic film. Unusual areas of uptake can be easily detected. The advantage of the method is the relative simplicity of technique, requiring no anaesthesia, arterial puncture, head-shaving or burr-holes, and it can be used on out-patients; its disadvantage is,

(a)

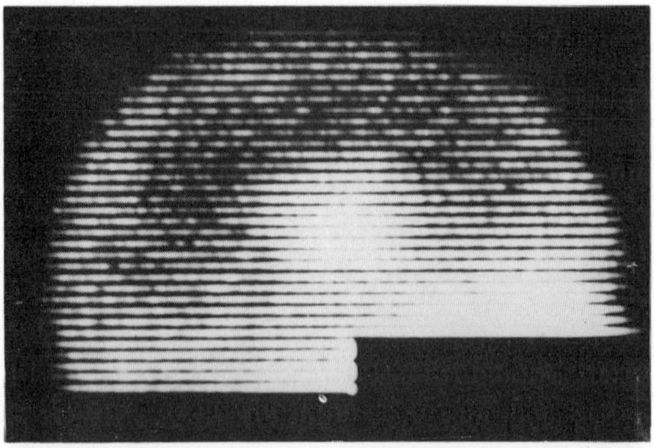

(b)

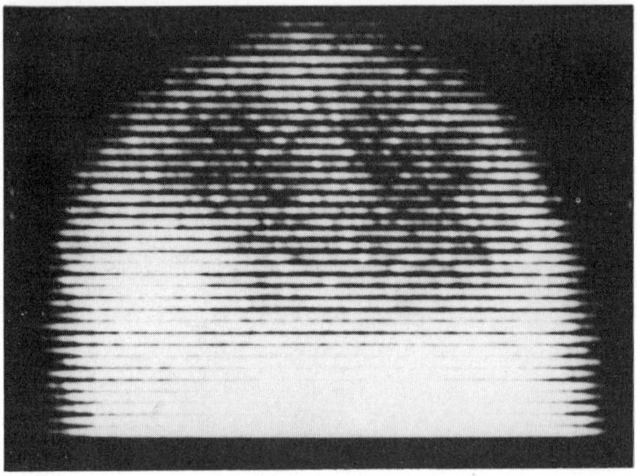

Fig. 81. Print from gamma-encephalogram (a) lateral, and (b) anterior-posterior projections, showing rounded temporal lobe metastasis from cariconoma of bronchus.

like so many of these investigations, it needs rather bulky and expensive equipment with technical staff to run it; it does entail a radiation dose, though very small, and may not be used too liberally in children and needs care during the reproductive era; and in many cases confirmation of the nature of a positive finding still requires expert contrast radiography or CT scanning. Where this is available, the use of the isotope method has been almost completely replaced, but its use, especially by means of the gamma camera, can be valuable in general hospitals providing its limitations are fully appreciated.

The isotope technetium 99m is widely employed and prior to administration potassium perchlorate is given orally to block uptake by the choroid plexuses. With this isotope the scalp, dural sinuses, and face and neck muscles also show uptake, which helps to orientate the lesion in respect of its exact site in the brain, but unfortunately tumours near the base of the brain and in the posterior fossa are largely obscured.

The 'gamma camera', which is capable of producing a record of isotope uptake far more quickly than the scanner itself, has added a new dimension to brain scanning by allowing the performance of serial studies at intervals of a few seconds, and make it possible in some cases to distinguish one type of lesion from another. This applies to intracranial lesions, but the term 'dynamic scan' is often used to refer to a technique by which multiple pictures show the flow of isotope (and therefore that of blood) through the vessels in the neck, through the cerebral circulation and away through the veins. This enables differences on two sides to be compared in, for instance, carotid artery thrombosis. Sometimes this may obviate the need for arteriography.

The isotopes are best taken up by meningiomata, even, oddly enough, the avascular variety—but these are also best shown arteriographically, and the problem of the difficult small parasagittal meningiomata may be masked by the isotope concentration in the venous sinuses. Glioblastomata are the next most easily shown, and these may be picked up in the parieto-occipital area which is notoriously difficult to cover arteriographically, certainly from carotid injection alone. By demonstrating multiple metastases this type of scanning may make arteriography unnecessary. Blood clots, intracerebral and subdural, also take up the isotope, and the value of this in the elderly patient who is drowsy and confused following minor head injury is obvious.

Certain patterns of uptake, indicating cerebral infarction, can be recognised, and by repeating the procedure, it is possible quite harmlessly to watch the evolution and disappearance of an infarcted area in a way arteriography never achieved.

A negative isotope scan does not exclude anything but in general there are rather more false positives than false negatives. When this section was first written it was emphasised that the method was a valuable adjunct to the longer established methods of investigation, but had not replaced them. This is still true, but now isotope scanning is rapidly itself being replaced by much more informative measures.

RISA scans

Before the advent of CT scanning another use of isotopes was in the investigation of the so-called cerebral atrophies, which usually means a patient presenting with presenile dementia. The concept of low-pressure hydrophalus, and the ability to improve some patients' conditions by the use of the Spitz–Holter valve or similar device has made it important to differentiate these cases from those of widespread atrophy. Air encephalography, using small quantities of air, in either case merely showed marked ventricular enlargement, but in the true atrophy air could be seen filling the widened cortical sulci. If sufficient air had been used, and the sulci did not fill, this was an indication for introduction at a later date of radioactive iodinated serum albumin (RISA) either into the lumbar or the cisternal theca, followed by serial scanning over the next 48–72 hours. Indium, often introduced cisternally, could be used in the same way. The isotope will enter and remain in the enlarged ventricles in low-pressure hydrocephalus, but in other atrophic states it will follow the normal CSF pathways over the surface of the brain. RISA scanning, or alternatively, scanning using albumen tagged with radioactive technetium, which has a shorter half-life, can also be used to check the patency of ventricular shunts.

In attempts to determine the origin and source of CSF rhinorrhoea or otorrhoea the pathway followed by the fistula can be traced using these isotopes, serially scanning over twelve hours. This still remains a valuable technique.

Cerebral blood flow

The use of isotopes in the measurement of cerebral blood flow in practice can offer the comparison of flow through the two hemispheres, or parts of the hemispheres, and can be applied to such cases as carotid stenosis before and after endarterectomy. There are many problems, but by using multiple counters areas of increased or decreased blood flow can be detected, and it can be used to assess the value of methods aimed at improving cerebral blood flow generally. Needless to say any method of improving the investigation and treatment of cerebrovascular diseases is welcome, for this is probably the largest neurological problem. Applying these techniques to cases of migraine has produced a completely new attitude towards the mechanism of migraine attacks, and is going to be the basis of considerable controversy for some years to come.

COMPUTERISED AXIAL TOMOGRAPHY
(CT *or* CAT *scanning*)

This is a system of great complexity by which X-rays are passed through the skull in a series of horizontal planes and the degree of absorption of the X-rays by different tissues, is measured, recorded, computerised, and then reproduced on a display screen in the form of a horizontal section of the skull which can be photographed by a polaroid camera. The information can be transferred to a disc and placed in another display machine to produce larger images, and enable different tissues to be singled out for special study. The whole apparatus is calibrated to give different degrees of density to different tissues, so that water, or CSF, or oedema fluid, have a very low absorption, and show as a dark area on the screen, and bone or calcified structures have a high absorption and show as dense white areas. Intermediate degrees of absorption such as brain, will produce shades of grey, while abnormal tissues such as tumours, abscesses, cysts, infarcts, and haemorrhages will all show in differing degrees of density (Fig. 82). An infarct for instance will show as a dark area, and a haemorrhage as a denser area; oedema will show as a dark area, often spreading over a wide zone in the brain with finger-like processes extending from the central darkness. Meningiomata show as very dense tumours, and gliomata vary, but by the intravenous injection of certain substances such as urografin and rescanning the patient, tumours can be made to stand out clearly, and this applies to multiple secondaries as well. This enhancement will pick up the capsule of chronic abscesses and clarifies dubious areas which might or might not be abnormal.

Because of the system's ability to show the CSF pathways as areas less dense than brain, the ventricles and some parts of the cerebral sulci can easily be shown. Ventricular enlargement can thus be vividly demonstrated, and if due to obstructive hydrocephalus, the size of the IIIrd and IVth ventricles and the aqueduct can be seen in different slices, and the site of obstruction assessed. In cerebral atrophic states the sulci may be seen clearly to be greatly enlarged, even at times in the absence of ventricular enlargement, though both frequently co-exist. This was previously only possible to demonstrate by the uncomfortable process of air-encephalography, and it takes only a fraction of the time, and needs neither anaesthesia nor admission to hospital. The tips of the temporal horns and the cerebellar sulci are not so well shown as in air-encephalography so that it does not replace it entirely. Children, or patients who cannot keep still, may need an anaesthetic purely for the purpose of obtaining excellent pictures.

A special feature of this type of scanning, which was perhaps a little unexpected at first, is the excellent views obtained of the orbits. The globe of the eye, the optic nerves, and of course any intra-orbital mass, can be demonstrated better than by any other easily available method.

Further elaboration of techniques has made it possible to some degree to reconstruct images in the vertical planes, and this has been particularly valuable in picturing extra-sellar pituitary extensions and other space-occupying lesions in the chiasmal and IIIrd ventricular areas.

Combining CT scanning with the use of intra-arterial or intra-thecal contrast gives good definition of vessels and cisterns while serial scanning in cases of intracerebral abscess has greatly reduced the need to introduce radio-opaque substances to be taken up by the walls of the abscess, reduces the need for frequent repeated tapping, and clarifies the possibilities of total excision.

Initially CT scanning concentrated on the head, but the whole body scanners, capable of imaging horizontal sections through virtually the whole body and all internal organs, can be applied to examination of the spinal cord, the thecal spaces, and the vertebral bodies, and with enlargement techniques good pictures can be obtained of various forms of extrathecal and intrathecal pathology. Greater clarity of information can be obtained by scanning following the introduction of contrast media into the CSF, and

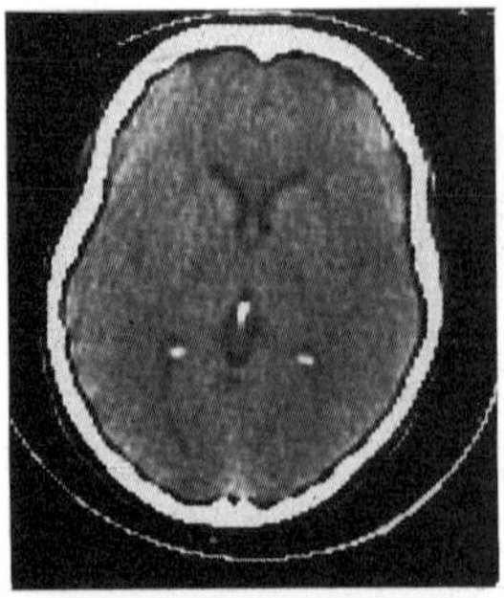
(a)

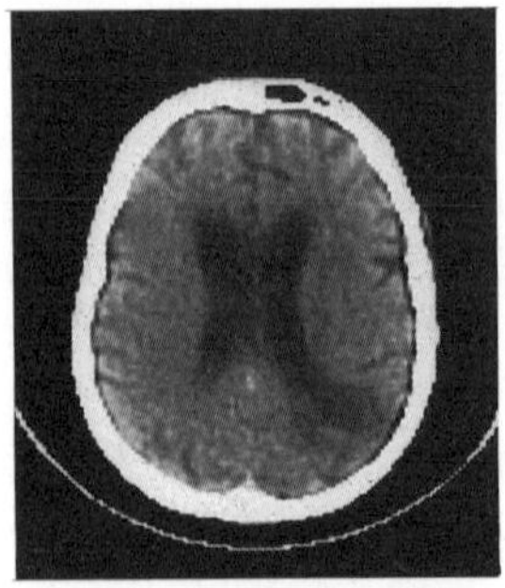
(b)

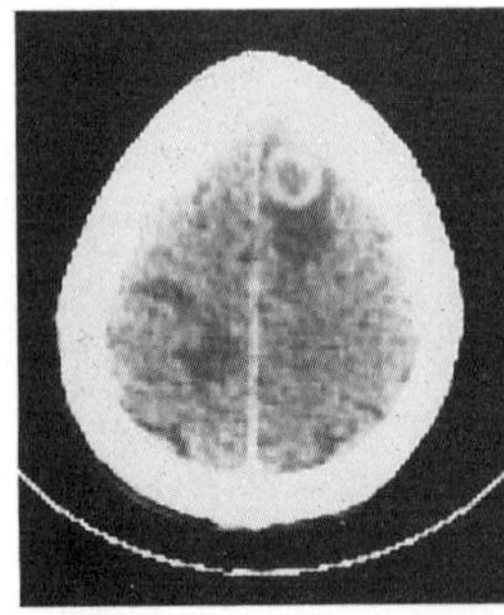
(c)

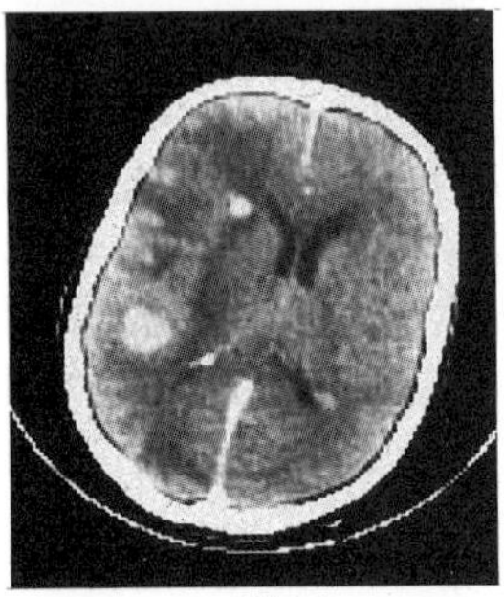
(d)

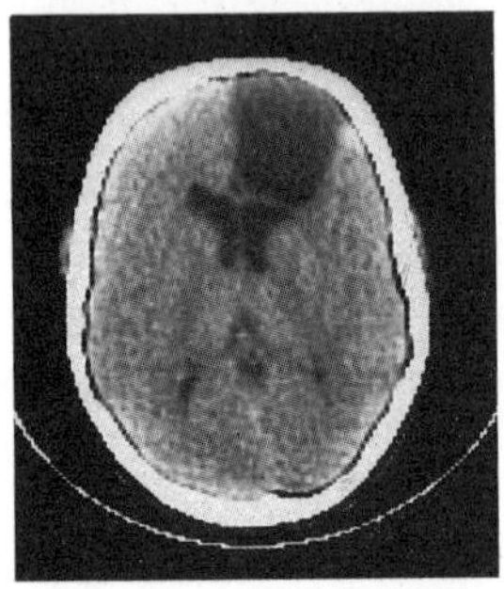
(e)

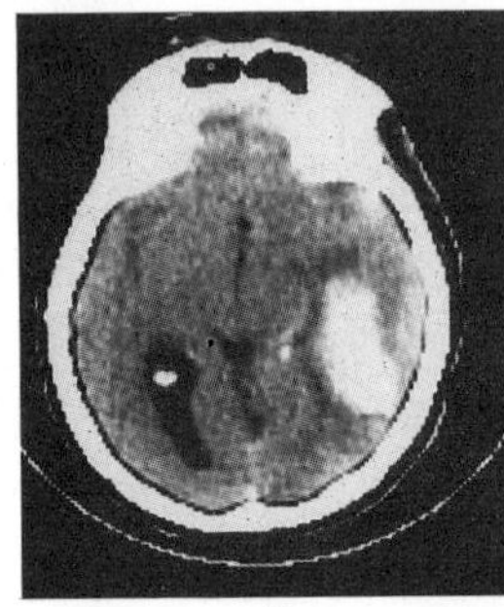
(f)

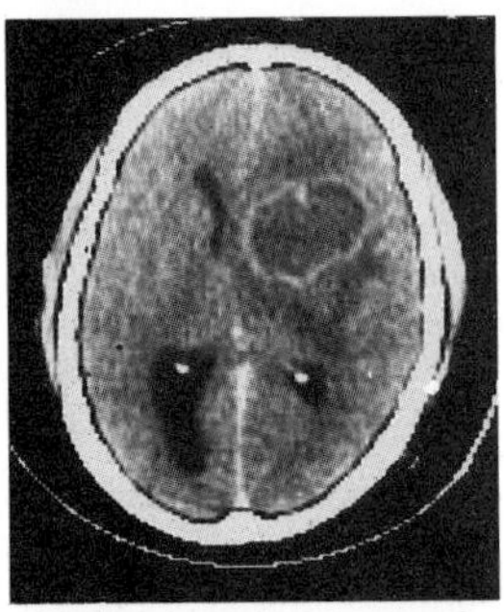
(g)

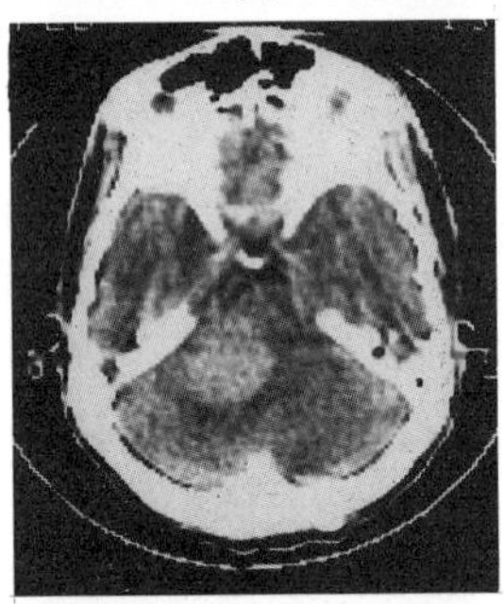
(h)

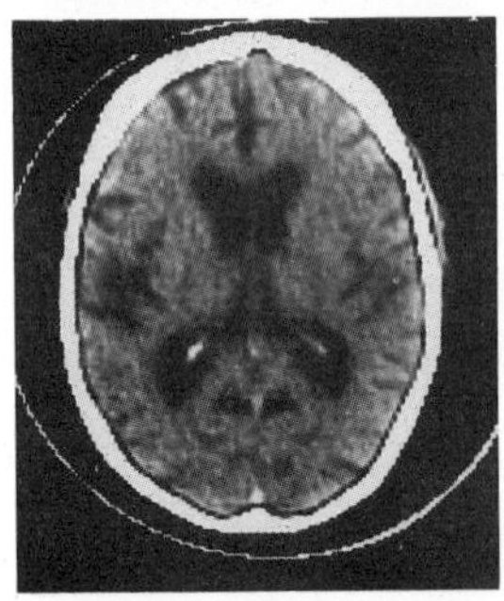
(i)

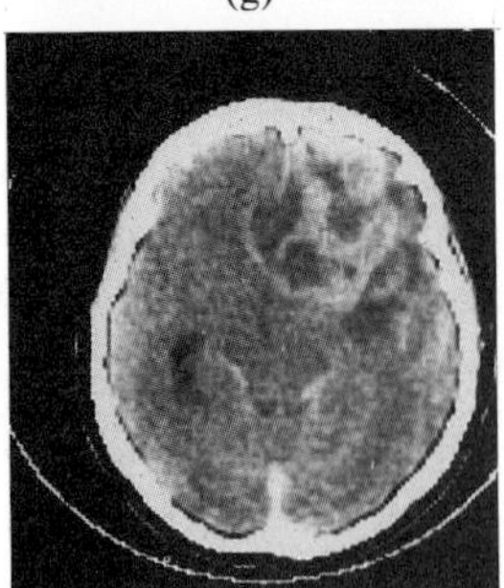
(j)

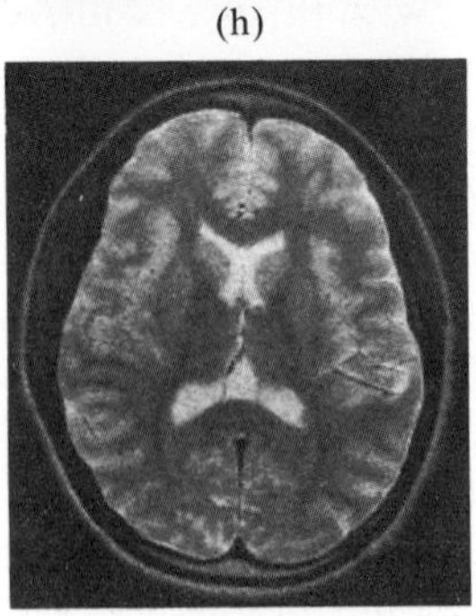
(k)

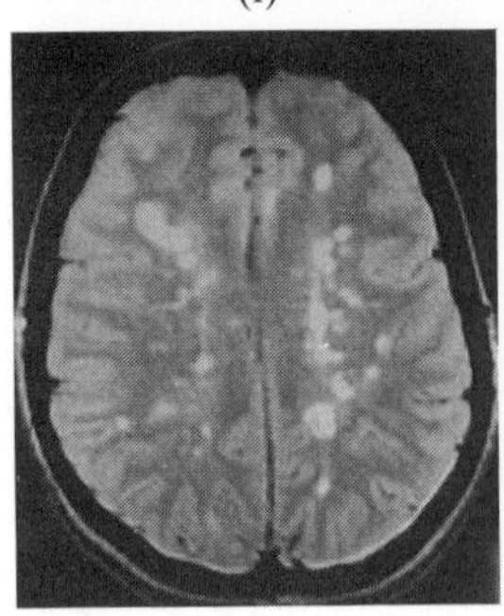
(l)

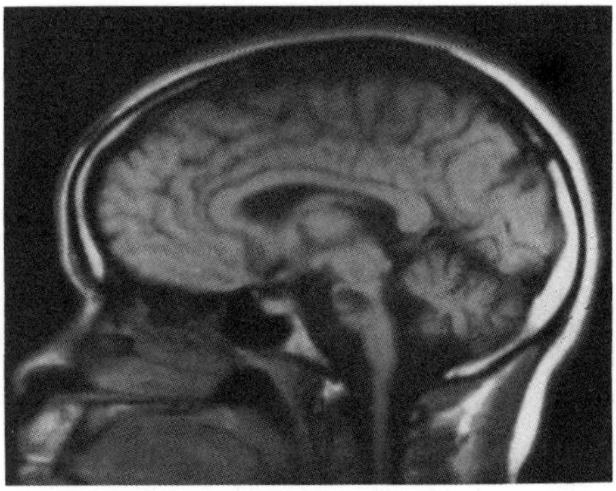

(m)

Fig. 82. Examples of CT and NMR scans.
(a) Normal scan, showing small lateral ventricles, normal subarachnoid space, calcified and central pineal and two calcified choroid plexuses.
(b) Enlarged ventricles, widened sulci and a translucent infarcted area in the right posterior cerebral territory.
(c) Two metastases, right frontal and left parietal, with surrounding oedema. Note the ring-like appearance of the deposits.
(d) Glioblastoma left hemisphere with massive oedema and displacement of ventricular system to right.
(e) Large congenital porencephalic cyst right frontal region.
(f) Right parietal intracerebral haematoma.
(g) Right posterior frontal abscess with surrounding oedema.
(h) Left acoustic neuroma.
(i) Cerebral atrophy shown by widening of the sulci, especially in the Sylvian fissure, and symmetrical dilatation of the ventricles.
(j) Multi-cystic glioblastoma right frontal lobe.
(k) Normal NMR scan. Compared to CT scans the bone is not shown, the ventricles in this view are shown white, and the distinction between grey and white matter is clear.
(l) NMR scan of hemispheres showing many areas of demyelination in the white matter, in a case of multiple sclerosis.
(m) NMR scan reconstruction in sagittal section, showing cerebral hemispheres, corpus callosum, brain stem, cerebellum, and upper cervical cord. A post infarct cyst is clearly seen in the pons. Technical variation shows CSF pathways black.

though not yet replacing myelography completely is rapidly becoming a great adjunct to it.

By now, in both brain, cord, and whole-body scanning, radiologists and clinicians have re-orientated themselves to looking at horizontal sections, previously an unfamiliar exercise to all but pathologists.

NUCLEAR MAGNETIC RESONANCE (NMR)

Also known as magnetic resonance imaging (MRI), the abbreviation NMR is used in this edition.

It was predicted in the last edition that NMR would soon become a familiar term, and this indeed has been the case. Again the precise mechanics of the procedure are beyond the ken of the average clinician, but the results obtained are in many conditions even better than CT scanning. There are two main reasons for this—bone is not a major hindrance to the imaging procedure, so that excellent pictures of the posterior fossa, the brain stem, and the foramen magnum region can be obtained, and it is possible to construct sagittal sections more easily so that one can see the whole brain stem and upper cervical cord in one slice. The spinal cord itself at other levels can also clearly be shown. Tumours and vascular lesions of the brain stem and cord, IVth ventricular tumours and cerebellar lesions are much better shown than by CT. Again the optic nerves, the orbits and the globe of the eye are strikingly clear.

All the advantages of CT imaging apply to this procedure, but in addition areas of demyelination can be picked up much more vividly, and can be detected in both the brain stem and the cervical cord, so that for the first time one is able, in life, to demonstrate the presence of multiple lesions in suspected multiple sclerosis rather than relying purely on one's clinical acumen. The prognostic value of this in a patient presenting, say, with just retrobulbar neuritis and nothing to suggest more than one site of a lesion clinically, is of course obvious. The profession is, however, going to have to come to terms with how best in their patients' interest to deal with this newly obtainable knowledge.

Apart from the nervous system, NMR can also be applied to the muscles, and while still in its infancy in this respect, may become of great additional benefit in muscular dystrophies and other diseases.

POSITRON EMISSION TOMOGRAPHY (**PET** *scanning*)

Whereas the previously described scanning techniques show clearly alterations in the structure of the brain and the presence of abnormal tissue, the PET scan can show the differing metabolism of the brain in health and disease. This has been very informative in studying the evolution of cerebrovascular accidents, in delineating different types of cerebral atrophy, and in some primary metabolic diseases of the brain. At the time of writing this is mainly a research tool, the scans are hard to interpret unless one has gained great experience in the field, and there is need to have easy access to a cyclotron. It is therefore at the moment of limited availability but the technique offers considerable hope in the future for clarification and classification of many of the more diffuse disturbances of brain function.

The great advantages of the scanning procedures described are of course the dramatic clarity of the pictures that can be obtained, the relative lack of discomfort, at virtually no risk to the patient, and the elimination, in many cases, of hospital admission for investigation. They are already altering to a considerable degree the pattern of neurological practice.

Their two main disadvantages are, firstly, economic. The initial installation, especially of NMR equipment, is very costly in money and space and upkeep is considerable. In many countries only a few selected centres are able to afford them and their positioning may be governed more by geographical consideration than by the size or sophistication on the units selected. The other disadvantage is rather a subtle one, yet of great importance. As the ease of access to these investigations becomes more widespread there is a danger that less attention will be paid to the fundamental processes of clinical bedside diagnosis, both in practice, and even more important, in teaching. The doctors first seeing a patient will need to be able to do this until the end of time, unless diagnosis becomes totally computerised, when there may be no need for doctors at all. This is probably what people said after Roentgen's discovery, but we still seem to be around.

Chapter 38
The Clinical Value of Electroencephalography

The first edition of this book stated that though the electroencephalograph has proved to be of utmost importance in neurophysiological research, its practical value in clinical neurology needed to be reviewed, revalued, and most warily assessed, and the reader was warned against the mushroom-like growth of inadequately staffed EEG departments, and the quite unwarranted diagnoses, and recommendations for specific treatment, which were sometimes made from, or read into, EEG reports. In the last 25 years such reassessment has in fact taken place in most areas, and in the minds of most people. As a result of this, the type of information which is regarded as being obtainable from the EEG is now settling into proper perspective, and what was always potentially a valuable investigation is more often being used in a manner which brings out its true value. This is not true everywhere, however, and one is appalled to see specific drug therapy recommended on EEG reports by individuals whose only knowledge of the patient is their tracing.

Again it is still necessary to remember, however, that its value in producing an actual diagnosis is very limited. The fact that a right frontal lobe tumour causes slow waves to arise from the right frontal lobe does not mean that slow waves arising from the right frontal lobe necessarily means the patient has a right frontal lobe tumour, or even that he is most likely to have one. Again a tracing can be quite normal in a patient suffering from unequivocal epilepsy, so that it cannot be used to 'exclude' epilepsy, or indeed anything, but the index of probability of certain conditions (e.g. herpes encephalitis or a cerebral abscess) can be drastically reduced by a normal EEG.

The purpose of this chapter is to help the reader to clarify in his own mind the circumstances under which truly useful information can be obtained. These circumstances are many, but an EEG is not a short cut round, or a substitute for, (*a*) a complete history from the patient and relatives, (*b*) a complete neurological and general physical examination, (*c*) the radiographic, biochemical or surgical investigations which may be required as a result of (*a*) and (*b*). A single normal tracing means very little and gross structural disease may be present with insignificant EEG abnormalities. It has to be stated once again that CT scanning has enormously reduced the use of the EEG in those centres fully equipped. In fact it appeared that the future of electroencephalography in such centres might well become confined to its use in epilepsy, cerebral infections, and certain degenerative disorders. However,

D.F. Scott, in a timely article in the *Journal of Hospital Medicine* of July 1987 draws attention to the role of the EEG as part of the general spectrum of clinical neurophysiology. No one would argue about its use, if well performed, in the diagnosis and monitoring of epilepsy, providing its limitations are realised. The modern ability to take ambulatory records on tape throughout 24 hours or more, and play them back at leisure has an increasingly important place in the differentiating of transient minor seizures, be they true petit mal, short focal attacks, attacks of temporal lobe origin, or of no organic origin at all. This type of recording can now be combined with video-recording of the patient, so that the physical and EEG events during transient seizures can be studied, without the observer having to be with the patient throughout the whole period.

The EEG is a vital instrument in the recording of evoked potentials (see p. 330) be they visual, auditory or somatosensory, and assists greatly in detecting lesions in the nervous pathways hidden to routine bedside examination, and has special value in detecting clinically 'silent' lesions in multiple sclerosis.

Then there is the still controversial area of brain death, in which the EEG is one of several measures capable of assisting the clinician in one of the most difficult decisions of modern medicine—the discontinuation of 'life' maintained purely by artificial means.

Bearing all these considerations in mind the indications listed below make no attempt to ally particular abnormalities with particular disease states, but are aimed at giving a general picture of the ways in which electroencephalographic examination can be of clinical help, especially in general hospitals where the more sophisticated imaging techniques may not be available. It is of course also cheaper

Indications for electroencephalography

(*a*) *In the investigation of a patient complaining of attacks of disturbance of consciousness.* The main purpose of the request should not be a vague hope that the EEG will decide if the patient has epilepsy. This must come from a detailed clinical history, correlated later, perhaps, with any abnormal EEG findings.

The aim should be to learn if there is *any* abnormality, whether it is mild or severe, spasmodic or continuous, showing a constant single focus of origin for the abnormal discharge (suggesting structural disease), or the characteristics of a petit-mal attack (almost certainly 'idiopathic'); or if, by comparison with previous tracings, in a patient under treatment, an assessment of greater electrical stability can be made. Any treatment must be known and stated clearly in the request, for certain drugs can fundamentally alter the EEG.

(*b*) *In the investigation of sudden unexplained episodes of disturbed behaviour*. A localised abnormality in the temporal lobe may suggest that these are episodes of what used to be called psychomotor epilepsy—an excellent and much lamented term.

(*c*) *In the investigation of children showing brief periods of detachment from their surroundings*. The EEG can give confirmation that the child has true petit-mal attacks, or may show abnormalities which suggest that they are minor grand-mal episodes.

(*d*) *In the investigation of a comatose patient whose physical signs are not of localising value*. A strong constant focal discharge will indicate the area towards which further investigative procedures must be directed.

(*e*) *In the investigation of suspected intracranial infection*. A strong focal discharge can indicate the site of a cerebral abscess with considerable accuracy, and may even be able to locate multiple abscesses. Clear slow wave temporal lobe abnormality very predominantly unilateral is a feature of herpes simplex encephalitis. A completely normal tracing would be strong evidence against an encephalitis, viral or bacterial.

(*f*) *In the investigation of suspected hypoglycaemia*. Recording tracings after prolonged starvation (often needing to be up to 72 hours), and if abnormal, repeating the examination during and after the administration of glucose may give diagnostic results. The return of a greatly abnormal record to normal within a few minutes is dramatic.

(*g*) *In the investigation of unexplained intellectual deterioration*. This especially applies to children. A focal discharge will indicate the site to which further radiographic studies should be directed at any age. On occasions, in children, prolonged subclinical epileptic activity may be shown, or petit-mal attacks of such frequency may be seen that the child can hardly ever be fully in contact with his surroundings. Very rarely the typical tracings of a subacute sclerosing panencephalopathy, or a hepatic encephalopathy can be distinguished. In progressive dementia in adult life metabolic encephalopathies can be shown, and the findings in Jakob–Creuzfeld disease may be diagnostic.

(*h*) *In the follow-up of a patient recovering from a diffuse cerebral disturbance such as an encephalitis*. The gross diffuse slow activity of the acute stage can be seen to decrease, and normal features to appear sometimes a little before clinical improvement is certain, and this helps greatly in prognosis.

(*i*) It can also be of value in operating theatres, monitoring depths of anaesthesia, assessing cerebral function during by-pass procedures, and may give a warning of impending cerebral complications.

What an electroencephalogram will not do

(*a*) It will not exclude organic disease.

(*b*) It will not exclude epilepsy. It can be normal even while a patient is having some form of fit. It will not decide fitness to drive a car.
(*c*) It will not exclude a cerebral tumour, nor decide whether a tumour is benign or malignant.
(*d*) It will not show whether a patient has a psychoneurotic or psychotic illness.
(*e*) It will not, by itself, diagnose any disease condition although it may suggest very strongly petit-mal epilepsy, sub-acute sclerosing panencephalopathy, the Jakob–Creuzfeld syndrome or, in infancy, infantile spasms.

Contra-indications to electroencephalography

(*a*) If, by waiting for an EEG report, treatment for epilepsy, or the radiological investigation of intracranial structural disease is likely to be delayed.
(*b*) If a seriously, or precariously ill patient has to be conveyed considerable distances for the examination.
(*c*) If the physician requesting the EEG is likely to be more influenced by a normal report than by his own assessment of the problem.
(*d*) If the physician reporting on the EEG is one who advises treatment or changes in treatment purely on the form of the tracing, without personal knowledge of the patient.

Technique of examination

Only a bare outline of a highly technical procedure will be given here, in an attempt to make the reported findings more comprehensible.

About 19 *electrodes* are held in place on the scalp, either by a cap of straps, or by 'sticking on' with collodion. They are usually placed in standard positions covering as much of the underlying brain as possible. A *lead* runs from each electrode to a headpiece and on to the amplifiers. Each recording pen is connected to two electrodes leading to one *channel* so that two channels record the activity from three adjacent electrodes, one electrode being common to each. The earlier machines had three or four channels only, but the use of at least an 8-channel apparatus is now obligatory, and 16-channel machines are becoming standard. Pre-set switching enables a large variety of recording patterns to be used, although in practice a relatively small number of standard patterns are routinely used.

Physiologial rhythms

Channels recording from electrodes over the posterior part of the brain usually show an *alpha* rhythm when the eyes are closed. This is the original activity recorded by Berger using a pair of electrodes, one frontal and one occipital. The waves occur in runs of varying length, now defined as between

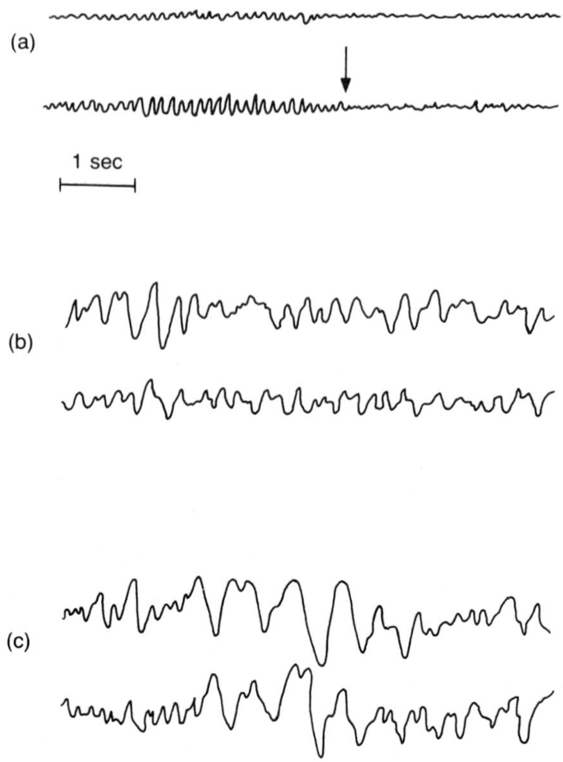

Fig. 83. Normal and abnormal rhythms. (a) Alpha rhythm. Note suppression on eye opening at arrow. (b) Theta rhythm. (c) Delta rhythm. (Paper speed 3 cm per second.)

8 and 13 cycles per second,* and these tend to disappear when the eyes are opened or during some form of thought process, such as mental arithmetic.

Theta activity runs at 4–7 c/sec, is seen in small amounts anteriorly, particularly in transverse recording patterns, and in children may be the dominant rhythm.

Beta activity is above 13 c/sec present at low voltage at random in most records, common in tense apprehensive subjects and prominent in patients on barbiturates.

Lambda waves are seen posteriorly, conventionally recorded as an upward deflection and present in many subjects when looking at a patterned field.

μ *activity* is complex, being a basic rhythm of about 10–12 c/sec with a harmonic component superimposed. It may represent the resting activity of

*Many European machines use the term 'hertz units' for cycles per second, abbreviated to Hz. As a result some EEG reports may use phrases such as 'a rhythm of 10 Hz'. This is the same as 10 cycles per second.

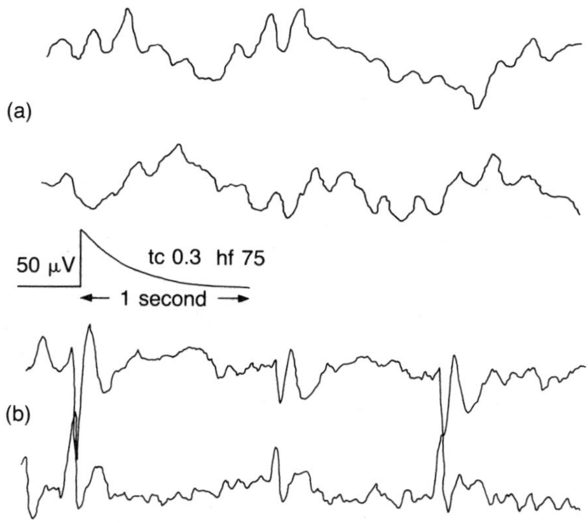

Fig. 84. Focal discharges. (a) Focal delta activity in a case of cerebral abscess. (b) Focal spikes in an old cortical injury. (Paper speed 3 cm per second.)

the motor and sensory areas, and can be blocked by movements or stimuli applied to the opposite half of the body.

K complexes, seen most commonly anteriorly, consist of one or more high voltage slow or sharp waves followed by a burst of rhythmic activity (sigma activity) and related to arousal stimuli during sleep, though not necessarily followed by arousal.

Abnormal rhythms

Excessive theta activity in adults is abnormal, and though often seen in deep-seated midline cerebral lesions, it occurs in a variety of conditions, and its evaluation is exceedingly difficult.

Delta activity consists of very slow waves, less than 4 c/sec and outside sleep its presence in adults is always abnormal. It can be generalised in many pathological processes and in long-standing epilepsy, but when localised is indicative of a local structural lesion.

Focal discharges (Fig. 84). If the deflections of an abnormal discharge are in opposite directions at the same moment in two channels having a common electrode, this is termed *phase reversal* and indicates that the origin of the discharge is near the common electrode (Fig. 84a).

Spikes (Fig. 84b). These are very sharp waves, usually of high voltage, looking somewhat like the QRS complex of an electrocardiogram. They are always abnormal and if persistent at one site may indicate a focal cortical discharge.

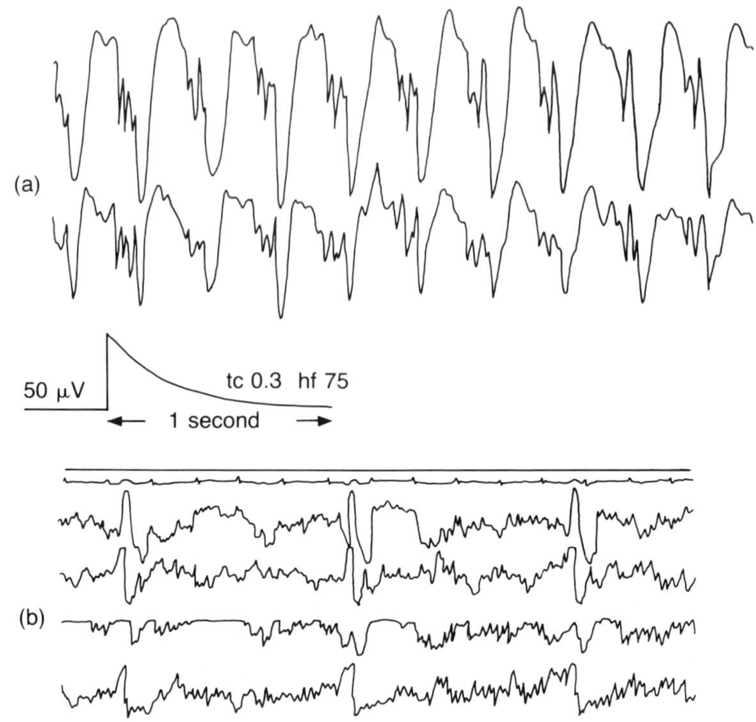

Fig. 85. Characteristic EEGs. (a) Petit-mal attack—regular 3-per-second spikes and waves (paper speed 3 cm per second). (b) Inclusion body encephalitis. Regular periodic high voltage complexes throughout record (paper speed 1.5 cm per second).

Spike and wave discharges. These consist of a spike followed by a large delta wave, or vice versa. They may occur in isolation, in runs of irregular size and speed, or in completely regular runs of abrupt onset and cessation, three complexes occurring each second (Fig. 85a). This last is the classical activity associated with petit-mal epilepsy, but atypical spike and wave runs of irregular frequency are common in all forms of epilepsy, and may consist of one or more spikes, associated with irregular slow waves and biphasic waves, and usually occurring episodic bursts.

Myoclonus. In myoclonic attacks the EEG shows sudden sharp wave complexes, perhaps 4–6 together, with associated slow waves, but often with several sharp waves to one slow one. The runs are very much shorter and more irregular than in petit-mal.

Hypsarrhythmia is a term given to a grossly disorganised record showing high voltage spikes and slow waves, and it is almost confined to children suffering from infantile spasms or 'salaam' attacks—a non-specific clinical picture which may also occur in metabolic disorders such as phenylketonuria, or in tuberose sclerosis.

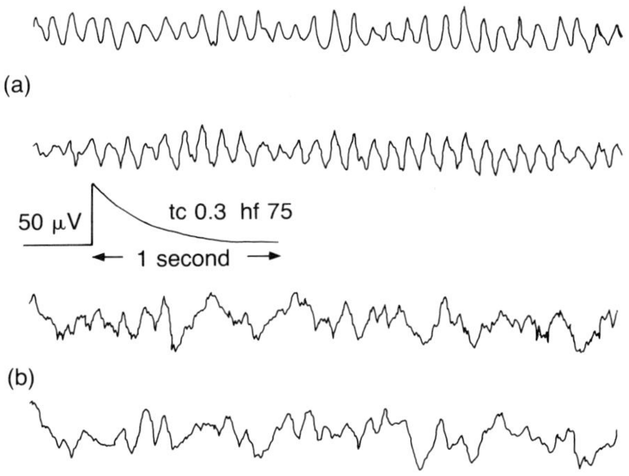

Fig. 86. Effect of hyperventilation. (a) A normal resting record. (b) Abnormality after 2 minutes overbreathing.

Periodicity. In certain sub-acute encephalitides (inclusion body encephalitis or sub-acute sclerosing leucoencephalopathy) sharp followed by large slow-wave complexes appear at regular intervals throughout the record (Fig. 85b). Regular periodic groups of slow waves are sometimes seen in the lipoidoses, and in a variety of other conditions.

Methods of stimulation

One of the problems of electroencephalography is that abnormalities may not be present at the particular time that the tracing is being taken. Various ways have been evolved by which abnormalities may be evoked or slight abnormalities made more obvious and more clear cut.

Hyperventilation

The patient breathes deeply and vigorously for about three minutes, or less if he cannot tolerate it. This may convert a dubious tracing into one that is definitely abnormal (Fig. 86). It may, however, produce deviation from the normal in apparently normal subjects, but this is usually transient. It is particularly significant if the abnormality persists for over a minute after stopping the hyperventilation and a very exaggerated response may be seen in hypoglycaemia, even in the absence of a low blood sugar. This can be abolished by oral or intravenous sugar in such patients. In epileptics it may change a relatively normal record into one which is very unstable and abnormal. In the majority of patients suffering from untreated petit-mal runs of spike and wave activity occur during hyperventilation. There is also always the chance of producing a classical grand-mal fit, so that enthusiasm should be tempered with caution.

The stroboscope

Intermittent flashing lights placed in front of a patient's closed eyes may, in some cases, produce abnormal discharges, sufficient even to cause a full-scale fit. Individuals are often susceptible to particular frequencies. It is of particular value in petit-mal, and in myoclonic attacks, and a rate of 17–25 flashes per second will usually produce EEG abnormality in patients presenting with 'television' epilepsy or other forms of photogenic epilepsy.

Some patients intensely dislike the subjective effect of flashing light, and if this is the case, and the resting record has shown adequate information, there is no purpose in persevering with it.

N.B. One needs to be careful in using this machine. The senior author's technician was once carrying out stroboscopy on an epileptic patient, who had a nurse in attendance. When the flash was switched on the nurse had a full-scale epileptic attack.

Sleep and barbiturate records

Many epileptics, when drowsy, show in their EEG more marked changes or abnormality not present before. Cortical focal discharges may appear. In addition the method is of value in children and nervous adults by reducing the artefacts due to movement and muscle tension. Sleep can be introduced quite simply, in a quiet department, by a small oral dose of quinalbarbitone sodium or pentobarbitone sodium. Intravenous thiopentone sodium, to produce light anaesthesia, can have the same effect, and has the advantage of speed, for a sleep record may take most of a morning, a pentothal record half-an-hour. The same accentuation of abnormality may be seen, and used in conjunction with sphenoidal leads, the fast activity produced by the barbiturate may be suppressed on the side of temporal lobe damage.

Use of leptazol

Intravenous leptazol combined with stroboscopy at about 20 flashes per second is a very potent method of stimulating abnormal rhythms, and overt fits, or epileptic-type discharges in the EEG can be induced in normal subjects if a large enough dose is given. It is not a reliable method of distinguishing epileptics from non-epileptics, but it can emphasise local cortical discharges, and it can reproduce a fit during which clinical and EEG observations may produce information useful in the consideration of patients suitable for surgical treatment of their epilepsy.

More advanced recording techniques

SPHENOIDAL LEADS

Many methods have been used to place electrodes as near as possible to the inferior surfaces of the brain which are so far removed from the normal scalp electrodes. The most important areas, the inferior surfaces of the temporal lobes, can be approached by sphenoidal electrodes, introduced through the cheek, passing below the zygomatic arch and through the mandibular notch. Records are taken with pentothal administration, and in temporal lobe abnormalities unilateral spike discharges, focal slow waves, or suppression of barbiturate-produced fast activity may clearly reveal the side of the abnormality and may influence a surgeon towards carrying out electrocorticography, and possibly temporal lobectomy.

CORTICOGRAPHY AND DEEP ELECTRODES

This is the technique by which, during a surgical procedure, electrodes are placed directly on the surface of the brain, or inserted into the brain substance. The site of the maximum focus of abnormality can in this way be located in considerable detail.

The particular value of this method is in delineating the region of cortex responsible for the epileptic attacks, or in locating otherwise undetectable small cicatrices, neoplasms and hamartomata which are not uncommon in the temporal lobes. It is suggested by some that corticography enables a more limited amount of temporal lobe, or an unusually placed focus, to be excised than in standard surgical procedures, perhaps with better results.

Use the EEG with a specific purpose in mind, and with a specific request, giving the electroencephalographer and his technician adequate clinical details, so that they may be aware of the clinical problem, and if indicated may employ special recording techniques.

As shown earlier the EEG has applications well beyond the range of epilepsy, but it should not be thought that it can be used as a screening operation. It must not be expected to produce a diagnosis, except sometimes in the conditions mentioned earlier. It must not be used in isolation from full clinical study, but intelligently integrated into the clinical and therapeutic environment, it can be a great help in difficult problems.

The chapters entitled 'The value and limitations of electroencephalography' in L.G. Kiloh and J.W. Osselton's book *Clinical Electroencephalography* (Butterworth) and on the clinical use of the procedure in J. Laidlaw and J.B. Stanton's book, *The EEG in Clinical Practice* (Churchill Livingstone) were first written many years ago but they are recommended to clinicians as being very pertinent to modern practice.

Chapter 39
Peripheral Electrophysiology

There have been many advances in the field of peripheral neurophysiology in recent years. While a large part of the work of such departments is still concerned with electromyography and nerve conduction studies, the role of evoked potentials in clinical neurology has expanded considerably and now provides everyday help in patient management.

ELECTROMYOGRAPHY

The electromyograph (EMG) records the electrical activity of muscle. A concentric needle electrode, with an inner (active) wire and outer (reference) cannula, is used. The potential difference between the two parts is amplified and displayed on a cathode ray oscilloscope as well as being fed through a loudspeaker system. A camera is usually included in the apparatus which can photograph the oscillographic patterns for more leisurely study and permanent record and many modifications of the type of oscillograph have made tracings easier to see, record and analyse, while recording on tape for later playback and study at leisure is common practice.

Needle electrodes can record from single motor units or fibres, and are now available carrying multiple electrodes which can be attached to a multichannel oscillograph. Many adjacent parts of the muscle can thus be examined at one time.

Normal records

Insertion of the needle produces a burst of potentials which rapidly die away within 2–3 seconds. At rest there is no electrical activity. On slight voluntary movement, one sees single *action potentials,* which are biphasic sharp waves of 0.2–3 mV, firing at 5 per second and increasing both in speed and amplitude as voluntary activity increases. As the movement becomes greater, so many fire that a most complex *interference pattern* is obtained, but the biphasic, or at the most triphasic, character of the waves is maintained. Polyphasic waves may occasionally be seen normally, but are said to be less than 4 per cent of the total. Stimulation of the motor nerve over 12 times per second produces action potentials in the muscle which increase during the first 3–5 stimuli, and later show a temporary decrease in amplitude which then remains constant.

Abnormalities occur during insertion, at rest, or during activity. Insertion activity is prolonged in denervated muscle.

Most of the abnormalities occurring in resting muscle happen to be typical features of *denervation*:

(*a*) *Fibrillation potentials* are action potentials spontaneously arising from single muscle fibres. They are bi-phasic or tri-phasic spikes of short duration (< 5 ms) and low amplitude ($< 200\ \mu V$) and give a very characteristic clicking noise on the loudspeaker.

(*b*) *Positive sharp waves* are usually found with fibrillation potentials and consist of an initial positive deflection of about the same amplitude followed by a slow change of potential that forms a small, prolonged negative phase of 10 ms duration or more.

(*c*) *Fasciculation* in which motor unit potentials fire spontaneously and rhythmically when the muscle is at rest.

(*d*) *Altered interference pattern* as a result of the reduction of the number of functional motor units. However these surviving motor unit potentials become large, polyphasic and of long duration. This is the result of re-innervation of denervated muscle fibres by collateral branches from the nerves of surviving units.

Muscle disease

Primary abnormalities of muscle fibres (myopathies) are distinguished by a variety of characteristic changes in the EMG. However, these do not elucidate the cause of the muscle disease and some of the changes can also be found, for example, during reinnervation of muscle after neurogenic lesions (as above).

There is increased insertional activity and even, sometimes, abnormal spontaneous activity—both features more typical of denervation. Inflammatory muscle disease is particularly likely to cause these. But the changes in individual motor units and their pattern of recruitment is more definite. Characteristically, potentials are small, often polyphasic, and of short duration. The loudspeaker crackles in a typical manner. A full interference pattern may be seen, but the potentials may be seen to be smaller in amplitude.

Nerve conduction studies

We have seen how muscle sampling with a needle electrode evaluates the state of muscle itself. Nerve conduction studies and measurement of the amplitude of nerve or muscle action potentials constitutes the second approach in examining neuromuscular function. Surface electrodes are mostly used.

Motor nerve conduction velocity (MCV) is investigated by recording the muscle action potential (MAP) following stimulation of a given nerve at two variable sites. If the distance between the different sites of stimulation is measured, then this figure can be divided by the difference between the two action potentials ('proximal latency' minus 'distal latency') to give the conduction velocity in that particular 'segment' of nerve. This technique cannot be applied to the 'segment' between nerve and neuromuscular junction, the 'distal motor latency'. Normal values for this have been established for the main nerves most usually examined. Finally, one records the amplitude of the muscle action potential by placing a surface electrode over the muscle belly and then stimulating the motor nerve at various sites.

The latency and amplitude of the *sensory* action potential (SAP) can also be determined with the use of a surface electrode. Electric shocks are applied at specific sites to stimulate sensory nerve fibres, for example, stimulating the middle finger with a ring electrode and recording the SAP of the median nerve at the wrist.

Any of these parameters of peripheral nerve function can be affected by neuropathies or individual peripheral nerve lesions. *Demyelinating* conditions (Guillain–Barré syndrome, diabetes, carcinoma) cause profound slowing of conduction velocity. In contrast, neuropathies characterised by *axonal degeneration* do not. In these, whether caused by alcohol or other toxins, velocities seldom fall by more than 20–30 per cent. Local damage, for example by entrapment, will cause low conduction velocity in a particular segment of nerve. Both types of generalised neuropathy are associated with reduced or absent sensory and nerve action potentials.

It can be seen that the progression of, or recovery from, various nerve disorders can be monitored by these examinations. A distinction may be made between weakness of myopathic or neurogenic origin, and local or generalised abnormalities can be discerned.

Some particular indications for neuromuscular electrodiagnostic tests

THE INVESTIGATION OF PERIPHERAL NERVE LESIONS

These tests are hardly necessary for diagnostic purposes when the cause of a muscle weakness is obvious (e.g. old poliomyelitis or known injury to a peripheral nerve), but can be valuable in the assessment of prognosis and progress of recovery. Fibrillation potentials in the EMG as early as a week after the lesion suggest that recovery may be poor. Unfortunately, these findings are not always well correlated with clinical results. Median, ulnar and lateral popliteal palsies are the most common.

THE LOCALISATION OF A LOWER MOTOR NEURONE LESION

By correlating the muscles known to be supplied by particular spinal segments, anterior roots, or peripheral nerves with the muscles showing signs of denervation on the EMG, it is possible to differentiate the site in the motor pathway at which a lesion lies.

DISTINGUISHING NEUROGENIC ATROPHY FROM MYOPATHY

Clinically this may be difficult. As discussed, in neurogenic atrophy, the EMG shows the features of denervation. In early myopathy, the EMG should show the pattern of primary muscle disease. In polymyositis, the two major types of abnormality may be combined.

IN MYOTONIA

The diagnosis of myotonic dystrophy or myotonia congenita, should be possible clinically, but the EMG may show myotonia in apparently normal muscles, including the ocular muscles; can be used to assess the effects of treatment; and may also show myotonia in other muscular disorders, such as myositis. The features of voluntary activity are prolonged during an attempt to relax, and after percussing the muscle or moving the electrodes there are salvos of fast, variable-amplitude potentials, which rapidly die away, producing on the loudspeaker the well-known 'dive bomber' noise.

IN DEMONSTRATING MYASTHENIA

The falling away of voluntary activity on attempted sustained contraction and its recovery following neostigmine or edrophonium (Tensilon) injection can be clearly demonstrated, and again this may be found in muscles thought to be normal. Repeated stimulation of a motor nerve in a normal subject will produce a muscle potential of uniform amplitude if the rate of stimulation is slow, less than 30 per second. In myasthenia gravis, repetitive stimulation with rates of only 3–5 per second induces a reduction or *'decrement'* in amplitude. In contrast, rapid stimulation rates of 20–50 per second results in a decrement in normal subjects, but an increase or *'increment'* in amplitude in myasthenic (Eaton-Lambert) syndromes.

THE DEMONSTRATION OF ABNORMALITY IN OTHER MUSCLE GROUPS

If faced with an obvious lower motor neurone lesion (e.g. of the lower limbs), one is anxious to know whether this is part of a widespread polyneuropathy or due to some local lesion of the nerves or roots supplying the lower limbs. EMG patterns of denervation from the upper limbs in such cases may show that the disease is in fact widespread. Conversely, the finding of denervation in the presence of upper motor neurone signs can support a diagnosis of amyotrophic lateral sclerosis.

THE DEMONSTRATION OF ANTAGONIST ACTIVITY

If there is some doubt as to the correct relaxation of antagonists for a given voluntary movement, e.g. in extrapyramidal disease, or even in hysterical weakness, EMG recording from the antagonists, which should be silent, may show a great deal of electrical activity.

EVOKED POTENTIALS

Very small electrical potentials are 'evoked' in the cortex or spinal cord following stimulation of the special sense organs or peripheral nerves. The use of digital computers to provide electronic 'averaging' now means that surface electrodes can be used to investigate these small 'evoked potentials' so as to provide a non-invasive, objective test of various nervous pathways. The recording of evoked potentials now has an established place in clinical neurophysiology alongside EEG, EMG and nerve conduction studies.

The *visual, auditory* and *somatosensory* potentials are the most widely used, and it is in the diagnosis of *multiple sclerosis* (MS) that they have found their main application. Clinically suspected lesions can be confirmed, or subclinical ones detected. For example, the ability to establish the existence of optic nerve disease in a case of paraplegia reduces or avoids the need for myelography.

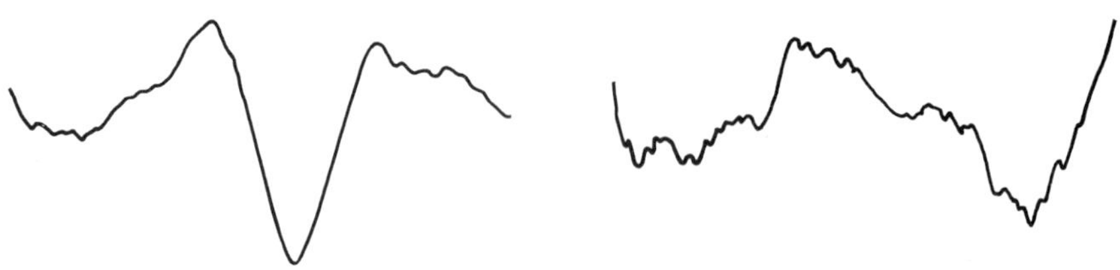

Fig. 87. Visual evoked response (VER). Left tracing normal. Right shows delayed, prolonged, distorted response with lowering of amplitude. A case of multiple sclerosis with an optic nerve lesion.

The characteristic finding in the visual evoked potentials (VEP) in multiple sclerosis is an increase in the *latency* of the response. In acute optic nerve disease the amplitude of the VEP is greatly reduced also. This is in parallel with the decline in visual acuity and recovers accordingly with clinical improvement. The latency, however, recovers in only a very small number of cases and so can be detected at a later date thus providing objective proof of previous disease.

Ocular abnormalities and other forms of optic nerve disease will also affect the VEP, and so the examination, as with *all other* neurophysiological investigations, must be carefully interpreted in the context of the known clinical situation. A normal VEP, for example, in the presence of apparent blindness is of great assistance when hysteria or malingering are suspected.

Auditory brain stem (AEP) and somatosensory evoked potentials (SEP) can be used in combination with the VEP to increase the yield of detection of subclinical lesions in MS. But the AEP, although useful, is not so reliable as the VEP. The changes are less definite and tend to fluctuate, but do prove useful in the assessment of hearing in small children or suspected 'functional' cases.

The SEP, recorded either over the scalp or cervical spine, can reflect subclinical lesions in the posterior columns in MS, or be useful in the investigation of other spinal cord, plexus, or root lesions.

In studying EMG, nerve conduction or other neurophysiological investigation reports, the exact meaning of the terms used must be appreciated, lest too much is read into the findings. 'Myositis' and 'myelopathy' in an EMG report may not mean muscle inflammation or spinal cord parenchymatous disorder, but EMG appearances such as may be seen in these conditions. 'Demyelinating' conditions (p. 328) refer to the sheath of peripheral nerve, and does not refer to multiple sclerosis. To quote Professor J.A. Simpson: 'electrodiagnostic techniques should be used to explore the physiological properties of normal and pathological states of the lower motor neurone or muscle, and not to make a nosological diagnosis'. They share with electroencephalography the capacity for adding another physical sign to the patient's clinical picture.

Part VIII
Conclusion

Chapter 40
The Indications for Full Investigation in Certain Common Neurological Disorders

It has been stated several times earlier in this book that the majority of patients with neurological symptoms do not, in the first place, come into the hands of a neurologist or special unit. The general physician still sees a vast amount of neurological material and may feel the need for advice as to when to refer a patient for more extensive investigations, either as an out-patient or an in-patient, to units or departments with special facilities for scanning, sophisticated neuroradiology, electrophysiology and neurochemistry. The most common disorders are included, as obviously all and every condition cannot be covered, but one has learnt from experience that neurologists are more frequently consulted about those mentioned below than any others, and some general guide-lines are given.

'Full investigation' is intended to mean those studies which would necessitate the transfer of the patient to a specialised unit, department or centre, e.g. for scanning procedures, maybe arteriography, myelography, etc.

The controlling purpose behind such a move should be to obtain a specific piece of information which is *likely* to be obtained in that particular case, and the knowledge of which is genuinely likely to be profitable. There is no justification for allowing these complex, very expensive, and not necessarily harmless procedures to become part of a blunderbuss investigation to avoid overlooking something.

Headache

The problem is that of detecting an early cerebral tumour, or a vascular anomaly. There is probably no symptom for which it is more tempting to suggest a CT scan, and in an ideal world with full facilities at little cost this might well be done in each troublesome case. However, extensive studies have shown that if patients simply with headache are subjected to this very costly procedure the chances of showing anything *relevant* are minimal, and those that did were suspected anyway. Everyone will relate an experience in which a patient dying from a cerebral tumour had nothing but headache as a symptom until the terminal stages, but these are phenomenally rare, and under present conditions there cannot be justification in investigating every case. Certain indications are however very important:

(*a*) If the onset of the headache is both dramatic and of great severity,

especially if accompanied by vomiting and nuchal rigidity. This might suggest a subarachnoid haemorrhage.
(*b*) If a headache of gradual onset steadily increases over several days and is accompanied by true vomiting, such as occurs in rising intracranial pressure.
(*c*) If the headache is accompanied by loss of consciousness or by increasing drowsiness and slowing of the pulse—for the same reason as (*b*).
(*d*) If it is accompanied by progressive failure of vision—as in optic nerve compression, or chronic papilloedema.
(*e*) If it is accompanied by any abnormal neurological signs that were not present before, papilloedema being, of course, the most important.
(*f*) If it is accompanied by epileptic attacks not previously present.

It is essential to establish that the complaint is truly *headache*, and that an honest assessment is given of its duration and severity. The intolerable, agonising, constant headache, unremitting for 20 years, is not due to organic disease, but is a common reason for referral with a view to further investigation. Pestering by patient or by relatives is not an indication for carrying out these procedures. Remember—tension headache is still the commonest form of headache though the patients may prefer to think that they suffer from migraine and sometimes the distinction is very difficult.

Migraine

The problem here is usually whether a vascular anomaly, or very rarely, a tumour, might be present. Migraine may affect one side throughout most of a patient's life, but careful questioning will usually reveal that one or two attacks at least have affected a different site.

Further investigation is justified under the following circumstances:

(*a*) If any attack, prolonged for several days, is accompanied by true neck stiffness.
(*b*) If there is true loss of consciousness.
(*c*) If there are abnormal physical signs during or after an attack.
(*d*) If, at some stage, an EEG has been done and shown a constant focal discharge—remember EEGs are easier to come by than CT scans.
(*e*) If careful auscultation of the skull and the orbits has revealed an intracranial bruit. The investigation of choice here will be an arteriogram. A CT scan may strongly suggest an angioma, but it needs confirmation, and its vascular supply shown, for this is essential to the surgeon.

It is a curious paradox that after a proven subarachnoid haemorrhage due to a vascular anomaly, patients may retrospectively give a history indistinguishable from migraine, yet if patients with typical migraine are routinely investigated, it is quite exceptional to demonstrate any vascular anomaly.

Epilepsy

Epilepsy may, at times, be due to cerebral tumours, infections, vascular anomalies, or surgically treatable cicatrices.

The aims and limitations of electroencephalography are discussed in Chap. 37. The investigations should be carried further in the following circumstances:

(*a*) If the patient has no family history and has truly had the first generalised attack after the arbitrary age of 35. It is justifiable even in these cases to delay contrast radiography if full neurological examination, skull X-ray and EEG are quite normal, or if the EEG shows features common in 'idiopathic' epilepsy. When CT scanning becomes easily available this will obviate the need for admission to hospital, arteriography and air encephalography unless it shows a focal lesion which requires further clarification.
(*b*) If the fits are focal, at any age, unless clearly the result of perinatal cerebral damage. If they spread to affect increasing areas each time.
(*c*) If there is a residual Todd's paralysis after an attack.
(*d*) If the EEG consistently shows a solitary focus.
(*e*) If the type of attack indicates a temporal lobe origin, i.e. an olfactory or gustatory aura, *déjà vu* phenomenon, well-organised visual or auditory hallucinations, or psychomotor features.
(*f*) If fits occur in a patient who has a past history of subarachnoid haemorrhage for this story is common in angiomas.
(*g*) If there are any abnormal neurological signs on examination which are not obviously due to birth trauma. Even in cases of severe perinatal cerebral damage, if fits are of very great frequency, investigations may reveal a hemisphere so grossly atrophic that hemispherectomy may be carried out without increased hemiparesis, and with reduction of fits—*but only in an infant.*

Strokes

It has been accepted for some years, reluctantly maybe by some, that the clinician has utmost difficulty, at the bedside, in distinguishing between a small intracerebral haemorrhage and a large infarct. CT and NMR scanning have proved this to the hilt, and incidentally have given vivid support to the views of those who considered the treatment of cerebral 'thrombosis' by anticoagulants potentially lethal. Even the CT scan has difficulty sometimes, when the haematoma is isodense with brain. The differentiation is more than academic because there is an increasing tendency to utilise methods of draining haematomata.

CT scanning has however enormously reduced the need for arteriography, but it is still essential when a vascular anomaly is present, and of course if there is a possibility of improving cerebral blood supply, when the site and degree of an occlusion or stenosis is important—this applying mainly to the carotid artery tree.

All further investigations should be guided by the possibilities of some therapeutic process ensuing. The main features that would influence one in cases of stroke would therefore be:

(*a*) If the patient is unusually young (under the arbitrary age of 55), and is not hypertensive.
(*b*) If there is an accompanying history of fits.
(*c*) If there is any separate history of subarachnoid haemorrhage.
(*d*) If there is a 'staggering hemiplegia', each attack affecting a little more of that side of the body.
(*f*) If the 'strokes' are very transient, lasting only a few hours.
(*g*) If the 'stroke' has had a gradual onset over many days. This is probably not a cerebrovascular accident at all.

In (*d*), (*e*) and (*f*) when internal carotid stenosis might be suspected, arteriography should be considered up to the age of 65.

No apology is made for repeating that arterial studies should be considered only if the patient's age and general condition warrants it, for one should always be asking oneself what the purpose, regarding the future, of the investigation, is.

Subarachnoid haemorrhage

Practically all subarachnoid haemorrhages are due to vascular anomalies. CT scanning has become an important investigation here as well because though it may not show the minute detail of aneurysms, it will easily show any intracerebral haematoma that may be developing, except in rare exceptions, and it gives strong suspicion of an angioma. It also shows subarachnoid blood, and if there is blood in the ventricles. In addition it can differentiate between patients with expanding haematomata and those who develop a massive infarct, not uncommonly, a few days after the original bleed. The findings therefore influence the question 'Will arteriography in this case lead to some therapeutic procedure?' and that must be the ruling influence in those hospitals where CT is not available. The possibility arises these days in all who are not too elderly, too grossly hypertensive, or already moribund. Opinions differ on the optimum time for investigation and it depends on facilities and the particular preference of the surgeon who will have to do any operative procedure. It becomes urgent if the haemorrhage is accompanied by a hemiplegia in the young, if a hemiplegia develops after a few days, or if a patient, apparently initially recovering, begins to develop drowsiness. Rapidly repeated haemorrhages are of very dangerous significance and demand urgent investigation and treatment. Angiography is particularly important if there have been fits in the past, for this combination of symptoms may indicate an angioma.

Sciatica

One wishes to determine if there is a continued root compression from disc material, or if the syndrome is caused by a tumour. Myelography is indicated:
(*a*) If there is continued disabling pain despite a period of *absolute* rest of not less than five weeks, and if the distribution of the pain does not give a clear indication of which root is involved.
(*b*) If there is paralysis of any muscle which does not recover within a few days.
(*c*) If there is any disturbance of micturition—but this should be carried out on the same day on which operation is planned.
(*d*) If the pain is clearly in the distribution of a lumbar root, but is not accompanied by any stiffness of the back. This may be seen in spinal neurofibromata.

Spinal CT scanning with or without contrast media is often used in preference to conventional myelography. Those who have been converted to the process of discography will, one hopes, also wish to combine this with scanning.

Parkinsonism

The question is whether the patient truly has Parkinson's disease, or if it could be one of the familial disorders, or due to a cerebral tumour.

If the patient is in adolescence or if there is any family history, tests of the urine for amino-acid and copper output, slit lamp examination of the cornea for a Kayser–Fleischer ring, liver function tests and blood copper, copper oxidase, and caeruloplasmin estimations are essential, for Wilson's disease can now be very greatly improved by penicillamine treatment.

Neurological investigation is indicated if the tremor is *purely* unilateral and associated with contralateral headache, with fits, or with any sign of increased intracranial pressure. This syndrome may be caused by a remediable sphenoidal wing meningioma, though deeply situated gliomata can also be responsible and these may be *ipsi*-lateral.

In true Parkinsonism the widespread use of *l*-DOPA either alone or in combination with a decarboxylase inhibitor, has greatly reduced the need for surgical operations to alleviate the symptoms. There are, however, still patients who do not respond, are intolerant of the drug, or in whom a purely unilateral tremor on the non-dominant side makes thalamotomy the most helpful treatment. The patient should show no mental changes and no signs of bulbar involvement.

Herpes zoster

Though a very common condition, it is sometimes forgotten that it can occur in the skin dermatomes related to the site of:
(*a*) Extradural compression of the cord, usually when caused by metastases.

(*b*) A plaque of multiple sclerosis in the acute stage.
(*c*) The onset of polyneuritis or transverse myelitis.

Investigation is indicated if there is any paralysis *below* the level of the herpetic eruption. Paralysis in the motor zone corresponding to the level of the infection is not uncommon in the ordinary zoster.

Deafness

The problem is one of detecting a cerebello-pontine angle tumour. CT scanning is very helpful in sizeable lesions, but owing to the mass of bone in the area, not so satisfactory in small tumours, though it can show the internal acoustic meati for comparison. Into this field NMR is going to be invaluable, as it is not obscured by bone, and nowadays the ability to remove small tumours and save the facial nerve makes early diagnosis even more important. Deafness should be investigated neurologically if:

(*a*) It is unilateral and accompanied by pain or sensory loss over the first division of the Vth cranial nerve.

(*b*) If there is facial paralysis of *gradual* onset, or any cerebellar ataxia on the same side. Geniculate herpes may cause both VIIth and VIIIth nerve paralysis, but is of very rapid onset.

(*c*) If there is associated weakness or wasting of the tongue, palate, or paralysis of a vocal cord, especially if there is a polyp in the external auditory meatus. This will be due to a glomus jugulare tumour.

Visual failure

Most causes of visual failure bear no relationship to the nervous system. Loss of vision must be carefully investigated neuroradiographically if:

(*a*) It is accompanied by optic atrophy in the non-arteriosclerotic patient, especially if first affecting one side and then the other.

(*b*) If careful perimetry and scotometry have shown any field defect which could be caused by compression of the visual pathways.

(*c*) If there are any signs of endocrine deficiency.

(*d*) If the visual failure and headaches have developed concurrently.

(*e*) If there are any associated abnormal neurological signs.

This means that all cases of unexplained visual failure should be given a most careful examination. 'Optic atrophy' is not a diagnosis. It is a description of what the examiner thinks he is seeing, and the causes are legion.

No one can expect to go through his career and to be right all the time, but most errors arise from inadequate taking of history and inadequate physical examination – particularly the inadequate history. The physician who is careful with both will rarely have difficulty in deciding which cases come into the category where organic disease is a serious possibility and any such case is likely to require full investigation *if the results of that investigation will alter the management of the problem.*

Part IX
Appendices

Appendix A
Recording the Neurological Examination

Examiners differ in the order in which they elicit the physical signs. Providing they have in their minds a logical sequence which they religiously follow, this variation does not greatly matter, but in all cases the written record should be standardised. This not only ensures that nothing is missed out, but it also makes it easier to compare the notes of different examiners on different occasions from different hospitals.

Clarity, simplicity and precise terminology

These are as much keywords for a good record of physical signs as they are for a good history.

Put one fact on one line and never compress details into corners. The wording in the record should be such that a doctor unaccustomed to neurological work could easily understand the findings.

Avoid abbreviations unless they are ubiquitous in use. R. and L. for 'right' and 'left', or K.J. and A.J. for 'knee jerk' and 'ankle jerk' are so well recognised as to be acceptable, but statements such as LoSoKoo* or O = L & A†, mean nothing to the uninitiated, yet are not infrequently used.

Do not make vague statements, such as 'Some weakness of the right arm', or irrelevant, irritable, or potentially libellous comments. Remarks such as 'This is the most stupid patient I have examined this year' may have a transient cathartic effect, but read badly at follow-up.

It is perfectly justifiable to record facts of importance such as 'Sensory tests unreliable owing to patient's confusion' and it is justifiable to put simply 'normal' if one is quite satisfied that this is the case.

The position of the patient

For descriptive purposes the patient is always considered to be standing facing the examiner with the arms slightly abducted and the palms facing forwards. Records are made as if the patient's outline was so drawn on the case sheet, i.e. his right-sided reflexes are recorded on the left side of the case sheet. Sensory abnormalities should be described briefly in the text and

---

*Liver, spleen and kidneys not palpable.

†Pupils central, equal, react to light and accommodation.

drawn accurately on sensory charts, using a code for the various types of sensation, being ready to use several charts if superimposing on one should produce too confused a picture.

A simple scheme for recording a neurological examination

This must be preceded or followed by a well-documented examination of the other systems, with particular reference to examination of the heart, blood pressure and peripheral pulses, the lungs, breast, glands, abdomen, prostrate and rectum and, of course, the urine.

1 HANDEDNESS

2 CONSCIOUS LEVEL, ORIENTATION, and DEGREE OF CO-OPERATION

3 Presence or absence of NECK STIFFNESS and KERNIG'S SIGN

4 SPEECH DEFECT—general description. Detailed analysis at the end of examination.

5 CRANIAL NERVES

I	
II	Visual acuity
	Visual fields
	Examination of fundi
III, IV, VI	Pupils
	External ocular movements
	Nystagmus
V	Motor functions
	Sensory function and corneal reflex
VII	Motor function, upper and lower face
	Taste
VIII	Whispered voice
	Rinne's test
	Weber's test
IX, X	Motor functions (including vocal cord examination)
XI	Motor functions
XII	Motor functions

6 THE MOTOR SYSTEM (arms, trunk, legs)

(*a*) Position of limbs and deformities.
(*b*) Muscle bulk and presence of wasting.
(*c*) Presence or absence of fasciculation.
(*d*) Involuntary movements.
(*e*) Muscle tone.
(*f*) Muscle power with detailed analysis of any weakness.

7 THE SENSORY SYSTEM (describe briefly and draw on chart)
(*a*) Pain sense.
(*b*) Temperate sense.
(*c*) Sense of light touch.
(*d*) Position sense and sense of passive movement.
(*e*) Vibration sense.
(*f*) Stereognosis and graphaesthesia.
(*g*) Two-point discrimination.

8 THE REFLEXES (insert other reflexes if applicable in appropriate position)

Jaw jerk Biceps jerk Supinator jerk Triceps jerk Finger jerk Abdominal reflexes Knee jerk Ankle jerk	0 = absent ± = diminished + = normal ++→++++ = degrees of exaggeration
Plantar reflexes	↓ = flexor ↑ = extensor

9 CO-ORDINATION and analysis of ataxias

10 STANCE AND GAIT

11 SKULL—inspection, palpation, percussion, auscultation

12 SPINE—inspection, palpation and mobility

13 STRAIGHT LEG RAISING, in degrees

14 CAROTID PULSES—palpation and auscultation

15 DETAILS of APHASIA, APRAXIA, AGNOSIA and DISORDERS OF BODY SCHEME
Probable location of lesion(s).
Differential diagnosis.
Proposed relevant investigations.

A scheme such as this, long though it may seem, if consistently repeated can eventually be completed quite quickly, and sets a standard which is easy to read, to understand and to remember.

Appendix B
First Examination in the Out-Patient Department or Consulting Room

A complete neurological examination takes a great deal more time than is likely to be available in a busy out-patient clinic. A scheme for initial testing is thus required which is rapid enough to be applied to many patients in the course of one afternoon, but sufficiently comprehensive not to overlook important abnormalities. Patients can in this way be singled out for examination in detail either at a later time or following admission to hospital.

History and general examination

The history must always be full. With experience it is possible to help patients, without leading them, to concentrate quickly on those aspects of their story which are going to be of greatest value to the physician.

Each patient must have heart, lungs and blood pressure, abdomen, breasts, glands, and femoral pulses examined.

Speech

Note the presence of any speech defect and try to decide its main type (see Chap. 28), reserving more detailed analysis until later.

Cranial nerves

Examine the fundi, the visual fields by confrontation, the pupils, the eye movements.

Test pain sensation over the face.

Test the strength of the upper and lower facial muscles.

See how easily the patient hears the whispered voice.

Make him open his mouth, say 'ah' and put out his tongue.

Ask him to raise his head from the pillow against slight resistance.

Motor system

Examine for deformities of the limbs, wasting, and fasciculation of muscle.

Test the grip, the strength of biceps, triceps, and deltoid; dorsiflexion and plantar flexion of the feet; and flexion and extension at hip and knee. Tell him to tighten his gluteal muscles.

Reflexes

The jaw jerk, biceps, supinator and triceps jerks, the knee and ankle jerks, the abdominal and plantar reflexes, should be tested in each case.

Sensation
Test with a pin the face, the tip of the shoulder, the outer and inner aspects of the forearms, the median, radial and ulnar areas of the hands, three levels on the trunk, the middle third of the thigh, both sides of the tibia, the dorsum of the foot, the little toe, and the gluteal region.

Co-ordination
Carry out the finger–nose and heel–knee tests, and make the patient perform rapid alternating movements.

Stance and gait
Observe the gait and stance both when the patient is aware that he is under observation and when he is not.

Such an examination need take only 10 minutes and can be written down in another 3. An experienced neurologist may be able to locate a lesion and make a probable diagnosis as quickly as this, but the vast majority of patients do not have their first examination carried out by an experienced neurologist and this shortened scheme cannot be expected to supplant the need for a detailed examination at greater leisure if abnormalities are discovered. If, however, it is conscientiously carried out in all patients, including those whose symptoms are not primarily neurological, it will be uncommon for any vital abnormality to be missed.

Appendix C
A Suggested Scheme for the Examination of Higher Cerebral Function

Attention	Affect ....
Appearance	Hallucinations ....
Behaviour	Delusions ....

ORIENTATION

Name	Age	Address
Date	Month	Year
Where are you?		Who am I?

LANGUAGE

Spontaneous	Fluent Non-fluent
Comprehension	Yes/No questions Pointing to command Object placement
Repetition	
Naming objects	
Reading	Sentences, letters words, 'auditory'
Writing	Weather, job, dictation
Calculation	Serial 7's, sums

PRAXIS

1 Put out tongue, blow out match, smell a rose, suck through straw, close eyes
2 Make fist, wave goodbye, salute, point. Imitate use of comb, toothbrush, scissors
3 Light cigarette, play piano, violin, drive a car
4 Dressing

5 Construction . . . Command and copy cube, clock, house, flower, star, matches, Koh's blocks

GNOSIS AND BODY SCHEME

Right/left orientation

Finger gnosis

Visual
- Topography (draw plan of ward)
- Objects (singly and mixed)
- Colour recognition and significance
- Picture to describe
- Faces
- Expression and eye movements

Auditory

Neglect/denial phenomena
- Anosognosia
- Autotopagnosia
- Localisation of touch
- Tactile inattention
- Two-point discrimination
- Graphaesthesia

MEMORY

Immediate recall
- Digit span

Recent
- Three unrelated words
- Fictitious name and address
- Babcock sentence
- Current affairs, interests
- Events in hospital

Remote

REFLEXES

Pout, grasp, Glabellar tap

Corneomandibular, palmomental, nuchocephalic

Appendix D
The Glasgow Coma Scale

COMA SCALE	Eyes open	Spontaneously											
		To speech											
		To pain											
		None											
	Best verbal response	Orientated											
		Confused											
		Inappropriate words											
		Incomprehensible sounds											
		None											
	Best motor response	Obey commands											
		Localise pain											
		Flexion to pain											
		Extension to pain											
		None											

In each square is marked the 'score' for each test on consecutive examinations – annotated either as a figure on a Scale 1–4, or simply by a tick.

Index